The Multiplayer Classroom

The Multiplayer Classroom
Game Plans

by Lee Sheldon

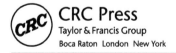

CRC Press
Taylor & Francis Group
Boca Raton London New York

CRC Press is an imprint of the
Taylor & Francis Group, an **informa** business

CRC Press
Boca Raton and London
First edition published 2021
by CRC Press
6000 Broken Sound Parkway NW, Suite 300, Boca Raton, FL 33487-2742
and by CRC Press
2 Park Square, Milton Park, Abingdon, Oxon, OX14 4RN

© 2021 Taylor & Francis Group, LLC

Library of Congress Cataloging-in-Publication Data
A catalog record has been requested for this book

ISBN: 978-0-367-24904-5 (hbk)
ISBN: 978-0-367-24901-4 (pbk)
ISBN: 978-0-429-28501-1 (ebk)

Typeset in Minion Pro
by KnowledgeWorks Global Ltd.

For Erin

*My love, thank you for teaching me so
much in the reality game of life.*

Contents

Chapter 32 ■ Episode 6 – Wolves in Sheep's Clothing   271

Preface

IN THE SUMMER OF 2009, I began designing classes that I taught at Indiana University in Bloomington as games. In 2011, I wrote a book called *The Multiplayer Classroom: Designing Coursework as a Game* about the beginning of this journey that I continued at Rensselaer Polytechnic Institute in Troy, New York. That book covered two courses taught at IU and two courses taught at RPI. In order to meet the publication date of the book in Spring 2012, I was unable to complete the story of the fourth class. I finally concluded the story of that interrupted course while at Worcester Polytechnic Institute in Worcester, Massachusetts, and add fourteen more from RPI and WPI for the second edition of that book published in 2020. While I was to use principles of the Multiplayer Classroom in many other courses, these were the main examples of the concept.

Simply put, the courses were constructed as narrative-driven non-digital multiplayer games, what are often called alternate reality games or ARGs. These were designed by me and played by my students in the real-world in real-time. The game mechanics were no more elaborate than slides on a screen or interactions in the classroom. None of the courses in my multiplayer classrooms cost a penny to produce. It's a fact of which I am quite proud. Here was a way for teachers to introduce games into their classes without cost to them or their schools. Out of the sixteen case studies from other teachers in the two editions of the book, some chose to spend a bit more than zero, but still not very much at all. In fact, multiplayer classroom games do not need slides or computers or even classrooms. They can be taught anywhere indoors or out.

In parallel to these multiplayer classrooms, however, I have been privileged to work on other game-based learning projects, sometimes collaborating with other teachers at the institutions where I taught, sometimes in collaboration with educators and subject-matter experts from other schools. These games, far from being free, were supported by grants or other funding, and they cover a diverse list of topics I could not begin to teach on my own. Even before I designed my first classroom as a game, I had worked as a designer or writer or simply as a consultant on games applied to combating drug addiction, teaching literacy, algebra, statistics, and business ethics. I worked on games teaching Arabic to soldiers in Iraq, recreating jazz clubs of the 1940s and 1950s in Oakland, California, teaching social responsibility and environmental awareness to 4th through 6th graders, and democracy to high school students. As I write this, I have just completed consulting on a NASA grant-based physical game, an "escape room in a box" designed to be played in hundreds of museums and planetariums.

All of these games were a team effort. Some teams were large, some were compact. In every case, we were a combination of designers, subject-matter experts, and facilitators, those who worked in plain view such as our actors and the puppet masters who worked behind the scenes. I have one admonition for you if you should find yourself a part of one of these teams. Trust each other. Designers make games. Trust us on gameplay. Trust subject-matter experts. They know more about what you are teaching. And trust your puppet masters, those who keep the experience running smoothly. They know more than anyone what is going right and what is going wrong. Just as we create puzzles for the players to solve, puppet masters must solve even more. Yes, this should be obvious. Unfortunately, more often than not, I've met too many who seem to think they can do it all, and if someone like that is in charge, your game may be doomed from the start. I am happy to report that this was not true of any of the four games in this book.

I often have been asked to reveal more about what goes into making these more elaborate educational ARGs: the planning, the collaboration, the structuring, and the running of them. Each required significant preparation and the foundation for the building of these games is a design document. In this book, I have included the design documents of four of these larger projects complete with introductions, annotations, and afterwords. My collaborators all provided forewords. In order of their completion, the games were designed to a) make players fitter and healthier, b) teach Mandarin and Chinese culture, c) teach an online class on culture and identity on the Internet, and d) teach two huge sections of a cybersecurity class.

Be on the lookout in this book for what I call collateral learning. Collateral learning occurs at the convergence of two distinct, undeniable forces: gameplay and storytelling and the human attributes that hunger for the best of both. I began using this term quite a while ago to describe what happens when we learn something without being explicitly taught. We touch a hot stove and learn touching hot stoves without mittens is a bad idea. We learn to bow in greeting when someone from another culture bows to us. In this book, you'll see students learning the way most mammals do: through play. I add storytelling to play. Good teaching *is* storytelling. It intensifies the pedagogical experience, as the students learn because *they want to find out what happens next.* They learn almost without realizing they're doing it. That is collateral learning. I'll occasionally point out examples of this, but there are many more to discover.

As I said above, these games are played in the real world in real time. And their nature must allow for and incorporate the unexpected. Designs change based on everything from weather to the time periods in which the games run to all of the complexities that occur when human beings interact.

Game design documents take many forms. Each document in this book was structured to give the production team access to elements that needed to be created and roadmaps on how, in a perfect world, the games would progress. We do not live in a perfect world. Adjustments were sometimes made on the fly without proper documentation. Some elements of the earlier games simply have been lost over time. I have done my best to logically fill in the gaps.

In *Skeleton Chase 2: The Psychic*, the only correlation between the game's purpose to promote physical activity and the narrative was to create a story as a reason for running around.

In *The Lost Manuscript*, the narrative was designed to complement and reinforce the language instruction. I have included *examples* of teaching from only a few class sessions, rather than detail all lessons. This was done to avoid repeating examples that were essentially similar from class to class. You do not need to see every Chinese phrase students learned to get the idea what lessons were taught and how they related to the narrative and gameplay.

In *Secrets: An Internet Mystery*, the story was directly tied to subject matter. The class lectures and assignments were included in the full design document. While I have edited these, I've also left in more detail to provide a continuity to the overall theme and its implications. They seem all the more relevant in today's world. Also, you will find lectures that relate directly to storytelling and game design such as the discussions on player identity and intrinsic versus extrinsic motivation.

For the last section, *The Janus Door*, everything was designed to tightly integrate all topics of the class and the gameplay. Professor Peterson structured his lessons for the design document like an outline. To include every level of detail would require readers to spend a lot of time searching for definitions and examples. While the material is fascinating and more than ever relevant today, I would suggest your own independent research if you have an interest to learn more. I have included only the higher levels of the outlines so again readers can make the connections between the subject matter and the narrative and gameplay.

The intention of this book is not to teach the subject matter of these courses, but to illustrate how, whatever the topic, that could be addressed in an educational setting designed as a game. While you cannot play these games, it is my hope that in reading this book the narratives and how they are connected to the subject matter will be clear. I also hope that you will not only get a good look at how they were constructed, but that you will also get a feel for what the experience playing each must have been like.

When I started this project, I thought I could simply reproduce four game design documents in their original forms. I soon learned to do so would have invited chaos. The documents were created for different types of projects at different times in my development as a designer of this peculiar hybrid of games and learning. I have chosen to reshape each of them into a similar structure so the reader will not need to learn where to find their information or comparisons between them. Where possible, redundancies have been reduced. The way *The Janus Door* episodes originally were constructed suffers a bit from this. It should be only a minor irritation. Annotations have been added where clarity or additional information is necessary. Some are simply anecdotes to help you get a sense for how the designer thinks and how it feels to be in the midst of the action when a multiplayer classroom goes live.

One final caveat. This book was a teaching moment for me in several ways. One of the most important of the lessons I learned, I pass on to you now: document everything! Don't plan to rely on memory. Memory is a fragile vessel.

These documents, with all their successes and missteps, complete the portrait of what a multiplayer classroom can be that I started over a decade ago. I encourage you to pursue and build upon these ideas as an alternative to simply buying video games for students, whether children or adults, to play in the classroom. If you are interested in trying to design one yourself, look around. You may find someone interested in funding it. All of these were funded by grants or schools.

I am writing this during the turbulent times for education we are facing due to the COVID-19 pandemic. I want to address that crisis. While only one of the classes included in this book was explicitly designed to be online, with a little imagination *all* of the classes could be translated into remote learning. I urge you to consider an alternate reality game. Get out from behind your virtual podium. Harness the power of an online multiplayer classroom.

In *The Multiplayer Classroom: Designing Coursework as a Game*, I strived for simplicity, how to create games that required only as much effort as teachers decided to make. In *The Multiplayer Classroom: Game Plans*, you will see what it takes when subject-matter experts and game designers work together and level up to much more challenging games.

Lee Sheldon
October 2020

Acknowledgments

SECTION 1 *SKELETON CHASE 2: THE PSYCHIC*

Dr. Jeanne Johnson, Dr. Anne Massey, Elizabeth Steward and all of our puppet masters, Chris Eller (Chris Debuc and official still photographer), Rin Ehlers Sheldon (Hope, Faith, and Quinn), Graham Ehlers Sheldon (Sam Clemens and video/sound production), Jeff Grafton (Steven Cartwright), and Dastoli Digital (flying saucer video).

SECTION 2 *THE LOST MANUSCRIPT*

Mrs. ShihChia Chen Thompson, Ben Chang, Mei Si, Jim Zappen, Prabhat Hajela, Anton Hand, Hsiong-Ming Chen (Inspector Pei), Rui Zheng (Tingting Lu), Lee-Hua (Lilly), Miaw (Mrs. Ling), Sui Duan (Dr. Chen), and all of our other cast members who brought our visit to China to life.

SECTION 3 *SECRETS: AN INTERNET MYSTERY*

Professor David Seelow, Dr. John Prusch, Mark Oppenneer (web development), Dr. Scott Dalrymple, Dr. Joshua L. Smith (Dale Kenyon), Mary O'Donnell (Audra Casey) and all of our other cast members both onscreen and offscreen, and Focus Eduvation (video production).

SECTION 4 *THE JANUS DOOR*

Dr. Zachary Peterson, Nick Gonella (TA and cast member), Kyle Mulligan (web development) and, yes, again: Rin Ehlers Sheldon (Verita Menzo and video production) and Graham Ehlers Sheldon (Nicholas Menzo and video production), and Stand Up Productions (video production).

And last, but certainly not least, my incredibly patient editors at CRC Press and Taylor & Francis, Sean Connelly, and Jessica Vega.

About the Author

Lee Sheldon began his writing career in television as a writer-producer, eventually writing more than 200 scripts ranging from *Charlie's Angels* (writer) to *Edge of Night* (head writer) to *Star Trek: The Next Generation* (writer-producer). Having written and designed more than forty commercial and applied video games, Lee spearheaded the first full writing for games concentration in North America at Rensselaer Polytechnic Institute and the second writing concentration at Worcester Polytechnic Institute. The second edition of the companion book to this one, *The Multiplayer Classroom: Designing Coursework as a Game*, was published by CRC Press in March 2020. The second edition continues the story of multiplayer classrooms from elementary schools to post-secondary classrooms, designed and taught by Lee and sixteen other educators. The third edition of Lee's book, *Character Development and Storytelling for Games*, a standard text in the field, is also forthcoming from CRC Press in 2021. He is a regular lecturer and consultant on game design and writing in the United States and abroad. His most recent commercial game, the award-winning *The Lion's Song*, is currently on Steam. For the past two years, he has consulted on an "escape room in a box," funded by NASA, that gives visitors to hundreds of science museums and planetariums the opportunity to play colonizers on the moon. He is currently writing his second mystery novel.

Contributors

Jeanne Johnston has a PhD in Human Performance. She is a Clinical Associate Professor in the School of Public Health at Indiana University, Bloomington, and the Coordinator of the Physical Activity Masters of Public Health Degree Program at the school. Her research focuses on utilizing physical activity as a means to prevent chronic disease, improve function in chronic diseased populations, and improve quality of life across the lifespan. Populations of interest include college students, work site, master athletes, older population, and the cancer survivor population. In addition, she has expertise in physical activity assessment methods and utilizing technology as a means to influence physical activity. Her favorite breed of dog will always be the golden retriever.

ShihChia Chen Thompson was born in Taipei, Taiwan. She studied Art Education and Fine Art in National Changhua University of Education and was a High School Art teacher for several years in Taiwan. After moving to New York State, she received her Master's Degree for teaching Mandarin Chinese from Union Graduate College. ShihChia taught Chinese to American students in different schools. Her students ranged from preschool age to college students. Over many years of teaching, her students showed their interest in learning Chinese culture and using Chinese language in real life situations. It is her passion to integrate her Art Education background into her Chinese classroom. She currently lives in Houston, Texas with her husband and they raise their two children with bilingual education. Her children always enjoy their trips to Taiwan with her and are able to use Chinese language on their visits.

David Seelow teaches at the College of Saint Rose in Albany, New York. He founded the Excelsior College Online Writing Lab, The Center of Game and Simulation-Based Learning and the Revolutionary Learning blog. He holds a Master's degree in English from Columbia University and a PhD in Comparative Literature from Stony Brook along with several public school licensees. His book *Radical Modernism and Sexuality: Freud/Reich/DH Lawrence & Beyond* was published by Palgrave Macmillan in 2005 and he edited *Lessons Drawn: Essays on the Pedagogy of Comics and Graphic Novels* published by McFarland in 2018. He is about to finish editing *Teaching in the Game-Based Classroom: Strategies for Grades 6–12* to be published in 2021 by Routledge's Eye on Education series and he is working on a book for CRC Press tentatively called *Play/Games/Sports: Interpretations* *of Modern Culture*. Currently, Dr. Seelow's favorite games are tennis, *Hellblade: Senua's Revenge* and tug of war with his beloved pug Roderick.

Zachary N.J. Peterson is an Associate Professor of Computer Science at Cal Poly, San Luis Obispo, California. His technical background is in applied cryptography, particularly as applied to storage systems. He also has a passion for creating new ways of engaging students of all ages in computer security, especially through the use of games and play. He has co-created numerous security games, including [d0x3d!]: a network security board game, and explored the use of interactive fiction and alternate realities for education, in and out of the classroom. He is a Cybersecurity Policy Fellow at New America, a Cyber Security Fulbright Scholar, and the recipient of multiple National Science Foundation awards to support computer security education.

SECTION 1

Skeleton Chase 2: The Psychic

CHAPTER 1

Introduction to Section 1

Skeleton Chase 2: The Psychic is an alternate reality game (ARG), the sequel to *The Skeleton Chase*, an ARG that ran from September 23 to November 12, 2008.

Dr. Jeanne Johnston was the Principal Investigator and subject matter expert on the grant. Dr. Johnston is in the Department of Kinesiology at Indiana University where she is a Clinical Associate Professor and the Coordinator of the Physical Activity Masters of Public Health Degree Program at the school.

Dr. Anne Massey from IU's Kelley School of Business and I were Co-Principle Investigators. Dr. Massey is now Dean of the University of Massachusetts at Amherst's Isenberg School of Management. At that time, I was an Assistant Professor at the Department of Telecommunications, Indiana University, Bloomington. It was my first academic appointment.

This was the era of the *Wii Fit* and *Dance Dance Revolution*. Most researchers were focused on those devices to replace the monotony of treadmills. But any repetitive game experience that relies solely on activities that are unchanging from week to week and offer no real context for those activities can get old fast. This entire ARG, with an ongoing narrative full of surprises and suspense, and all of the puzzles and challenges, was designed to give students a reason to exercise rather than simply the exercise itself. The hope was that participants would be so caught up in the gameplay they would willingly, and for the most part without even conscious effort, meet their weekly step goals in a way that was more fun than spending hours of repetitive activities only one step removed from working out on a treadmill or circling the track.

Collateral learning in action! Or more accurately: collateral exercising?

As you will see, we provided both extrinsic and intrinsic rewards. Some were awarded for gameplay successes. Others were random awards to ensure that all teams would be motivated to continue play, even those who weren't solving as many puzzles or winning specific contests.

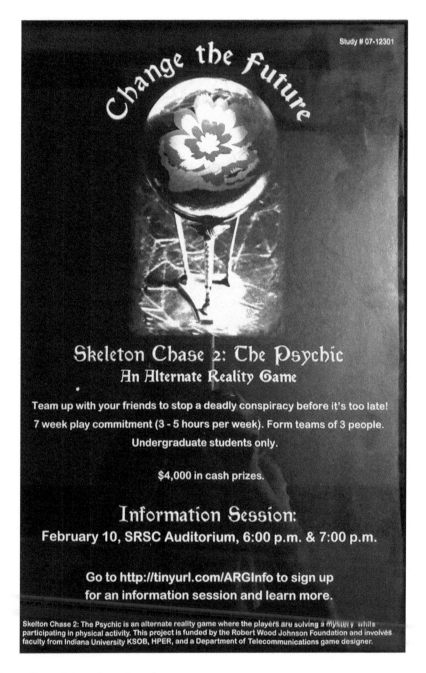

The *Skeleton Chase 2* recruitment poster.

With Institutional Review Board (IRB) permission acquired, the game was adver-tised widely on campus from January 12 to January 26. Advertising included informa-tion at the Recreational Sports booth, posters, emails to lists and classes, word of mouth from participants in the first game and more. The Call Out meeting on January 26 was packed. The presentation included an explanation of what an ARG was, materials from

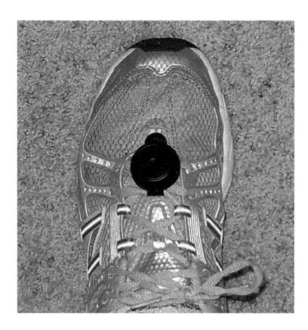

ActiPeds were worn on the shoes of players.

the first game, responsibilities and expectations, parameters of play and what would be required from students.

These requirements included a $25 deposit to cover replacement costs for the ActiPeds students would need to wear. ActiPeds were an accelerometer that measured step count, distance traveled and activity time and wirelessly uploaded the data to a website where participants and researchers could track activity levels remotely.

Players had to be able to receive Twitter messages. They signed an informed consent, setting dates for baseline testing and post-testing and students were asked to complete a survey at the end of the game.

Players could sign up as teams or individuals. There was a second meeting on February 2 where twenty-six teams were given final instructions. Several teams dropped out early in the game. Twenty-two finished. Baseline testing was held on February 5, 6, 9, and 10. The game was launched on February 23 with the trailhead announcement in the Indiana Student Daily newspaper of a psychic coming to Bloomington and the opening of pre-game content on game websites and blogs. This gave students a chance to find background information they would need about the game's narrative and characters before gameplay officially began on February 23.

The first game was the lab component of a required course for first semester first year students at Indiana University's Bloomington campus. That story introduced Sarah Chase, an assistant professor of Kinesiology and Folklore who had vanished after announcing a major discovery. Others were also missing: a former Assistant Instructor of Sarah's, Sam Clemens, and his former girlfriend Stacey. Over the seven weeks of gameplay, students learned that an unethical company called the Source Corporation was testing Sarah's discovery, a drug derived from the skeleton plant on human beings without their knowledge. The plant, also known as a purple dandelion, is not nearly as scary as its name might suggest, quite lovely in fact. Source wanted to get it to market as swiftly as possible since Sarah's formula appeared to dramatically prolong life. At the end of the game Sarah was found. Sam was in hiding, attempting to prove that the skeleton plant was actually an oracle that could foretell the future. Sarah had been kidnapped by Source when she was about to blow the whistle on their scheme. The drug, tested on Stacey with disastrous results, was tested on Sarah as well, and she was last reported under treatment at a hospital in Skeleton Canyon, New Mexico. Source's point man in Bloomington, Steven Cartwright, fled, vowing revenge on Indiana University and the students who had thwarted his plans.

You may have noticed that the initials of so many names in the story are SC. It's not a coincidence, just a deliberate red herring some attentive players might wonder about. And yes, Skeleton Canyon is a real place on the Arizona/New Mexico border. It was the site of Geronimo's surrender in 1886.

Skeleton Chase 2: The Psychic picks up where the last game ended with several of the characters returning.

DIFFERENCES FROM THE FIRST GAME

The following list was created as we prepared for *Skeleton Chase 2*.

- Players of the first *Skeleton Chase* game were first year, first semester students, and some found themselves overwhelmed by the puzzle-solving and critical-thinking components of the game. Recruitment for *Skeleton Chase 2* is open to all university students, twenty-five years old or younger.

- The first game was tied to a specific class. This imposed a weekly structure of storytelling and a hint line manned by puppet masters during the day and early evening to help lagging teams keep up with the story. *Skeleton Chase 2* is not tied to a weekly structure and therefore will evolve at a pace set by its players. Progress will be monitored by puppet masters three times a day, and adjustments in pace and content made accordingly. Puzzles can be added, made more difficult, or easier, on the fly, depending on player progress.

- Instead of a dedicated website for the game, we are using Oncourse CL, the Indiana University learning and participant connection tool for many classes and projects.

- Texting in *SC* was accomplished through cell phones tied to the characters. In *Skeleton Chase 2* texting will be handled by Twitter, greatly simplifying the chore of spamming many teams simultaneously.

- Player photography has replaced back and forth texting as a way to gauge player progress in *Skeleton Chase 2*. Players will email photographs of certain locations to characters as part of the storyline, so puppet masters can confirm they are completing required game content.

Adding photography as a principal game mechanic worked extremely well to keep the players on track, to let us know they were completing the puzzles and giving them an overt reason to be creative. It also explains why there are so many images in this section!

- Geo-Caching has been added as a gameplay element. While *Skeleton Chase 2* retains the idea that players will participate for a short time each day several days per week, we have added timed events we call "sprints" where players must locate hidden objects in a short period of time using GPS tracking.

This game ran before GPS and accelerometers were standard on cell phones. Garmin handheld devices were used to ensure all teams had the same access to GPS.

- ActiPeds, the accelerometers used in the first game, are again being used to track player steps. To upload the data they collected, they will wirelessly sync to dedicated receivers connected to the ActiHealth database on a computer. In the first game all players resided in the same student housing, and the ActiPeds would upload their physical progress every time they returned home. In *Skeleton Chase 2* players will be required to check in at a desk in the School of Health, Physical Education and Recreation once per week for the wireless link.

ActiPeds were accurate, state of the art devices at that time.

- Prizes have been made more attractive and the chances of one or two teams dominating play have been decreased. Chits can be collected for participatory rewards.

Due to the nature of the physical fitness grant that funded the research, this ARG had far more real-world activities and interactions than typical ARGs that exist primarily on the Internet.

What follows are all of the design documents for *Skeleton Chase 2: The Psychic* that could be recovered. Some documents, such as repetitive instructions, have been removed to reduce the length of this section, and in some cases, material has been rearranged to make it easier for a reader to follow. The non-player character section was added to help introduce the characters to the reader.

To learn more of the underlying research goals and results, please consult the chapter on the first *Skeleton Chase* game, entitled *Influencing Physical Activity and Healthy Behaviors in College Students: Lessons from an Alternate Reality Game* that was published in *Serious Game Design and Development: Technologies for Training and Learning* (Janis A. Cannon-Bowers and Clint Bowers, 2010, IGI Global).

CHAPTER 2

Foreword to Section 1

Jeanne Johnston

SKELETON CHASE 2: THE PSYCHIC was funded by a grant from the Robert Wood Johnson Foundation. The grant was sufficient to build and run two iterations of the game called *The Skeleton Chase* and *Skeleton Chase 2: The Psychic*. A third iteration, funded by the Coca-Cola company, was called *Skeleton Chase: Warp Speed*. It was designed to be played in two and a half days.

The initial *Skeleton Chase* game ran for eight weeks in the fall of 2008. Players for both the game and control group were first-year students at Indiana University in Bloomington, Indiana.

That game was designed to supplement the School of Health, Physical Education and Recreation's P-105 class that was part of the Living and Learning Center at Briscoe Residence Hall on the Indiana University Bloomington campus. All first-year students were required to take P-105, a class intended to teach them healthy behaviors. Students were divided into two sections. Both were required to attend lectures and complete homework assignments. One section of the class would play the game which would also be designed to illuminate the class topics as part of its narrative. The second section would be the control group, following the regular workout program using fitness equipment.

Details on the research and educational goals for this project are beyond the scope of this book. The research question we explored was if by simply playing the game students would become more motivated to be fitter, healthier, and wiser about life choices that affect fitness and wellness than the control group.

Our results bore out the thesis. While I remember one student who early on decided stationary bikes and treadmills were just fine for her, and a couple of others just wanted puzzle solutions given to them, the great majority of students who played the game not only enjoyed the experience but were indeed fitter and healthier.

This second iteration of the game was not tied to a class and was not a requirement. Students volunteered for the chance to play. The game was not without its speed bumps. We had to deal with obstacles like spring break and last-minute complications like a worldwide physical activity event that was sandwiched into the storyline. Running a game like this would have been impossible without the tireless dedication of a wonderful team who took this project on in addition to their own classes and regular duties.

You will see in the design documents included here only a few photographs of students playing out of the hundreds taken. The seriousness with which they attacked the puzzles, searched for clues, and offered their theories on aspects of the mystery indicates how immersed they were in the experience. And again, the results indicated that students who participated in *Skeleton Chase 2* were measurably fitter and healthier at its conclusion and challenged and entertained throughout its run.

CHAPTER 3

Design Document

GAME INTERFACES—ONCOURSE GL

At the time Oncourse GL was the Indiana University learning management system for classes and projects. It provided participant lists, announcements, resources, a wiki, and links to related topics. All of the interfaces were handled through Oncourse. The system was retired in 2016.

Skeleton Chase 2 will be using Oncourse as its primary tool for connecting to players.

There will always be a need for "official" communications between those running the game and all players, sub-groups, and individuals. There are also mechanisms important to the game's progression like hints or exams. While convenient to route everything through a central hub, as was done here, try to keep as many as possible within the world of the game to preserve the illusion of the fourth wall.

The "fourth wall" is a term derived from a play performed in a traditional theater where the setting is often enclosed by a back wall and two side walls with the actors pretending a fourth wall separates them from an unacknowledged audience. Speeches such as Shakespeare's soliloquys "break" the fourth wall because the actor addresses the audience directly.

This is probably hardest in any game-based learning experience than any other type of game. You won't be able to do it all the time. But it's worth the effort to try. Just keep in mind the balance between learning and the fun that immersion within the game world provides. You will see a couple of examples in the following episodes: one type of communication that felt intrusive, and one where it was necessary to resolve an issue satisfactorily for the players.

An Oncourse site will be established with the following links:

Websites

Quinn Morgan
> Link to Quinn Morgan, Psychic website.

Celebrity Sheet
> Link to Celebrity Sheet Online.

IU Security Public Website
> Link to IU Security public website.

IU Security Internal Site
> The Internal IU Security website can be accessed from the public website with a password.

Sarah Chase
> Link to Sarah Chase's HPER faculty webpage. Her blog can be accessed from this page.

Blogs

Quinn Morgan
> Quinn Morgan's blog can be accessed from this website.

Hope Johnson
> Hope Johnson's blog also contains a Secret Page (accessed via a hidden link).

Sam Clemens
> Link to Sam Clemens' personal blog.

Sarah Chase
> Sarah Chase's blog is not regularly updated.

Announcements
> General announcements for all players.

Email Archive
> Archive of all emails sent to skeletonchase@oncourse.iu.edu.

Wiki
> Contains a list of all player Twitter IDs.

Resources
> Copies of information session PowerPoint presentations, designer notes, game instructions.

Forums
> For inter-team discussion.

Chat Room
> For real-time communication.

Roster
   Listing of all players, their user IDs and email addresses.

Site Setup
   Tools for setting up the Oncourse *Skeleton Chase 2* site.

Home
   Home page of the site.

Help
   Documentation for how to use the site.

GAME LOGIC FLOWCHARTS

Given the limited time between the first two *Skeleton Chase* games, flowcharts were the easiest, and fastest, way to track, all on one page, the game elements (narrative, encounters, puzzles, objects, bottlenecks etc. that would control the course of the gameplay. These were the primary tools used to illustrate the game structure and logic.

You may notice what appear to be dead ends in the flowcharts. To use a reverse arrow would suggest that players needed to retrace their steps to follow another line, whereas the links being digital allowed players to directly access other links as jumping between emails in a mail program or websites in a web browser.

Every *Skeleton Chase 2* episode begins with a game logic flowchart. Each flowchart illustrates all of the main pieces that comprise that episode and how the game progresses from one to the next. The legend for the flowcharts follows.

Legend
Definitions

- Physical Location/Document/Object represents something tangible existing in the real world.

- Phone: Voice/Text indicates phone calls, either live or recorded, and SMS text messages generated through Twitter.

- Webpage/Email refers to standard internet content and communication.

- Puzzle/Clue/Riddle covers actions players must take to proceed and instructions on how to accomplish those actions.

- Decision marks a point where players may decide between one course of action or another.

- Off-Page Link indicates the connection between the current episode's flow chart and other episodes.

Legend

☐	Physical Location/ Document/Object
☐	Phone: Voice/Text
☐	Webpage/Email
☐	Puzzle/Clue/Riddle
◇	Decision
▽	Off-Page Link

Game logic flowchart legend.

There are deliberate roadblocks where the progression in the game is entirely at the control of the puppet masters. These are usually puzzles. They allow us a fluidity of response in reaction to the pace of gameplay. The step following a roadblock is not offered to players until the puppet masters are ready for players to advance.

NON-PLAYER CHARACTERS (NPCs)

Students from the IU Department of Theater and Drama (renamed in 2013 to the Department of Theater, Drama and Contemporary Dance), played the various non-player characters with the exception of Chris Debuc, who was a telecommunications graduate student and a professional photographer. Characters are identified as either being new to *Skeleton Chase 2: The Psychic* or returning from the previous semester's *The Skeleton Chase*.

Quinn Morgan (New)

Reclusive psychic who has built a reputation while remaining a total mystery. Direct contact with Morgan, even by those who are helped, is handled by phone calls (Morgan uses an electronic speech-altering device), emails, and text messages. No photograph of Morgan is known to exist at the beginning of our story. In fact, Morgan is a true psychic named Faith Pierpont, working for the NSA.

Hope Johnson (New)

Enthusiastic new investigative reporter for Celebrity Sheet Online, a gossip and scandal website similar to TMZ. Hope is glamorous and bubbly. But this exterior is an act. Hope Johnson is one of the many public roles Quinn Morgan takes on when interacting with other people.

Sam Clemens (Returning)

Sam was Sarah Chase's graduate assistant. During the previous game Sam studied a plant called a skeleton plant that Sarah was using in her research for the Source Corporation. He became obsessed with the plant to the point where he broke into the school's cyclotron and bombarded the plant with subatomic particles, causing the plant's basic structure to be altered. He is currently hiding somewhere on campus, watching the plant undergo some bizarre changes…

Milton Mars (Returning)

The grouchy chief of Indiana University's Security, Mars is concerned that Steven Cartwright, an executive for a company called the Source Corporation, has returned to Bloomington to exact revenge on those who ruined his plans. A student, Stacey Cassell, died. These events were covered in the first *Skeleton Chase* game. His two loves in life are Gilbert & Sullivan and his dog, Beartrap, who has just had three puppies.

Steven Cartwright (Returning)

Revealed as the Source Corporation point man on Sarah Chase's kidnapping, and the illegal testing of her drug on unwitting subjects, Cartwright is now on the run from police. He has vowed revenge on the people that thwarted his plans, and may in fact be returning to exact that revenge, as his trail seems to lead to Bloomington.

Sarah Chase (Returning)

Assistant Professor of Kinesiology and Folklore who discovered properties within the skeleton plant that seemed to indicate it could retard aging to a great degree. Unfortunately, she was the victim of the Source Corporation's illegal human testing before the formula was safe. She is now recovering in a hospital in Skeleton Canyon, New Mexico and is reported to be doing well enough that she may return to her research in a few more months.

Faith Pierpont (New)

A professional, no-nonsense NSA agent. She adopts the personas Quinn Morgan and Hope Johnson to hide her true identity.

Chris Debuc (New)

Chris is the Celebrity Sheet Online staff photographer. He has an uncanny knack of showing up to photograph main events in the storyline and record the progress of the student teams.

Photographs of players taken by Chris were one of the intrinsic rewards student teams received for their accomplishments throughout the game. The photographs were displayed on various websites and blogs for all to see. An intrinsic reward is internal, such as personal satisfaction for a job well done. An extrinsic reward is bestowed, such as a good grade. Unlike an intrinsic reward, an extrinsic reward is less fulfilling and may even make the task feel more like just work.

PRE-GAME CONTENT

Certain content needed to be ready and waiting for players before the trailhead was published. The Pre-Game Content section covers it. We also made sure that the email and Twitter accounts for the various characters were available to be found by players when needed.

Quinn Morgan's Website
My Methods

If only I could explain. If only I could teach what others have called my "gift." It is no gift, my friends, but a terrible burden destiny has placed on my shoulders. I accept it.

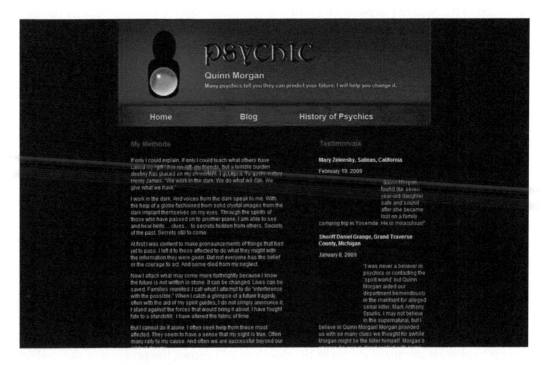

Quinn Morgan's preproduction website.

To quote author Henry James: "We work in the dark. We do what we can. We give what we have."

I work in the dark. And voices from the dark speak to me. With the help of a globe fashioned from solid crystal, images from the dark implant themselves on my eyes. Through the spirits of those who have passed on to another plane, I am able to see and hear hints… clues… to secrets hidden from others. Secrets of the past. Secrets still to come.

At first, I was content to make pronouncements of things that had yet to pass. I left it to those affected to do what they might with the information they were given. But not everyone has the belief or the courage to act. And some died from my neglect.

Now I attack what may come more forthrightly because I know the future is not written in stone. It can be changed. Lives can be saved. Families reunited. I call what I attempt to do "interference with the possible." When I catch a glimpse of a future tragedy, often with the aid of my spirit guides, I do not simply announce it; I stand against the forces that would bring it about. I have fought fate to a standstill. I have altered the fabric of time.

But I cannot do it alone. I often seek help from those most affected. They seem to have a sense that my sight is true. Often many rally to my cause. And often we are successful beyond our wildest dreams.

I'm often asked how I do what I do. I do not do it alone. I have help both from this world. And beyond.

Watch my blog for warnings of impending danger. Answer my call for help. Together we can push back the dark and restore light to the world once more.

Testimonials

"Quinn Morgan found our three-year-old daughter safe and sound after she became lost on a family camping trip in Yosemite. He is miraculous!"—Mary Zelensky, Salinas, CA.

"I was never a believer in psychics or contacting the 'spirit world' but Quinn Morgan aided our department tremendously in the manhunt for alleged serial killer, Mark Anthony Spurlis. I may not believe in the supernatural, but I believe in Quinn Morgan! Morgan provided us with so many clues we thought for a while Morgan might be the killer himself. Morgan's answer: he was in direct contact with some of the victims!"—Sheriff Daniel Grange, Grand Traverse County, Michigan.

"You can imagine how we felt when Quinn Morgan contacted us with the news that a tornado would touch down near our home within two hours. But his sincerity and concern convinced us, and luckily, we were able to convince other neighbors to evacuate as well. The result can be seen in the attached photograph."—Hugh Cawley, Hampton Roads, Virginia.

"My Uncle Henry left us $12,000 in cash in his will but died before he could tell us where he hid it. Quinn Morgan found the money in less than an hour, buried beneath the doghouse."—Daisy Bernanke, Olmsted Falls, Ohio.

CELEBRITY SHEET ONLINE

shamless celebrity indulgence

Feb 24

Nicky Hilton makes a citizen's arrest outside an IHOP

Tue, Feb 24, 2009 9:47 AM - Nicky Hilton is quite the badass. Not something I ever thought I'd say about a Hilton – male or female – but it appears to be true. Last night, for reasons completely unknown, Hilton was outside an IHOP. I'm guessing she probably just walks by there to mock the regular people who can't afford to pour platinum syrup on their diamond-encrusted pancakes or something.

While outside the IHOP, a homeless man accosted her, and Nicky took him down. Actually, he pushed her over, and Nicky got right back up. And then placed him under a citizen's arrest. See, totally badass.

Feb 24

Madonna fails to bring Jesus Luz to Oscar after parties

Tue, Feb 24, 2009 8:23 AM - Madonna was reportedly going to officially introduce her boy toy, Jesus Luz, at the post-Oscars Vanity Fair party, but instead she surprisingly showed up alone. She did, however, bring him to pre-Oscar parties, including the Grey Goose bash, where they sucked face the whole time. Reports had originally said that Madonna was really looking forward to introducing Jesus as her new boyfriend at the Vanity Fair party, one of the bigger, more public bashes.

Featured Reporter

Hope Johnson is Celebrity Sheet's newest investigative reporter. And keeps her own personal blog.

While most of our staff concentrates on the famous, the rich and the powerful, Hope digs out stories on people who are even more interesting!

While other reporters follow Angelina and Brad or governors from Alaska or the mothers of octuplets, Hope travels to distant lands to find people whose achievements are always amazing, and often totally unique!

Celebrity Sheet Online preproduction website.

Celebrity Sheet Online
RSS Feeds

General celebrity news from real websites.

The website that supposedly employed Hope Johnson. RSS feeds can be included in any website to provide updated content such as news or other matters of general interest to the site in a standardized format. The RSS feeds quickly established exactly what kind of website this was, and it was a way to bestow an aura of authenticity to a fictional website with little effort. The RSS feed updates itself on a regular basis.

IU Security Public Site
Passphrase Reminder

All students are reminded to use passphrases instead of passwords to increase security. IU Security has been creating and changing passphrases every quarter to ensure absolute security for the department's internal site, meant for the use of security officers and staff only. We understand that a passphrase can be more difficult than a simple password. In

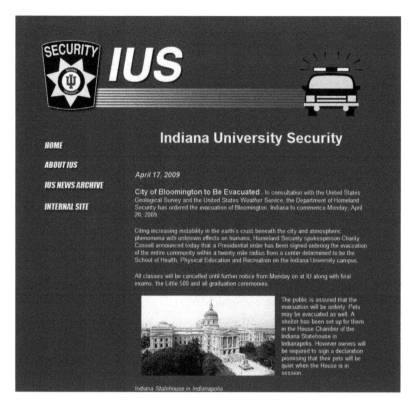

IU Security Public website.

fact, Chief Mars had to remind security personnel that the current passphrase should be entered with its three components separated by a single space only, no other punctuation. However, he points out, the increased difficulty is more than offset by the safer, more secure campus it promotes.

Beartrap Is a Mom!

IU Security Chief Milton Mars is pleased to announce that his miniature pinscher, Beartrap, has given birth to three adorable puppies, all girls. He reports that mother is doing fine and is remarkably relaxed with the new family. Beartrap's composure he attributes to the fact that he played Gilbert & Sullivan's "The Mikado" for her during the birth. He has not publicly revealed the names of the pooches, but he hints that their names are entirely in keeping with the blessed event.

On the public website there is a button labeled Internal Website that immediately attracted interest. The two posts above, Passphrase Reminder and Beartrap Is a Mom! and Chief Mars' photograph were all clues to figuring out the passphrase that unlocked the IU Security Internal Website. We wanted to make sure players could access the internal site as soon as possible. The actual steps to solving the puzzle are listed under the Episode 1 Puzzle Detail section at the end of this chapter.

IU Security Internal Site

No photograph of the internal website could be found. It was in the same style as the public website and all internal website text in this game plan is the original.

Who Is Quinn Morgan?

We, of course, take all threats to IUB seriously. Whether this man is a charlatan or not, several other law enforcement agencies appear to endorse both him and his unorthodox methods. For now, we should all be vigilant. In the meantime, we've asked for more details on Morgan. At least what he looks like. Electronically altered voices and cryptic emails are not how this department conducts its business.

Sarah Chase Recuperating

A phone call to the local authorities confirms that Sarah Chase is recuperating at Skeleton Canyon Hospital in Grant County, New Mexico. Thanks to her treatment, a combination of HMG-CoA reductase inhibitors and vitamin water, she is making great strides. Doctors are confident that she will be able to make a complete recovery and will hopefully be able to return to her duties as Assistant Professor of Kinesiology and Folklore at IU, her ordeal finally behind her.

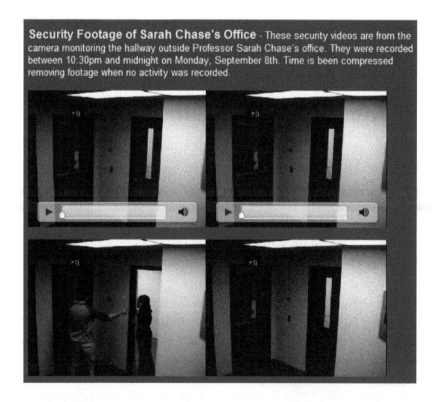

Professor Chase's abduction last semester caught on security camera.

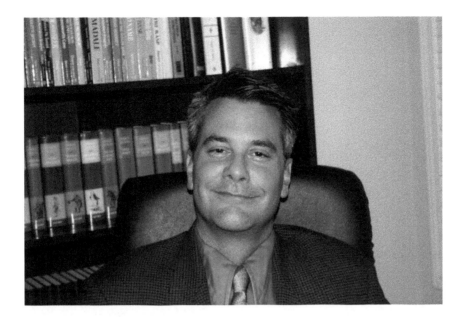

Steven Cartwright before his criminality was unmasked.

Time IS been compressed??? Has been compressed??? Sigh.

Steven Cartwright Still at Large

Steven Cartwright, the man responsible for numerous criminal acts committed last semester on the IU Bloomington campus has thus far eluded a nationwide manhunt. Cartwright, a security officer with the Source Corporation, threatened revenge against those who thwarted his plans. Therefore, all officers have been issued with photographs of Cartwright, and have standing orders to take him into custody should he return to Bloomington.

Sam Clemens Believed to Be on Campus

Sam Clemens, a former Assistant Instructor to Assistant Professor Sarah Chase, has begun to make entries to his blog again. No one takes his ravings seriously. He is obviously in need of psychiatric treatment. We are carefully monitoring his postings for clues to his location.

Dated February 12

i'm still here. right under their noses. living in my new lair. comfy. just me and my plant. junk food and my four demons keep me going just fine. lots of empty bottles everywhere. looking at most of them you'd think i've gone all russian! i promise to recycle. need more cheetos though. can't survive without my cheetos!

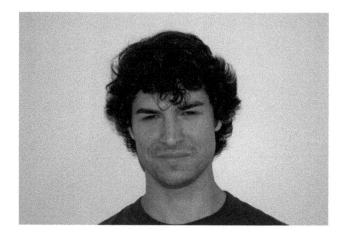

Sam Clemens on a happy day.

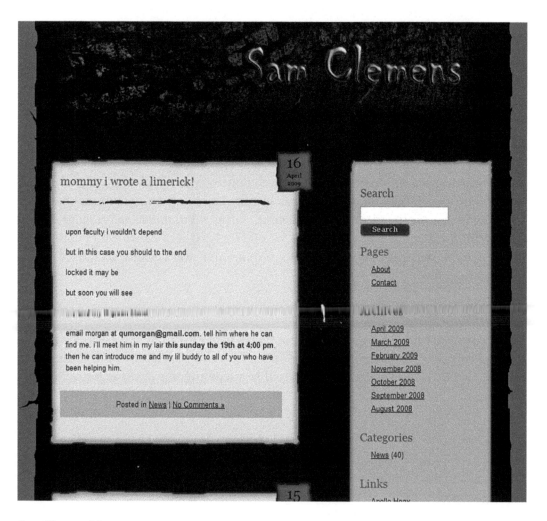

Sam Clemens blog.

Sarah Chase's faculty page, Sarah Chase's blog and the Source Corporation website were all active in the first *Skeleton Chase* game and were accessible to players in *Skeleton Chase 2* for context and backstory. Only Sarah Chase's blog was updated once in *Skeleton Chase 2* with the February 17 entry in later text.

Sarah Chase's Faculty Page

Note on Page

"Currently on leave. Personal updates here." There is a link to Sarah Chase's blog.

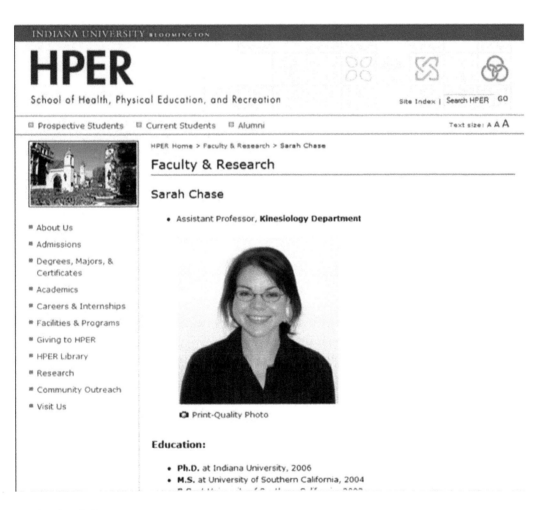

Sarah Chase's faculty page.

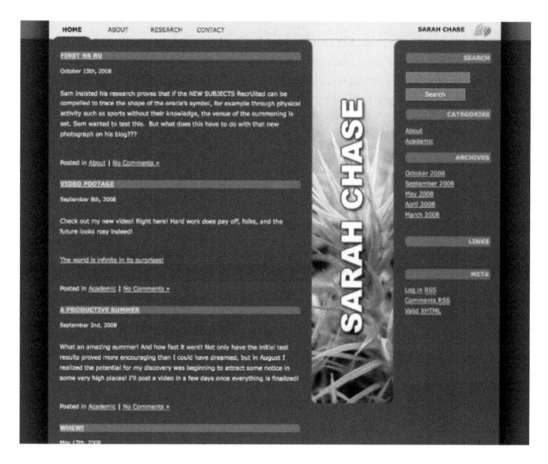

Sarah Chase's blog.

Sarah Chase's Blog
Dated February 17

A shout out to all my friends and colleagues back at IUB! I just wanted to tell you that I'm recovering wonderfully. I hope to be back on the job by next semester! Thank you for all of your good wishes. See you all sooner than you think!

Source Corporation Website

No links active. Banner across page reads: "Closed per order of the Justice Department"

POINT OF ATTACK

Every ARG begins at what is called the "rabbit hole" or the "trailhead." This is the moment, often very subtle, when the game announces its presence. It can be anything from an internet link in an advertisement to a flash drive found in a restroom. Some games have multiple trailheads to ensure that they will be discovered. If no one can find your game, no one will play it. The trailhead for *Skeleton Chase 2: The Psychic* appeared in the Indiana University Bloomington daily student newspaper, appropriately titled the *Indiana Daily Student*, on February 23, 2009. It was a small, but hopefully intriguing announcement with a link that sent readers to the website of our fictional titular psychic.

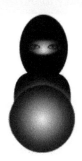

Quinn Morgan

Internationally renown psychic drawn to Bloomington.

Many psychics tell you they can predict your future.

I will help you change it.

I have worked with police departments, government bodies, and private citizens to find what is lost, save lives, and alter the very fabric of time itself.

quinnmorgan.com

Quinn Morgan's ad is *The Skeleton Chase 2* trailhead.

Of course, it doesn't help to begin your game with a misspelled word! Since this was to be a research project the students who were to play had already signed up and formed teams. They knew to look for the trailhead and follow the link. Did it attract any additional interest? Well... yes...

I had met with the university's Chief of Police. We used the word "security" instead of "police" for our fictional campus law enforcement. He cleared all that we planned to do, both for the story and the physical aspects of the game and promised to notify his officers. I warned him that at one point there may be reported sightings of unidentified flying objects. He laughed and said they received reports like that all the time.

However, clicking on the trailhead, Quinn Morgan's card, took anyone, not just our players, to the psychic's website where they found a warning that the university was in danger from an unknown source and there was a possibility that the town might need to be evacuated. Our campus police department got a frantic call from a member of the university's staff, asking what the danger was. The chief phoned me to let me know and to caution us that this was not as funny, and he wouldn't want to shut us down. Luckily that one staffer was the only call like that he received during the run of the game.

EPISODES

The game, divided into seven episodes, was played over seven weeks from February 23 to April 19, 2009 with an intermission for spring break from March 14 to March 22. As you'll see, the seven episodes do not directly map one episode to one week.

Each episode begins with a flowchart. These were the primary foundation the game was based on. This was both a good idea and a bad idea. It was good because the flow-charts gave us a roadmap of how both the narrative and the game progressed. It was a bad idea because those routes will change. It could be due to unexpected behavior on the part of players, or circumstances we didn't anticipate, like the addition of the WPA observance on April 8, 2009. We produced new documentation ad hoc: a file here, and email there, and failed to update the flowcharts or the chronology. As a result, when I began comparing the charts to the chronology of events for this book, I found at times major discrepancies between what was planned and what actually occurred. I have updated the flowcharts for this book and worked to adjust both their content and the content in the individual episodes. Any errors in fact or continuity are strictly my own. My advice is heartfelt: use all the tools at your disposal to make your game plans as complete and accurate as you can. And always update everything as close as possible to when a change is made.

I have been asked why all of these games are divided into episodes instead of weeks or lessons or chapters. I suppose the answer is I began my career as a TV writer and have written over two hundred episodes of various TV series. I think in episodes.

CHAPTER 4

Episode 1 – Trailhead

EPISODE 1 GAME LOGIC FLOWCHART

February 23–February 28

CHARACTERS

Quinn Morgan, Hope Johnson, Milton Mars, Sam Clemens, Chris Debuc

It's impossible to document all of the places photographer Chris Debuc turns up in each episode. I won't list him again. Just assume he is always nearby, camera ready, when our players are active.

NARRATIVE

Narrative strength, often overlooked, particularly in applied (serious) games is critical to creating an experience that will hook players and keep them playing. Whether the raison d'etre for the game is simply entertainment, or more serious in its intentions as are all four of the games covered in this book, I have preserved the narratives so you can see how they provide the important spine that supports both gameplay and learning. *Skeleton Chase 2* and its other two incarnations, was unique in that while there was some cognitive instruction it was designed as a direct attempt to increase the health and physical well-being of players who were not Big 10 athletes attracted to a specific sport, but ordinary students at Indiana University that could also benefit from a way to exercise that was more engaging than a treadmill.

Quinn Morgan arrives in Bloomington warning of an impending, but unspecified danger. Morgan indicates on his website that he accepts the help of others to "intercept the future" and change it. Morgan has alerted IU Security.

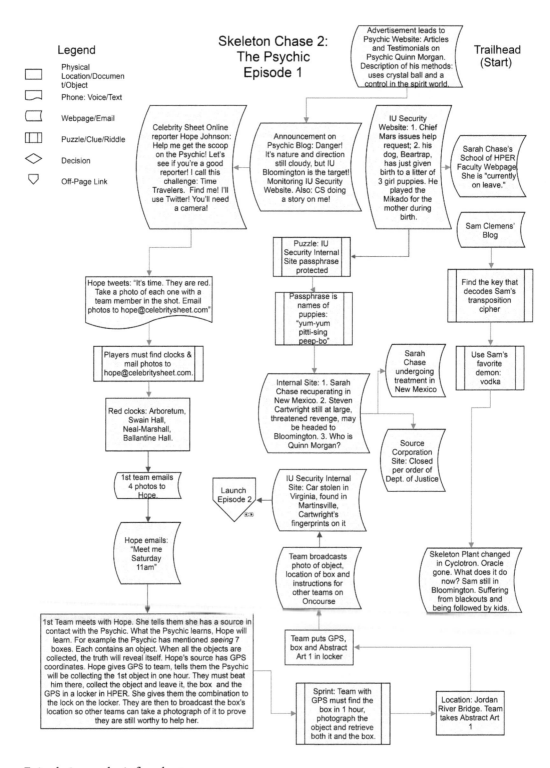

Legend

☐ Physical Location/Document/Object

⬢ Phone: Voice/Text

☐ Webpage/Email

☐ Puzzle/Clue/Riddle

◇ Decision

▽ Off-Page Link

Skeleton Chase 2: The Psychic Episode 1

Trailhead (Start)

Advertisement leads to Psychic Website: Articles and Testimonials on Psychic Quinn Morgan. Description of his methods: uses crystal ball and a control in the spirit world.

Celebrity Sheet Online reporter Hope Johnson: Help me get the scoop on the Psychic! Let's see if you're a good reporter! I call this challenge: Time Travelers. Find me! I'll use Twitter! You'll need a camera!

Announcement on Psychic Blog: Danger! It's nature and direction still cloudy, but IU Bloomington is the target! Monitoring IU Security Website. Also: CS doing a story on me!

IU Security Website: 1. Chief Mars issues help request; 2. his dog, Beartrap, has just given birth to a litter of 3 girl puppies. He played the Mikado for the mother during birth.

Sarah Chase's School of HPER Faculty Webpage She is "currently on leave."

Sam Clemens' Blog

Hope tweets: "It's time. They are red. Take a photo of each one with a team member in the shot. Email photos to hope@celebritysheet.com"

Puzzle: IU Security Internal Site passphrase protected

Find the key that decodes Sam's transposition cipher

Passphrase is names of puppies: "yum-yum pitti-sing peep-bo"

Players must find clocks & mail photos to hope@celebritysheet.com.

Sarah Chase undergoing treatment in New Mexico

Use Sam's favorite demon: vodka

Red clocks: Arboretum, Swain Hall, Neal-Marshall, Ballantine Hall.

Internal Site: 1. Sarah Chase recuperating in New Mexico. 2. Steven Cartwright still at large, threatened revenge, may be headed to Bloomington. 3. Who is Quinn Morgan?

Source Corporation Site: Closed per order of Dept. of Justice

1st team emails 4 photos to Hope.

Launch Episode 2

IU Security Internal Site: Car stolen in Virginia, found in Martinsville, Cartwright's fingerprints on it

Hope emails: "Meet me Saturday 11am"

Team broadcasts photo of object, location of box and instructions for other teams on Oncourse

Skeleton Plant changed in Cyclotron. Oracle gone. What does it do now? Sam still in Bloomington. Suffering from blackouts and being followed by kids.

1st Team meets with Hope. She tells them she has a source in contact with the Psychic. What the Psychic learns, Hope will learn. For example the Psychic has mentioned *seeing* 7 boxes. Each contains an object. When all the objects are collected, the truth will reveal itself. Hope's source has GPS coordinates. Hope gives GPS to team, tells them the Psychic will be collecting the 1st object in one hour. They must beat him there, collect the object and leave it, the box and the GPS in a locker in HPER. She gives them the combination to the lock on the locker. They are then to broadcast the box's location so other teams can take a photograph of it to prove they are still worthy to help her.

Team puts GPS, box and Abstract Art 1 in locker

Sprint: Team with GPS must find the box in 1 hour, photograph the object and retrieve both it and the box.

Location: Jordan River Bridge. Team takes Abstract Art 1

Episode 1 game logic flowchart.

Also new to Bloomington is Hope Johnson, a reporter for Celebrity Sheet Online. On her blog, Hope writes that she is determined to discover whether Quinn Morgan is real or fake and reveal to the world who this reclusive man really is.

On the IU Security public webpage Chief Milton Mars mentions a potential threat announced by an unnamed psychic. There is a story about his dog Beartrap giving birth to a litter of three puppies.

Discovering the passphrase that unlocks the IU Security Internal Site, players learn that Chief Mars has ordered his officers to be on the lookout for signs of danger. One obvious sign that IU Security is already concerned about is the fact that Steven Cartwright is still at large and threatening revenge on the Bloomington community. Mars also wants to know more about Morgan.

Sam Clemens, hidden away in a new lair on campus since the previous game, has begun posting on his blog again. His first post, in code, reveals he still has the skeleton plant in his possession, and that it is mutating. He thinks he is being followed by some kids. He also says that he is suffering from blackouts.

Hope announces on her blog that she is looking for help in her exposé of Morgan. She announces a challenge she calls "Time Travelers" for people to prove they have what it takes to be good reporters. First, they are asked to find four landmarks on campus, and send photographs of them to her. The landmarks are all large red clocks.

Meeting with the team who sent her photographs of all four clocks first, Hope reveals that she has a source close to Quinn Morgan. The psychic has mentioned seeing images of seven boxes. Each contains an object, but Morgan can't determine what they are. What Morgan has seen are coordinates that would allow a GPS device to lead someone to the first box. Hope tells the team they must beat Morgan to the first box and get away without being seen by him. This will give Hope leverage to get Morgan to cooperate with her story. They are to photograph the object, then put it, the box, and the GPS in a HPER locker.

We needed a series of lockers available to the game in HPER, the School of Health, Physical Education and Recreation. While we informed HPER—indeed our principle investigator Jeanne Johnson was a professor there—we felt an additional method was needed to ensure the game's locks remained on the game's lockers and were not removed by a staffer who had not been informed of the game. After getting permission for the lockers we needed, we printed up tags to identify these lockers that could not be assigned. They were removed when players would be present, but otherwise left on. This might sound like overkill, but we had reason to have more than one layer of protection.

In the first *Skeleton Chase* game, we wanted to create a lair for our wayward grad student, Sam Clemens, in a little-used boardroom at the top of the Indiana Memorial Union. We approached the university staff in charge and received permission and made certain everyone knew of our intentions. It wouldn't be a problem because the room was rarely used and always locked. We received a key to the room and on the day of the puzzle created a "nest" for Sam in a corner of the room. It was comprised of a sleeping bag, the remnants of junk food and candy wrappers and several empty liquor bottles, his "demons."

The puzzle went live. Players found an unusual addition behind Sarah Chase's office nameplate. It was a series of directions and the huge number of paces to take from that door to find Sam's lair. We had paced out the steps carefully for a six-feet two-inch man, the height of the actor playing Sam. There were a *lot* of steps, ending with multiple flights of stairs in the tallest building on campus to the room. The first team to make the effort found the room pristine. Even though the door had been locked, Sam's lair had vanished. During gameplay there was always a puppet master on duty in our lair in the basement of HPER, and there was a phone number to call, if there was a serious glitch in gameplay. That day the puppet master on duty was Elizabeth. The team of students called her. She went to the union and found the room was indeed spotless. She went back downstairs to the union office. At first no one could figure out what had happened. Then it dawned on someone. No one had informed the custodial staff...

A search of the custodial assignments gave them the name of the person responsible for the room and luckily, she was still in the building, probably in the basement. Elizabeth, clearly getting her fitness challenge for the day, tracked the woman down. And there on her cart were all of Sam's props in a plastic bag. Did the custodian hand them over? No, she thought our puppet master was the person hiding in that room, drinking all that liquor. Eventually Elizabeth convinced the custodian, lugged the bag of props back up to the top of the tower where there were now three teams waiting. She quickly set things up again and staggered off down the stairs.

The moral to this story? In a controlled environment, there are few chances for unwary intrusions from people with no knowledge of the game. However, it is not always possible to control all game locations! In order to keep actual university personnel from doing routine tasks that might disrupt this game, it was necessary to post warnings to the university's personnel. We put tags on our padlocks, and none were disturbed.

Once the team has placed the photograph of the object in the locker, they give directions of the location where the box was found to the other teams working on the challenge. The team does as it is instructed.

Sometime soon after, a new item appears on the IU Security Internal Site: A car stolen in Virginia with Steven Cartwright's fingerprints on it, has been found in Martinsville, only twenty miles north of Bloomington...

EPISODE 1 CONTENT DELIVERY CHRONOLOGY

The third regular section of each new episode of *Skeleton Chase* 2 in this book will be the New Content Delivery Chronology. This is the order in which students received information from the game. This might be in the form of character website updates, blog posts, emails, tweets, or personal appearances. These were constantly updated based upon player actions. For example, players might send unsolicited messages to the characters that required answers. At other times characters thanked teams and players for their efforts or congratulated them on their most recent achievements. These intrinsic rewards maintained the fourth wall as intact as it could be, and kept the players engaged by assuring them they were making a difference. Communications from the game will be grouped on the day they went live. Some were announced. Others had to be discovered by players.

Monday, February 23

This was the game's official opening day. The advertisement for Quinn Morgan appeared that day, and we began adding new content.

Quinn Morgan Blog

Seven days ago, I awoke in the night sweating and disoriented. A voice, a shriek of warning, had broken through my restless dreams. "Danger," it said. "Revenge!" And "All are threatened!" An image filled my head. Stone gates. A Castle? A mansion? It has taken me this long to identify them. They are Sample Gates, the entry to Indiana University, Bloomington.

Last evening, I stood before them. Somewhere nearby is the heart of the danger. But what form will it take? From what side will it strike? And who is responsible? There is intelligence at work. An angry intelligence that wants to make an example for some wrong. The rest is cloudy. My crystal ball remains dark. I am monitoring the IU Security website for clues. A potential distraction: a reporter from some cheap scandal website. I must find a way to ensure she cannot interfere.

Hope Johnson Blog

I've arrived in Bloomington. And I'm looking for help in getting the scoop on Quinn Morgan. Want to lend a hand? You can follow me on Twitter. My username is "celebrity-sheet." Wandering around the IU campus here in Bloomington, I've thought up a challenge for you to see if you've got what it takes to be a reporter. Your assignment: Find ME!!! I'll tweet you soon with your instructions. That means I'll be using Twitter to contact you, but if you didn't know that, it's time you joined the 21st century! Oh, and you'll need a camera! TTFN!

Who Am I?

My name is Hope Johnson. I am Celebrity Sheet's newest reporter. And I can't tell you how excited I am about investigating the world for YOU! While most of our staff concentrates on the famous, the rich and the powerful, I dig out stories on people who are even more interesting! While other reporters follow Angelina and Brad or governors from Alaska or the mothers of octuplets, I travel to distant lands to find people whose achievements are always amazing, and often totally unique!

My Background?

I have a degree in Journalism from the University of Louisville. I began my professional career writing for the Louisville Courier-Journal before moving to their website. That gave me a taste for the fast action of today's internet news. Since then I've worked for the online division of WISH-TV in Indianapolis, then TMZ and Perez Hilton. Now here I am with my own website and blog courtesy of Celebrity Sheet Online. And I couldn't be happier!

Current Assignment?

Quinn Morgan, Psychic. Reported to be one of the most accomplished psychics on the planet. His website lists some of his most notable successes. Yet his name rarely appears in news stories when a lost child is found, or a tornado strikes precisely where he predicts. And now Morgan claims that not only can he predict the future but change it as well. Using a technique he describes as "interception of the possible," he claims to have averted kidnappings, murders, even natural disasters.

But who is Quinn Morgan? Psychics have never been known to be so shy about their achievements. He rarely gives interviews, and only under the most stringent of conditions, and only via phone or email. Asked about his birthplace, he only gives coordinates: 39°29′30″N 91°47′23″W! Asked about his age, he claims to be "younger than Rasputin when he died."

No one has yet managed to turn up a single photograph of him at any age. It's difficult to call him a "famous psychic" because so few of the general public have ever heard his name. Yet those he has helped, including law enforcement agencies around the world, have praised his tireless efforts on their behalf.

And now he has announced his next challenge: an unknown threat to the quiet college community of Bloomington, IN. Check his website, www.quinnmorgan.com. You won't find many details of this danger, or what he intends to do about it. But I plan to apply whatever leverage I can to lift the veil from this man of mystery.

Who is Quinn Morgan? With my faithful readers' help, that's what I plan to discover!

Watch my blog for the latest developments as I track down The Psychic!

Reward Offered!

Want to help break a major news story? Want your name on a byline with Hope Johnson, intrepid girl reporter? Help me get the goods on Quinn Morgan, and if possible, a picture of him! Heck, even get his phone number! Fame and glory will be yours!

IU Security Public Site

Chief Mars Issues Help Request

IU Security has been contacted by a person claiming to have psychic abilities. This person further claims that the IU Bloomington campus, and possibly the entire city of Bloomington is in some danger which he refuses to define. While this department in no way endorses the man or his methods, we ask all students, faculty and staff, to email IU Security (iusecuritytipline@gmail.com) with any information that may confirm or dismiss his claims.

In addition to monitoring the official communications required of players, we would also need to create ad hoc responses to unsolicited private messages, such as the one that follows. Even though the replies were sent only to a single student, this kept them personally involved in the narrative and occasionally gave them something special they could share with others. Both are intrinsic rewards.

Letter from Chief Mars

Hello [Student Player Name],

Thank you for volunteering to help us. We have asked for information on this psychic from several law enforcement agencies who have worked for him. But they can provide almost no details. Check back on the IU Security website for updates. We've also learned there is a reporter in town doing a story on Morgan. We're keeping an eye on her blog. I'm of the opinion that if there is a threat, it comes from a wanted felon who committed a shopping list of crimes on the IU campus last semester. Right now, we've concentrated our efforts on locating him.

Thank you again for your efforts!
Milton Mars
IU Security Chief
P.S. Aren't my new puppies adorable?!

Players immediately began contacting characters with offers of help:

"Hello Mr. Mars,

My name is Player 1, and I believe I may have information regarding Sam Clemens' whereabouts.

He has talked about 'his plant' several times while also mentioning his 'lair.' This leads me to believe he is hiding out in the the new Physical Power Plant on Range Road.

I also read the report that there has been evidence that students are squatting and living for free at this building.

I have information that Sam Clemens may leave behind several bottles of alcoholic beverages, most likely rum, vodka, whiskey, and tequila bottles. If you find these, you may be in Sam's lair.

Good luck, and let me know if there is anything else I could do to assist in the investigation."

One player was already a double agent. To Quinn Morgan he wrote:

"I have heard that you have seen danger at IU, and are seeking people to help prevent it, I would like to help you in any way that I can, just let me know what it is that I can do."

—Player 2

And to Hope Johnson he wrote:

"You mentioned that you wanted the goods on Morgan, and what I can give you now is his email (qumorgan@gmail.com), blog (http://quinnmorgan.wordpress.com/), and Twitter account (qumorgan). He seems like he is interested in making contact with people around campus, so I plan on doing that. On the other hand, in the blog he makes it clear that he wants nothing to do with you. You clearly need an intermediary to get any real information, and I may be available. Hope to hear from you soon."

—Player 2

To respect their privacy, the real names of student players will be replaced with the clever pseudonym "Player" and a number. That number will differentiate players in a single communication. Player name numbers will not be universal throughout. For example, Player 1 may not be the same person from one communication to another.

Hope Johnson Blog

Time to recruit some intrepid reporters to help me! The word on the street is you've already formed teams to find out what's up with the psychic and the danger to Bloomington. Then this should be easy! I'm going to issue a challenge, a little test called "Time Travelers." I'll tweet what you need to do to win. Find my four time travelers and take a photo of each one with a team member in the shot. This Sunday I'll meet with the first reporters to send me all four photos. Ready to give it a try? I'll tweet you a clue. Good luck!

Sam Clemens Blog

i'm being watched. followed. the usual. but i have a new lair. very secure. i'm at home here with my four favorite demons. find my current favorite. let me count the letters. they bring me down. they loop.

i've encrypted the rest of this post. not sure why. but if you're smart enough to decode it, email the answer to me. i'll start writing more blog entries. here it is:

NFZGZJI KGVIO XCVIBZY DI XTXGJOMJI. JMVXGZ BJIZ. RCVO YJXN DO YJ IJR? IZR VYQZIOPMZ DI NVH'S GDAZ: WGVXFJPON. ODHZ GJNO. API.

okay, I know it's easy, but I want to tell all. decode it! email me what it says: saclemens1910@gmail.com.

Hope Johnson Tweet
Okay, it's time. They are 4. They are red.

Tuesday, February 24

Hope Johnson Blog

Wow! The response has been awesome! Getting to the bottom of this mystery should be easy! And over half of the teams have already completed my challenge! I'll be posting a couple of pictures soon: one from the first-place team, Free Tibet, and one that I just thought was fun from Button Mashers!

> Publicizing accomplishments, even just team activities, are easy intrinsic rewards that keep players playing.

The Free Tibet team won this first part of my challenge only 1 minute ahead of the second-place team, TBD! Whew!

Remember! **Everybody** needs to complete this part of my challenge! Without help from all teams I'll never dig up the dirt on Quinn Morgan, and you won't be eligible for fame and fortune.

For the rest who are still playing (this includes you, BHB): here again are the clues to my challenge. Ready? Okay, it's time. They are 4. They are red.

Take a photo of each one with a team member in the shot. Email the photos to hope. celebritysheet@gmail.com!

Figure out what four red things on campus have to do with time. I'll bet you pass at least one of them every day.

In the meantime, look for the winning photos and my first story on Quinn Morgan tomorrow!

> Once a puzzle was solved by one team, giving more explicit clues to solving that puzzle to the other teams kept everybody from getting too far behind. Also, teams that solved puzzles were encouraged to help other teams. A rivalry was established early between two of the major NPCs, Quinn Morgan and Hope Johnson. Teams decided which one they would help. A couple more players became double agents and surreptitiously worked for both.

Wednesday, February 25

Quinn Morgan Blog

Several of you helping to find a name to the danger that I sense threatens Bloomington have privately expressed your fear to me that we seem no closer to the truth. To my friends I say: do not despair! Remember, we are only a few days into our search. I feel the forces allied against us, and they are powerful. But we will defeat them, I promise you.

I have three items to report.

First, there is a cloud upon this town, its origin unknown: a psychic fog that is troublesome to me, and my contacts in the world beyond. We are in touch, but their efforts to aid me are made more difficult. So, I must rely even more on you, my friends, who have rallied to my side. Your help is all the more important now.

Second, one of you—and you know who you are—claimed you wanted to help me. Yet you have given information to the reporter investigating me. Know that I'm aware of this.

> Here is another example of reacting directly to player actions and adjusting the narrative accordingly. Puppet masters were of course aware of all communications, so we saw that one player pretending to help both Morgan and Hope. Therefore, our psychic could "sense" their duplicity! We talk a lot about player agency when we design games. It's the player's belief they have control over their decisions within the game. This can sometimes be an illusion, but the player's conviction that anything they do in a game's world is meaningful is very powerful. This is often difficult to accomplish in a video game. In an ARG, it is much easier. It's the difference between a game that is immutable and one that is alive and aware of unscripted player actions.

Finally, and this is the most important: despite the psychic fog that dims the light, I have seen something. It is the number 7. Clear and glowing in my crystal ball. And something forms around it. A shape as yet unclear.

When I see more, I will post it here. Be vigilant. Be strong.

Celebrity Sheet Online

Quinn Morgan arrived in Bloomington, Indiana with very little fanfare on Monday, February 23. The only official announcement of his arrival was a small ad in the Indiana University student newspaper, appropriately named the Indiana Daily Student.

After I announced on my blog that I planned to find out all I could on the reclusive psychic, I received an email from Player 2, apparently a student at the university. He passed along to me Morgan's Twitter account name (qumorgan) as well as his email address: qumorgan@gmail.com. Thanks, Player 2! It's a start!

That gave me the idea to see if I could find more allies at the university, since Morgan claims to have seen IU's Sample Gates in his crystal ball. So, I devised a little challenge to see if I could locate some more students to help me out. I asked them to follow some clues

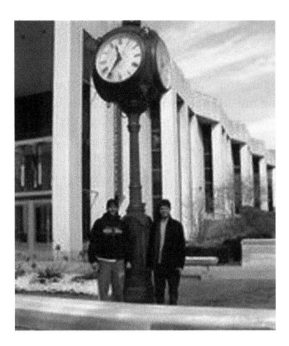

Team Free Tibet triumphs!

and send me photographs of certain landmarks around campus. And wow, my inbox is still getting deluged with photographs! Students who wanted to help have even formed teams!

I didn't get nearly this much help when I tracked down Max Adrian, a professional celebrity stalker, who charges fans astronomical amounts of money for personal photographs of their favorite stars. Of course, Max is in jail now for trespassing, reckless endangerment, and who knows what all. Sorry, Max, but what you were doing was awfully illegal!!

The team who emailed me their photographs first call themselves Free Tibet. That first photograph is one of theirs. Another team, Button Mashers, weren't first, but I liked their photographs. So, the second one is from them. Points for jois de vive!

> Team names are the actual names. Here is another example of providing players with an acknowledgment of their efforts and again maintaining the fourth wall so as not to pull them out of the world of the game.

I'm going to meet up with Free Tibet in a few days and give them their next assignment. They will share what they uncover with all of us. Promise!

In the meantime, I need everybody who has not photographed the "landmarks" to do so and send me their pictures! Let's make this story on Quinn Morgan a huge group effort!

Hope Johnson Email

Free Tibet! Just a reminder! We have a rendezvous this Saturday, February 28th at 11:00 am. You should know where by now. Our little secret!

Thursday, February 26

Sam Clemens Blog

so okay! so a lot of ya figured out my cipher! i know i screwed up a letter. one letter! not bad since i've been enjoying my demons' company a lot lately. so okay grats and toast of the vodka bottle to team banana stand! one minute behind you were somebody called psychic busters. a couple hours later and team thunderfly came through. Since then over a dozen more! i told ya it was easy!

so wait wait. team? you're in teams? why are you a team? what's goin on? somebody drop the low down on me.

so okay. here's the decoded cipher for anybody else tunin in:

SKELETON PLANT CHANGED IN CYCLOTRON. ORACLE GONE. WHAT DOES IT DO NOG?

NEW ADVENTURE IN SAM'S LIFE: BLACKOUTS. TIME LOST. FUN.

noG, Player 3? really? psychic busters figured out I meant noW. no sweat. you were numero uno.

so, my life in a nutshell, folks. enjoy!

I screwed up that letter. Don't blame Sam.

more good news: I only go out at night, right? and the lighting isn't really good. but I see okay. and I'm being followed. they look like two kids. young kids who shouldn't be out that late. and when I look back, they take off. happened now three nights running. what's up with that?

Hope Johnson Blog

Another informant, Player 1, tells me that the coordinates I mentioned where Quinn Morgan claims he was born, are the birthplace of Mark Twain, whose real name was Samuel Clemens. Player 1 told me there is someone here on campus *named* Sam Clemens, and he was an important part of some strange events that occurred at IU last semester. I had a look at his blog. There's a new update, if you haven't seen it: www.samclemensblog.com.

This is one sick puppy. A plant that he claims was once an oracle, but is now "changing" as he put it? Maybe he just isn't watering it enough! And what's all that about being stalked by kids? From reading his blog, it sounds like he's more likely a stalker!

But the fact that this skeleton plant was supposed to be an oracle, and now we have a psychic claiming to be able to see into the future (and even change it, uh huh). AND both Quinn Morgan and Sam Clemens' namesake were born in the tiny town of Florida, Missouri??? Nine—count them it won't take long—nine people lived there in the year 2000. That's... odd...

I see two possibilities and neither of them is coincidence. First, there is some real connection between them. Maybe they are the same guy. Or it's just more of the smokescreen Morgan conjures up around him like that psychic fog he wrote about in his latest blog entry. He could have been born in Olmsted Falls, Ohio for all I know!

Anyway, thanks Player 1! It sure is interesting!

Friday, February 27

Hope Johnson Blog

Okay, heads up! IF Team Free Tibet can't help me on Saturday at 11 am, I need a backup. Team TBD was in second place, so they're on deck. I'll send them an email around noon on Saturday, if their services are needed. If THEY can't help me, it'll be the Third Street Hooligans who'll get a chance. If THEY can't do it, I'll do it myself! So, gear up and be ready on Saturday!

> We chose three teams for each of the seven major sprints: the winners, second place teams and third place teams of the qualifying challenge, in this case the four red clocks. This deliberate redundancy was because these sprints were consequential events and we wanted to be sure they were not missed. If the first team failed, the second would run the sprint. If they failed, then the third team was ready to go. There was only one case where the second team was needed. No sprints required the third.

Saturday, February 28

Live Performance—Hope at Beck Chapel (11:00 am to 12:30 pm, hopefully no longer)
Hope is waiting at Beck Chapel at 11 am on Saturday, February 28.

> This was our first sprint. The beginning of this first sprint also included a personal appearance by Hope Johnson.

"You found me, excellent! I'm Hope Johnson, what are your names? [writes names in her notebook] I'll give you credit on my blog and in my Celebrity Sheet articles for your efforts! You'll be famous! Here's the skinny: I have a source in contact with Morgan, even though he's never seen him. That source is willing to help me because he doesn't believe in Morgan's psychic abilities and wants to help me find out what Morgan is really up to.

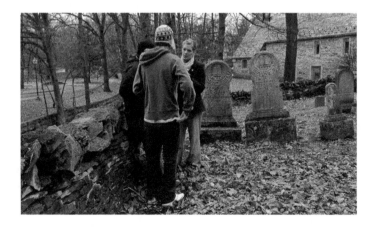

Hope Johnson is our first live actor appearance.

"Morgan has told my source that he has seen seven boxes in his crystal ball. Each contains an object of some sort. When all seven objects have been collected and examined, the truth will reveal itself. Every so often Morgan receives hints concerning the locations of the boxes. These hints are longitude and latitude. Morgan plans to use a handheld GPS device to track them.

"I have my own GPS! I'm going to give it to you. Photograph the object and email that photograph to me: hope.celebritysheet@gmail.com. I'll post it on my blog. Take the box with the object inside and this GPS to locker #165 in the HPER building. The combination to open the lock is 38-20-26. Leave the padlock locked on the locker when you go.

> Photographs of locations and objects and successful teams communicating with the other teams were essential to prove a team had located a box and so they could share their information with all players. Everyone then had the information they needed to continue in the game.

"Then you need to email the photograph to the other people helping me and give them very good directions to where you found the box, not just GPS coordinates. Most of them won't have GPS devices! In the email tell them to take a photograph of that location and send it to me so I know everybody helping me is on the same page.

"You should also fill them in on what I've told you about my source and Morgan's visions of the seven boxes.

"Morgan plans to collect the first box in one hour, so that's all the time you have. You need to beat him to the box!

"Can you remember all that? Anything you want me to repeat? [repeats as needed]

"All set? [gives them the GPS] You turn it on by pressing this button. Move the thumb stick here to highlight the main menu icon; and click like this. Highlight Find and Go and click. Now just follow the arrow! It even shows you how far you have to go! Now hurry! You only have an hour to beat Morgan to that box!"

> In a live performance where the "audience" has no script, you cannot write one for the encounter. Players do not have a script. Actors needed to be ready to respond in character and within the limits of the narrative no matter what the players decided to say, or what questions they might ask. So, documents like the above were written to make certain the actor knew the important points they needed to hit to move the game and the narrative forward, and to subtly give hints on what players might say or ask. The genuineness of the experience relied on the actors' ability to improvise.
>
> Live performances were special occasions, few and far between. They served as rewards for player progress and aided the willing suspension of disbelief. The game was structured so all teams were able to experience them. Puppet masters observed from a safe vantage point so they could intervene, if necessary. Happily, we never needed to protect our actors. It helped considerably that players were focused on gameplay and the competition, but many also enjoyed the roleplay and treated the

characters as if they were real. A glitch did occur during the performance. Another of our actors joined the puppet masters near the spot where Hope Johnson's performance was occurring. He was seen by the players taking pictures and when the sighting was later reported by them to other NPCs, they wondered who it might be as if it were a part of the narrative. Welcome to games played in the real world in real time! You will see how we worked the sighting into later episodes.

Hope Johnson Blog

Last day of February and we're off and running! At least Team Free Tibet was! Thanks to them we beat Quinn Morgan to the first of seven objects he has seen in his crystal ball. All of my reporters should have received a copy of the photograph Free Tibet took of the object they found. What is it? A piece of really bad abstract art? Part of a larger picture? Could be too soon to tell. Check out Celebrity Sheet Online on Monday for their photograph.

I wanted to give a shout out to the second-place team, TBD, too. They were standing by if Free Tibet had fallen down on the job. And here's some irony: not only did Free Tibet beat them by one minute in the red clock phase of my challenge, but TBD emailed me to say that the box was located only 60 feet behind their dorm! So close and yet so far away!

And to Team **3 Amigos**, I had to publish one of your photos, too. Talk about going above and beyond the call of duty!

My congratulations to Free Tibet and my thanks to everybody who is helping me! If you have any ideas about what the objet d'abstract art might mean, email me. I'll share the most interesting ideas in another blog!

Enjoy the rest of your weekend. What am I going to do? Shoot off an email to Mr. Psychic and let him know he'd be better off cooperating with us than fighting us! Then I'll start writing up today's adventure for Celebrity Sheet Online. Look for it in a day or two. TTFN!

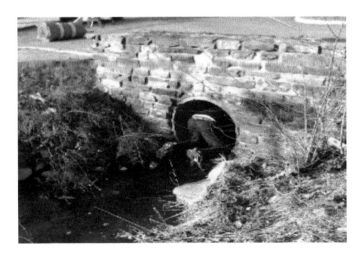

One of the three Amigos boldly going where no one has gone before.

IU Security Public Website

All officers check the internal site for an important update.

IU Security Internal Site

A car reported stolen in Virginia has been found twenty miles from Bloomington. It was discovered yesterday evening out of gas and abandoned in a parking lot in Martinsville with Steven Cartwright's fingerprints on it. He is undoubtedly trying to make his way here and must be considered a serious threat to this school.

PUZZLE DETAIL

In addition to the intrinsic rewards given to successful teams, extrinsic rewards were also handed out. This was true of all teams. Whether or not they were the first to accomplish a goal, all teams who completed puzzles were awarded with chits that could be accumulated for prizes. There were also cash prizes, contributions from local merchants, such as the gift certificates from the Game Preserve mentioned below, free pizza and other perks. The announcements of teams who won any of these awards incentivized all teams to participate even if they weren't solving the most puzzles. Prizes and awards were handed out a week after the game was complete. All teams received at least two.

These milestones also established a predictable rhythm for the gameplay that kept teams from getting confused or falling behind. The main puzzles, called sprints, required a reoccurring sequence of moves players had to make in order to progress in the game.

Here is a flowchart created for the kick-off meeting in February to alert all players what was expected of them and what clues were essential to solve the ultimate mystery posed by the game narrative.

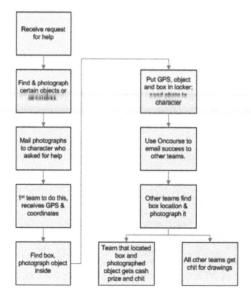

Main puzzle milestones.

There were seven sprints that formed the spine of the game's narrative. Sprints were timed special physical events. The first team or teams to complete them had a limited amount of time to use GPS coordinates to locate a plastic box with a clue inside.

But sprints were not the only puzzles in the game. A variety of peripheral puzzles, some very easy, others more difficult, ensured that all teams had a chance to solve at least some of them and contribute to the solutions of multiple mysteries. Here are three lists of the detailed steps puppet masters consulted for three early puzzles in Episode 1 to track player progress and offer hints.

Time Travelers

1. Hope announces on her blog a test called "Time Travelers." The word "time" is a clue.

2. Hope tweets: "Okay, it's time. They are 4. They are red. Take a photo of each one with a team member in the shot. Email the photos to hope@celebritysheet.com!" The word "time" is again a clue, as are the number 4 and the color red.

3. Players are to photograph the four big red clocks on campus and email the photographs to Hope.

Character communications in the game, like "Take a photo…" above, were used to make sure players recorded their progress through photographs, tweets, documents etc. In addition to earning the chits that could be collected for prizes, this served three purposes. First, their communications would indicate successful completion of puzzles and challenges. Second, as mentioned above, it meant our non-player characters could publicly celebrate player achievements. Hope and Morgan would post team names, acknowledge their members and broadcast their achievements by publishing photographs and player communications on their websites and in their blogs and emails. Third, it increased active competition between the teams, all within the narrative context of the game.

Hack into IU Security Internal Site

1. Players must hack into the IU Security internal web page.

2. The IU Security public website features a story on passphrases. In the story are two clues: the internal page passphrase is composed of three parts and they are separated by spaces, not punctuation.

3. The public site also carries a story on Chief Mars' dog Beartrap, who has given birth to a litter of three female miniature Doberman Pinscher puppies. Mars is quoted as saying he played *The Mikado* to soothe Beartrap during delivery. The fact there are three puppies and that they are female are clues. *The Mikado* is a clue.

4. Googling "The Mikado" brings up many references. Several give the names of the three young women characters in the operetta.

5. In every reference checked the women are always listed in the following order: Yum-Yum, Pitti-Sing, Peep-Bo. The passphrase with spaces between the names instead of commas is "yum-yum pitti-sing peep-bo."

Sometimes puzzles in the game were simply suggested by content that was available to all teams. Hacking into the IU Security Internal Site is an obvious example of this. Were we worried that no one would notice the hints on the IU Security Public Website? We had hopes that there were enough clues to indicate hacking the internal site was possible. The button on the public website labeled "Internal Site" was a reasonably obvious attractor. And there is something agreeably naughty in hacking into an official site they weren't supposed to access. Wouldn't it be interesting to see what IU security doesn't want us to see?

That pretty much guaranteed that players of a game containing mysteries and puzzles would want to find a way into the internal site. We were not wrong. The passphrase was figured out in less than twenty-four hours, used, and shared among the teams.

The fourth game in this book, *The Janus Door*, is chock full of agreeably naughty opportunities like this since it's a game teaching cybersecurity.

Sam's Message

1. Sam's message is written in a simple form of code called a transposition cipher. Sam's blog contains the following clues:

   a. Find the current favorite of his "demons" i.e., alcohol. His demons are whiskey, tequila, vodka and rum. In a recent post on the blog he mentions his lair is littered with empty bottles, mostly vodka. So "vodka" is his favorite demon.

   b. "let me count the letters." There are 5 letters in the word vodka.

   c. "they bring me down." count down 5 letters from the letter that is transposed. For example, "M" in the cipher is actually an "H."

   d. "they loop." If the letter in the cipher is less than 5 places from the beginning of the alphabet, the count loops around, and continues at the end. For example, the letter "X" is actually a "C."

   e. Punctuation is correct.

   f. Players can also decode the cipher by trial and error, identifying the most common letters first.

CHAPTER 5

Episode 2 – Gimme Shelter

EPISODE 2 GAME LOGIC FLOWCHART

March 2–March 12

CHARACTERS

Quinn Morgan, Hope Johnson, Milton Mars, Sam Clemens, Steven Cartwright

NARRATIVE

Hope's first story on Quinn Morgan hints that in previous cases, Morgan has been accused of creating problems he could then solve. Morgan tweets to all students that he has learned students are helping Hope and then asks that they only pretend to do so.

Morgan is correct. Hope tweets to all students that the source helping her has learned Morgan can't locate the second box but can only see a structure like a "shelter" or a "gazebo." She asks students to email a photo of each campus gazebo or shelter. There are four. Hope's source will give the photos to Morgan to see what he can make of them.

> You will not find Morgan mentioning shelters and gazebos. This particular "source" did not exist. We wanted to plant the idea of rival teams spying for the character they wanted to help to enhance competition, so we invented someone doing it. As you have already read, we needn't have bothered. Several students from both sides had already decided to support either Morgan or Hope. And by this time, we had at least a few double agents. Many students decided to help whomever was looking for help at the time to reap the rewards.

On the IU Security Public Site, it's revealed that Morgan has contacted IU Security and agreed to help them identify the threat. One possible suspect has been spotted: Steven Cartwright. A man matching his description has been found in a tourist's photograph. It shows Cartwright furtively entering a building. The public are asked to identify the

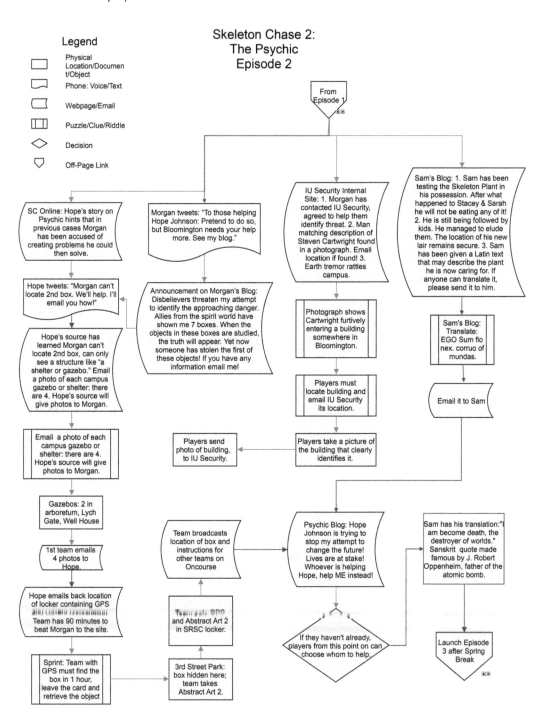

Episode 2 Game Logic Flowchart.

building if possible, by taking a photo that clearly indicates what it is. Students compete to find the building and send photos to IU Security. A third story concerns a small earth tremor that was felt in the Bloomington area…

Sam Clemens has been writing on his blog. He congratulates the players who solved the cipher by name. Thanks to their efforts, he will begin to blog again regularly. He has been testing the skeleton plant in his possession. After what happened to Stacey and Sarah, Sam declares he will not be eating any of the skeleton plant!

> This is a reference to Stacey Cassell and Sarah Chase drinking the Source Company's new formula, derived from skeleton plants, and injected into bottles of "vitamin water." Sarah became deathly ill with a variety of strange symptoms. Stacey, who drank more, was turned into an abominable snow person. Players never met her, but they heard reports of sightings of a large, hairy beast and of a strange howling heard in the dead of the night. Players got to hear the howling for themselves later in that game when they met with Sam Clemens in the university's greenhouse, disturbingly reminiscent of H.P. Lovecraft's "The Colour Out of Space."

Sam has again been followed. He has so far managed to elude whoever they are. The location of his "new lair" remains secure. Sam has been given a Latin text that may describe the plant he is now caring for. It reads: "EGO sum fio nex, corruo of mundus." He asks anyone who can translate it to please send the translation to him.

Morgan announces on his blog: "Disbelievers threaten my attempt to identify the approaching danger. My allies from the spirit world have shown me 7 boxes. When the objects in these boxes are studied, the truth of the danger threatening IU will appear. Yet now someone has stolen the first of these objects! If you have any information, email me!"

Students find the four shelters: two in the arboretum, one at the Lych Gate and one by the Well House. The first team to find all four emails photographs of them to Hope. Hope believes they are the key to the location of the second of the seven boxes Morgan has "seen." She emails the location of the locker and its combination to the winning team. The locker contains the Garmin GPS and instructions to beat Morgan to the site.

They are to leave the card showing they have taken the object inside. The box is hidden at the stage in the Third Street Park. The object inside is another painting, Abstract Art 2. The team puts the GPS and Abstract Art 2 in the locker and broadcasts on Oncourse to the other teams the location where the box was found and Hope's instructions.

Morgan angrily posts on his blog: "Hope Johnson is trying to stop my attempt to change the future! Lives are at stake! Whoever is helping Hope, help ME instead!" Players from this point on can choose whom to help.

Ideas about the translation are emailed to Sam. The text translates as "I am become death, the destroyer of worlds." This is a quote made famous by J. Robert Oppenheimer, father of the atomic bomb. Sam publishes the translation.

EPISODE 2 CONTENT DELIVERY CHRONOLOGY

Monday, March 2

Quinn Morgan Tweet (All Teams)

To those helping Hope Johnson: Pretend to do so, but Bloomington needs your help more. See my blog.

> In 2009 Twitter was new enough to many students that we needed to publish instructions on how to join. Tweets, then limited to 140 characters, were used in the game almost entirely as pointers to content on websites or in blogs. Although many tweets were sent, most carried no special information and for that reason some have been eliminated from this document. If this ARG were to be designed today, we would use texts. For *Skeleton Chase 2* private correspondence with more content was delivered in emails.

> A note on coordinating the tweets: first a blog or website would go live on the server. Once we knew it was successfully posted, we would add the tweet that prompted players to it. The original design documents were written that way. That sequence has been reversed in this document, otherwise you'd be reading the document *before* you read the tweet telling you to read the document.

Quinn Morgan Blog

There are those who threaten my attempt to identify the approaching danger. If they are misguided, or if they are actively aiding the forces that threaten us, they will not succeed.

Despite the psychic fog that increases around Bloomington, my allies in the spirit world showed me the shape behind the 7 in my crystal ball. It is a simple plastic box. 7 boxes. I gave this information to Chief Milton Mars of IU Security. I told him when the objects in these boxes are studied, the truth will appear. Yet the first box has been stolen. I don't want to think he has betrayed me. But I do not think that Hope Johnson is psychic.

Ms. Johnson promises to trade the contents of the box to me, if I will consent to a face-to-face interview. I do not respond well to blackmail. I call on those of you who are helping her to reconsider. Pretend to help her but instead send *me* the photograph of the contents of the second box when the coordinates are revealed to me.

> Here we continue to give players choices that will directly affect the game. In this case an offer to change loyalties. It was debated within teams and increased engagement and competition. I've used this quite a few times, both in my own multiplayer classrooms and those I have designed for others.

Celebrity Sheet Online

The Game Is Afoot!

Early last week I issued a challenge to Indiana University students to prove they had what it takes to assist in my investigation of self-proclaimed psychic Quinn Morgan. The response was overwhelming. I now have a team of crack reporters and paparazzi to help me find out the truth about Morgan. And just in time too!

On his blog Morgan claims to have seen the number 7 and a shadowy object of some sort in his crystal ball. Having learned that Morgan thinks the object is a small plastic box, and that Morgan was going to try and retrieve it; your intrepid reporter (Moi!) was determined to reach it before he did.

This past Saturday I came into possession of the coordinates to where the box supposedly could be found. I met my fastest team of reporters, Free Tibet, in the Beck Chapel cemetery on the IU campus. Team TBD was waiting to take over if Free Tibet failed. Why a cemetery? Frankly it was my photographer, Chris Debuc, who came up with that idea, and it certainly seemed to fit the occasion!

At the cemetery I gave them a handheld GPS receiver. I had already programmed the coordinates into it.

Knowing we only had an hour before Morgan would arrive to find the box, they took off running in the direction the arrow on the GPS indicated. Only minutes later, near a drainage outlet behind Ashton dorm, they found the box. Their photograph of the object inside is reproduced here. What is it? Amateurish abstract art? I've asked my reporters to send me their theories. And if it is only one of seven pieces of a larger picture as some suggest, what does it represent?

Team Free Tibet then took the picture, box and GPS to a locker in the Wildermuth gym at the School of Health, Physical Education and Recreation (HPER), where I picked them up.

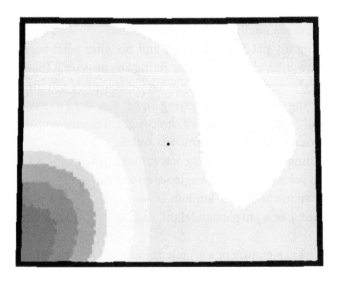

Many theories as to what this photograph means.

One unsettling moment came in the graveyard when we noticed someone taking photographs of my rendezvous with Team Free Tibet. It was difficult to get a good look at him since the camera covered his face, but he seemed young, tall and with a crop of unruly black hair. Since Chris (who took all of the pictures for this story) was the only photographer I had hired for my series on Quinn Morgan, what was I to make of this?

At first, I thought he was just a tourist. But he seemed only interested in us…

This was the beginning of the cover story we added for when the actor playing Sam Clemens was spotted near Hope's live appearance.

At any rate my fellow reporters and I are now one step ahead of Quinn Morgan. Hopefully he will now be willing to talk to me! More soon as this story continues to develop!

Hope Johnson Blog

Golly! Blogger War! Okay, I'll play. Mr. Morgan is lying. I did not attempt to blackmail him. I want to help. I sent the photograph of the object in the first box to him, some kind of simple abstract art somebody made on a computer.

I'll give him the second one when one of my reporter teams sends me a photograph of it. But I'm keeping the objects themselves. If he wants them, all he has to do is agree to meet with me. Ask yourselves? What is he trying to hide? Is he just afraid of being exposed as a fraud? Or is it something worse? Whine all you like, Mr. Morgan. My reporters are loyal to me. You want to challenge us? I know I speak for everybody when I say: bring it.

Tuesday, March 3

Sam Clemens Blog

who does hope johnson think she is anyway? last week she calls me a sick puppy then this week emails me and tries to make nice. go spy on criss angel. i'm no celebrity. i'm a gardener. i black out occasionally. so what?

so i've been testing my pet skeleton plant. and no, after what happened to stacey and miss high and mighty sarah chase, i won't be eating any more of it thanks. and no it doesn't need water, miss giggly reporter. the center, what we gardeners call the stigma, that's where the action is. it's getting darker, maybe getting bigger too, hard to tell.

those kids are still following me. one of these nights i'm goin to turn around and chase their skinny little bodies home to mommy. you watch.

hey, here's something: so i'm surfing the www, looking for some stuff any stuff on my pet skeleton plant. i run across this guy in england. an archaeologist. he's on some dig in some newly discovered roman ruins near london. he says they found a plant carved on a wall. he says it looks to him like a purple dandelion. that's a skeleton plant to you non-botanists out there.

so I email him. i want a picture or a sketch or something. skeleton plants love west texas where it's hot and dry, pardner. the only time it's hot and dry in England is when a pub runs out of smithwick's. probably just a daisy or something. i'll let you know.

Email to Chief Milton Mars

The following is another example of the real world in real time nature of an ARG and a taste of how carefully players were watching the game. A puppet master flagged this email from a player:

"Howdy Chief,
 I've noticed something in a recent post on Sam Clemens' blog that I thought would be of interest to you. He mentions being in contact with an archaeologist in England who is studying Roman ruins outside London, and has a link to a picture of the ruins. The picture is hosted on the website for the Source Corporation, the organization that Cartwright worked for as a security officer. If this archaeologist is in fact Cartwright, it may indicate his whereabouts outside the U.S., or perhaps another possibility. It's not much to go on, but it's something! Hope it helps!"

Player 1

I was notified immediately and responded in character:

"Thank you, Player 1! When you mentioned it I went and had a look. You were right! As you know the FBI closed down the site some weeks ago. I suspect Clemens was using it as a spoof address to conceal an IP that might help reveal his location. He probably noticed we were sniffing around and has now dropped it. Thanks for the tip. Sound detective work!
 Chief Milton Mars
 IU Security"

This was our mistake: a link from the previous game that should not be there. Throughout the running of an ARG expect the unexpected and be ready to cover your tracks!

Hope Johnson Email (All Teams)

As I told some of you on Saturday, I have a source who is in contact with Morgan. My source has learned the psychic can't locate the 2nd box. He can only "see" a structure. He describes it as a "shelter or gazebo made from limestone or concrete." I'm told there are four of these on campus, although one is more properly called a "lych gate." Email me a photograph of each one. Make sure one of your teammates is in each photograph for scale! My source will give the photographs to Morgan. Maybe that will help him to see more. Then I can ask for an interview in return for my assistance!

Wednesday, March 4

Hope Johnson Email (1st Team ONLY)

Great job, ZAM Squad! You've earned the right to try and recover the second box! I know Morgan expects to have the coordinates from his spirits (do spirits really need coordinates???) this Sunday morning, March 8th at 11am. I'll give you the exact instructions as soon as my source gets the coordinates for me.

Hope Johnson Blog

My investigative teams are living up to their advance press! **ZAM Squad** was the **first team** to send me four pictures. They are the four pictures I was looking for! However, read on...

I forwarded them to Mr. Morgan to prove I want to cooperate, not to coerce! He just emailed me and thanked me. But he added that none of ZAM Squad's pictures are giving him the image of a box he was expecting, nor has he yet received any coordinates from the spirit world. Where did I go wrong? More psychic smog, Quinn?

Okay, Hope, play nice. But if he's telling the truth, I'm not sure what this means.

In any case, everyone who has not yet done so, should send me the pictures of the three gazebos and the lych gate (remember, Google is your friend!) that I've asked for. Let's not try to second guess Mr. Morgan. When he finds out the coordinates, ZAM Squad has earned the right to track down the second box wherever it is.

In second place was **Team Thunderfly**. However, their pictures are too close in a couple of cases to tell if they are at the correct locations. I will give them a chance to take better pictures with less FACE and more location!

That would put **Free Tibet**, winners of my first challenge, in third position.

Psychic Busters were fourth, not far behind them. If Thunderfly can't get better pictures, they lose their slot and PB moves into third. For the record **TBD** was second fastest but had a location wrong. You'll still need to find that fourth location to complete the task. (Your pictures are also pretty close, be careful! As handsome as you are, I need to see *where* you are, as much as I need to see you!)

Now we wait until the psychic gets his psychical mojo in sync.

In other news, I've received an email from one of my reporters who thinks she knows who that mysterious second photographer might be. I'm not going to say it in public, yet.

Keeping the story of the mysterious second photographer alive.

We'll see how things develop...

Great job everybody!

Sam Clemens Blog

okay so here's a picture he took of the plant on the wall they uncovered. it's no daisy.

check out the one I chalked on the limestone near stacey's car when she disappeared last semester.

look at the center. it's dark like mine. he says there's also something written in ancient latin below the carving of the plant. "ancient latin?" it's a dead language dude. there's no such thing as modern latin. so it's taking them some time to expose because the stone is very fragile he said. he promised to send me a copy of the text when he gets it uncovered.

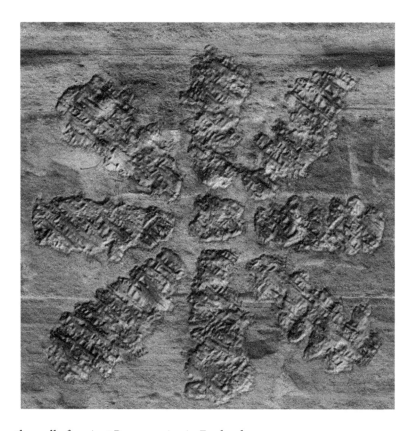

Carving on the wall of ancient Roman ruins in England.

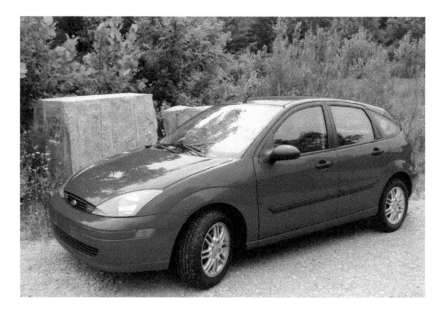

Sam's chalked image of a skeleton plant from the first game.

Thursday, March 5

Celebrity Sheet Online

The veil that surrounds man of mystery Quinn Morgan was lifted a bit today. Last week I reported on my blog a curious connection between Morgan and a young man named Sam Clemens. Clemens is reportedly hiding someplace on campus with a talking plant or something. Anybody remember *Little Shop of Horrors*??? Read more on my blog.

Now I can report I've uncovered what may be a significant key to unlocking Morgan's purpose here in Bloomington!

Read on…

You know all those glowing testimonials Morgan has on his website? Well, I've learned that at least one of them is suspect to say the least. The little lost girl Morgan claims to have located? The local authorities from Salinas, California tell me that Morgan rented a house in nearby Carmel three weeks *before* seven-year-old Tanya Zalensky went missing.

You with me so far?

Authorities now say that on the day before Tanya disappeared Morgan was stopped and given a traffic citation for a broken taillight right at the entrance to Golden Oaks, the subdivision where the Zalensky's live.

I'll bet you're ahead of me now!

Yep, in two of Morgan's successful cases that are NOT on his website, the authorities say they suspected he in fact created the incidents that he then stepped in to solve with his psychic powers!

Okay, but…

The Zalensky's, when told of this, reconfirmed their faith in Morgan's powers. They attributed his arrival on the scene before the little girl disappeared to his ability to see into the future. And Tanya's story has always been that she wandered off by herself and saw no one else until she was rescued.

And finally…

A traffic citation, Hope??? Well, golly! Can the officer who gave Morgan the ticket give us a description of Morgan? Here's a direct quote from Officer Ronald Crest of the Carmel-by-the-Sea Police: "Now that you mention it, that's a funny thing. I looked the guy straight in the face. I remember the guy was pleasant and courteous and apologized, but for the life of me when I try to picture his face all I see is a kind of *fog*…" More fog!!!

That's it from your intrepid reporter for now. I'm off to have breakfast at Runcible Spoon. I hear it is delish!

IU Security Public Website

Reclusive Psychic Promises to Identify Threat to Bloomington

Certain facts have come to our attention which indicate Quinn Morgan, the psychic who recently contacted local authorities, may be useful in discovering the nature of a threat to the university and the city of Bloomington. IU Security Chief Milton Mars is of the opinion that wanted fugitive, Steven Cartwright, is the source of the threat. While Mr. Morgan refuses to endorse that view until he is certain, he has provided local officials with convincing evidence of a plot against our community. So as not to jeopardize our ongoing investigation, details are being withheld from the public at present. But we want to ensure the public that there is no cause for immediate alarm. All law enforcement officers are working tirelessly to counter the threat. And we are confident of success. The following request for public assistance will greatly enhance our efforts.

Public Assistance Urgently Requested

This man is believed to be Steven Cartwright. Formerly an employee of the Source Corporation, Cartwright is now a fugitive wanted in connection with numerous crimes committed in Bloomington last fall. A federal warrant has been issued for his arrest. This photograph, taken by a Canadian tourist who no longer remembers the location, is believed to be in Bloomington. IU Security is asking all citizens to be on the lookout for this building. If you recognize this building, please photograph it. Email the photograph to iusecuritytipline@gmail.com. Include the building's address; and identify it by name if possible. Thank you very much for your cooperation.

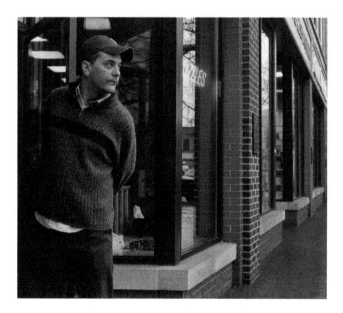

Fugitive Cartwright photographed in Bloomington.

Small Tremor Rattles Windows

The Indiana University Department of Geological Sciences has confirmed a small earth tremor shook Bloomington and surrounding areas at 4:17 this morning. Several campus residents called security, saying they had been awakened by dogs barking and windows rattling, but no damage has been reported. The tiny shake measured only 1.7 on the Richter scale. One unusual characteristic was that the temblor did not originate in the Wabash Valley Seismic Zone along the Illinois-Indiana border, source of most seismic activity in the area, including last April's 5.2 quake. In fact, the epicenter was almost directly beneath

Bloomington, 8.9 miles down. Another interesting feature was the apparent absence of any aftershocks whatsoever, although they may have simply been too small to measure. Geological Sciences are all very excited by this very local geological event, an absolute rarity, and are eagerly investigating what it could mean.

Friday, March 6

Hope Johnson Blog

A few days ago, **Player 1** from Team **Won and Done** emailed me with a theory about that **second photographer**. BTW, I'm surprised Team **Free Tibet** hasn't offered up a theory. I'm pretty sure they saw him too!

Anyway, Player 1 thinks it must have been Sam Clemens.

> Player 1 was right about the photographer. It was the actor playing Sam Clemens. He was photographing his girlfriend playing Hope Johnson. We later added a post where Sam (the character) admits it was he.

Player 1 also thinks Sam Clemens and Quinn Morgan are one and the same wacko. She supports the theory with the very reasonable question, "How many psychics can there be in Bloomington?" I'd have to agree with that. I mean Bloomington's a nice town, but it's not exactly Las Vegas.

However…

Sam, that silly boy, does say his pet plant is no longer an oracle. So, if he's telling the truth—I know BIG IF—there would still be only one, even if he isn't Quinn Morgan. My question to her was, "If he IS Morgan, why wouldn't he try to beat us to the first box instead of just taking pictures?"

And remember this: Sam claims he only goes out at night. This was Saturday morning.

Thanks, Player 1, for the food for thought!

Hope Johnson Email (All Teams)

ZAM Squad! Reminder! I need your help this **Sunday, March 8th at 11:00 am**. Expect a top-secret email from me Sunday morning with critical details.

And IF Team **ZAM Squad** can't help me on **Sunday at 11:00 am**, I need a backup team. **Free Tibet** was in second place, so they're next up. I'll send them an email by noon on Sunday, if I should need their help.

If THEY can't help me, it'll be the **Psychic Busters** who'll get a chance. And if THEY can't do it, I'll do it myself! So, I need these teams to be ready for action this Sunday!

> The team who won the right to participate in a sprint would be given detailed instructions of the steps they needed to take to complete the event. Teams that came in second and third during the qualifying puzzles would be also briefed to standby in case the first team failed.

Saturday, March 7

IU Security Public Website

Chief Mars Makes Plea for Assistance

On Thursday we posted the photograph of a man believed to be Steven Cartwright exiting or entering a building here in Bloomington. Despite all of the IU students who seem to be assisting the Celebrity Sheet Online reporter, Hope Johnson, and the psychic, Quinn Morgan, we've had very few responses! Please remember your own IU Security force needs your help too!

We have had a handful of photographs of what is believed to be the location. Once we can confirm this, we'll publish the results here. In the meantime, please remember long after the media spotlight has turned away from Bloomington to focus on some other popular story of the moment, we'll still be here requesting your assistance in keeping our community safe and secure.

Chief Milton Mars

IU Security

Hope Johnson Email (1st Team ONLY)

Greetings [team name]!

I'm busy following up another lead on Quinn Morgan. So, you'll have to do this on your own. But don't worry. The GPS and all the instructions you'll need will be in HPER locker # [TBD]" You'll have 90 minutes to find the box before Morgan, or one of his people, gets there. That should be plenty of time!

You'll probably run into my photographer, Chris Debuc. He's there to document the story. He'll have a BIG camera, so when you head out, try not to lose him!

Thanks for your help! I know you'll come through for me!

Hope

Sunday, March 8

Hope Johnson Email (1st Team Only)

"Okay, we're ready to rock. My source has obtained the coordinates of the second box. You'll have 90 minutes to beat Morgan to the site, find the box, photograph the object, email it to me at hope.celebritysheet@gmail.com and return everything to the locker. Then don't forget to email the photograph and directions to the box location to our other reporters. Good luck!"

Hope

Monday, March 9

IU Security Public Website

Cartwright Location Identified

ZAM Squad, a team involved in unraveling the mystery surrounding psychic Quinn Morgan's prediction of danger threatening our community, were the first to identify the location where fugitive Steven Cartwright was spotted last week in Bloomington. No one

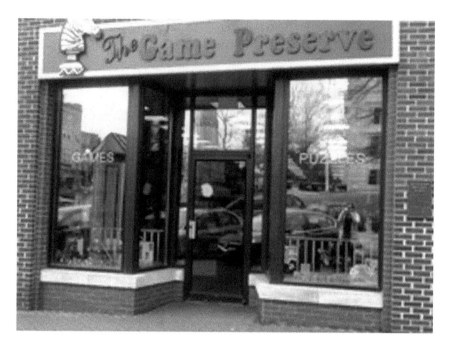

Cartwright was in the Game Preserve. Does he play D&D?

in the store, The Game Preserve on the square downtown, remembers Cartwright, or what if anything he may have purchased.

Our thanks also goes out to two other teams of concerned citizens: Psychic Busters and TBD who sent us photographs in a timely manner. Keep up the good work!

Chief Milton Mars

IU Security

Email from *Skeleton Chase* Team

Congratulations to Team ZAM Squad! They win a first-place bonus prize this week for being the first team to find the location of the photograph of Steven Cartwright posted on the IU Security website last Thursday.

Thanks to the generous support of the store in the photograph, The Game Preserve, they win a $35 gift certificate to the store!

In second place was Team Psychic Busters. They win a $25 gift certificate to The Game Preserve.

And last, but not least, Team TBD in third place wins a $15 gift certificate.

All three teams will be able to pick their prizes up at the regular check-in at HPER the week we're back from Spring Break.

Remember to solve *all* puzzles, not just the seven Milestone Puzzles. You never know when an additional puzzle will score you some extra prize goodness. And prizes will vary in value.

Great job everybody!

The *Skeleton Chase* Team

If you haven't already, you will soon realize that ZAM Squad were our stars, winning more first places than any other two teams combined. I have always tried to have as many intrinsic rewards as possible in my multiplayer classrooms. In the end there would always be a major extrinsic reward anyway: a grade. This game, unlike the others in this book and the first *Skeleton Chase*, did not have a captive audience looking for a grade. In a perfect world intrinsic rewards would be enough, and narrative and gameplay would provide them. Any teacher will tell you that education is not a perfect world. Above you see us crashing through the fourth wall to remind any players who might be straying, or not logging as many steps as possible, that there were pots of gold to be found at the end of this rainbow and they were somewhat easier to acquire. Rewards were never reserved for first place winners alone. Intrinsic rewards were doled out on this occasion by IU Security.

When we first thought of approaching local merchants to ask if they would donate prizes for our game, we had no idea how they would respond. We were surprised and delighted how many were happy to oblige. When you are looking for extrinsic rewards for a project such as this, I encourage you to reach out to the surrounding community. They are often eager to help. Not only was it good publicity, it was also fun for them to be included in the storyline. A later ARG designed and run by one of my classes at IU about a circus that used to winter in Bloomington was also successful in obtaining prizes for their players from Bloomington merchants.

Celebrity Sheet Online

Thanks to the heroic efforts of one of my teams of reporters, ZAM Squad, we have beaten Quinn Morgan to the second of the seven boxes he has seen in his crystal ball. Even though this time the coordinates took ZAM Squad off campus, they were still able to retrieve the box in just under an hour, barely beating our celebrated psychic! Free Tibet and Psychic Busters were standing by just in case, but ZAM Squad came through!

My photog, Chris Debuc, was there to record their efforts, as you can see. Chris reports no sign of the second photographer glimpsed last week at the graveyard. ZAM Squad's photograph of the object they recovered is reproduced here on this page. How it fits with the first I don't know. How this is a clue to the danger Morgan claims is threatening the peaceful college community of Bloomington, Indiana I don't know. But thanks to ZAM Squad I feel certain we are a bit farther along the trail to learning the truth.

Sam Clemens, the former IU grad student hiding out somewhere on campus has an interesting entry on his blog: a carving from some newly unearthed Roman ruins in the UK that looks a lot like the skeleton plant he supposedly is carrying for.

I can also report that the man **IU Security** suspects is the source of the danger, **Steven Cartwright**, was seen in Bloomington. A few days ago, IU Security published a recent photograph taken by a Canadian tourist (did she come here for the weather???) and asked

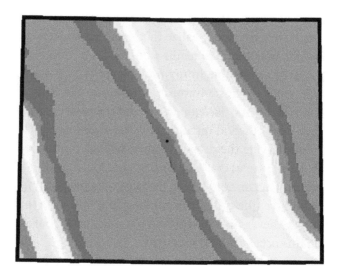

Another piece of abstract art?

citizens to identify its location and take a picture of the location. The man in the photograph certainly looks like Cartwright. I don't know if the location has been identified yet, but I've been wandering around Bloomington a lot lately, and it certainly seemed familiar to me!

Hope Johnson Blog

Thanks to the heroic efforts of one of my teams of reporters, **ZAM Squad**, we have beaten Quinn Morgan to the second of the seven boxes he has seen in his crystal ball. Even though this time the coordinates took a team off campus, they were still able to retrieve the box in just under an hour, barely beating our celebrated psychic! Free Tibet and Psychic Busters were standing by just in case, but ZAM Squad came through!

My photog, **Chris Debuc**, was there to record their efforts, as you can see. Chris reports no sign of the second photographer glimpsed last week at the graveyard.

How the second abstract art picture fits with the first I don't know. How this is a clue to the danger Morgan claims is threatening the peaceful college community of Bloomington, Indiana I don't know. But thanks to ZAM Squad I feel certain we are a bit farther along the trail to learning the truth.

Sam Clemens, the former IU grad student hiding out somewhere on campus has an interesting entry on his blog: a carving from some newly unearthed Roman ruins in the UK that looks a lot like the skeleton plant he supposedly is looking after.

I can also report that the man **IU Security** suspects is the source of the danger, **Steven Cartwright**, was seen in Bloomington. A few days ago, IU Security published a recent photograph taken by a Canadian tourist (did she come here for the weather???) and asked citizens to identify its location and take a picture of the location. The man in the photograph certainly looks like Cartwright. I don't know if the location has been identified yet, but I've been wandering around Bloomington a lot lately, and it certainly seemed familiar to me!

Tuesday, March 10

Sam Clemens Blog

okay, i admit i'm impressed. we've got some fancy gossip columnist running around campus, and a phony psychic, both asking for help from the local population. poor nobody sam clemens gives a call out and the response is sensational! overnight yet! almost restores my faith in humanity. almost. okay, scratch that last part entirely. but let's see how the translation machine is grinding along. we got.

> This puzzle brought out a tendency in college students to lecture. Here are a few of the thirteen opinions on the translation. The bolded comments are Sam's.

player 5: "i to be made deadly. to cut the throat of the whole."

player 7, college student: "The message you gave us was: EGO sum factus mortis. iuguolo of universitas. Now everyone knows Ego Sum is "I am" (at least, you know them if you know the famous words of Descartes: "Cognito Ergo Sum" = I think therefore I am.

    Since I do think, I used my sources to decipher the rest of the cryptic message. I came up with "I am (or have become) deadly. I will kill all [the masses].

    Now to me, this sounds like a threat. The fact that the message is in Latin, the "dead" language, isn't helping your cause." **or yours player 7. i'm not into women who go all brainy on me.**

player 9 (alpha team): "I am to become/made deadly. destroy the world. nice. looks like the apocalypse is sooner than we all think. by the way, it's not "real latin" because some phony who doesn't know latin just left a message using latin words- not latin itself. if you use the latin language this little message would be grammatically incorrect, fyi. that's why you can't translate the message as a whole- only the individual words."

more lectures! my archaeologist friend already suggested that it wasn't "real" latin. but assuming the romans from a thousand years ago knew real latin, who scratched this on their wall?

player 12: To the best of my knowledge it looks like a threat. Something to the tune of "I am the cause of death, destroyer of the world." Be careful Sam.

sam is always careful, Player 12. that's why he is still among the breathing.

Player 13: "I exist to become the death bringer. Butcher of the university"

Sam's blog continues: okay, so what do we know? it's not "real" latin. it hasn't been translated into real english either from the looks of it. it doesn't sound good, whatever it is. nasty apocalyptic stuff. and something else. this is gonna sound freaky, but it's familiar to me somehow. i never took latin. i don't know much about history. but those words. or not quite those words, but something really close. it sounds familiar, folks. i need to know why a thousand-year-old message written on a roman wall in not-so-real latin sounds FAMILIAR.

help me out here!!!

Wednesday, March 11

Quinn Morgan Blog

The psychic fog that is building around Bloomington has grown in intensity to the point where my regular control spirits can no longer penetrate it. However, I sense a local spirit trying to get through to me. The spirit is mischievous, as many are. He wants to help, but he apparently enjoys tricks and games.

I am asked to guess the identity of the spirit before he will help me locate the third box. The spirit promises that on March 23rd he will give me the means to identify him. I don't understand the need for delay, but the spirit seems to know that YOU will understand. I hope he is correct. Time is of the essence. I will contact you on March 23rd when I have learned what it is the spirit asks of me.

Until then remember you must choose to aid me or Hope Johnson. She is lying to you who help her. I do not believe she is after a story. She is trying to stop my attempt to change the future. Lives are at stake. I will not allow her to obstruct me again. Who will you believe? The search for the third box will split your ranks. Which side will *you* be on?

Thursday, March 12

Sam Clemens Tweet

"Ummm… see my blog…"

Sam Clemens Blog

okay…

player 1 from alpha team, player 2 from thunderfly, player 3 from tbd, player 4 from free tibet, player 5 from zam squad and player 6 from psychic busters…

you all tracked down the actual quote, and here it is: "i am become death, destroyer of worlds"

that's the one i was remembering… thanks… i guess…

so either these words etched on a thousand year old roman wall are from the *Bhagavad Gita*, a Hindu scripture written in sanskrit at least twenty-five hundred years ago and probably much older, or…

…they refer to j. robert oppenheimer, leader of the manhattan project, who quoted this when he saw the first test blast of an atomic bomb in 1945… or both…

what do we know? we know the inscription isn't proper latin… i'm pretty sure there were no hindu scholars running around ancient britain and i don't think the bomb blast sent dr. oppenheimer back in time…

so who wrote it there and why? and why was there a carving of my skeleton plant right above it???

tiny points of light have begun to appear in the dark center of my plant…

this is freaking scary…

Depending upon how your game is positioned within your class, consider cliffhangers at the end of a single class or a week of classes. Cliffhangers are those punctuation marks at the end of an episode in a Netflix TV series that encourage us to see what happens next. But cliffhangers are as old as the end of an act in drama, or a chapter in a novel. Giving students something to look forward to, other than reading the next chapter in their textbook, can motivate them. Here we had to deal with a ten-day vacation, but we did our best.

There was no scheduled gameplay from March 13 to March 22 due to Spring Break. The game resumed on March 23.

CHAPTER 6

Episode 3 – Stardust

EPISODE 3 GAME LOGIC FLOWCHART

March 23–March 29

CHARACTERS

Quinn Morgan, Hope Johnson, Milton Mars, Sam Clemens

NARRATIVE

There are new posts on the IU Security Public and Internal websites. Bloomington police have staked out the building where Cartwright was spotted. Chief Mars believes Morgan is on the wrong track. IU Security is also investigating Hope Johnson.

It's clear from Sam's blog that he is growing more frightened and paranoid even though his pursuers appear to be just children. He managed to lose them before they found his lair. The skeleton plant is getting very strange. It has a faint glow in the dark, and the center is changing shape. He wonders if his blackouts are related to the plant.

There is an announcement on Morgan's blog. Morgan's usual control is having trouble penetrating a psychic fog that is building around Bloomington. Morgan wants to pass control to a local spirit trying to get through. He needs to know the spirit's name before he can contact it. The only clue to the spirit's identity is that he is one of ten human statues outdoors somewhere on campus or in the surrounding community. Morgan needs help to locate the correct statue. He's sure he'll recognize it when he sees a photograph.

Morgan telephones Chief Mars to tell him that he has had a vision of Steven Cartwright near a four-sided scoreboard.

Hope tweets "Help me expose Morgan! He's a fraud. Or worse. Send pictures to me!" The teams helping Morgan will locate the ten statues and send photographs of them to Morgan. The teams helping Hope will locate the statues and send photographs to Hope. This sets up a competitive sprint with four teams taking part.

Hope receives the ten requested photographs from one of her teams and tweets "Tell me who the statue is! Don't tell Morgan!" Soon after, the ten statue photographs are sent to Morgan from one of his teams. He tweets that one of the statues triggered "a snippet of song"

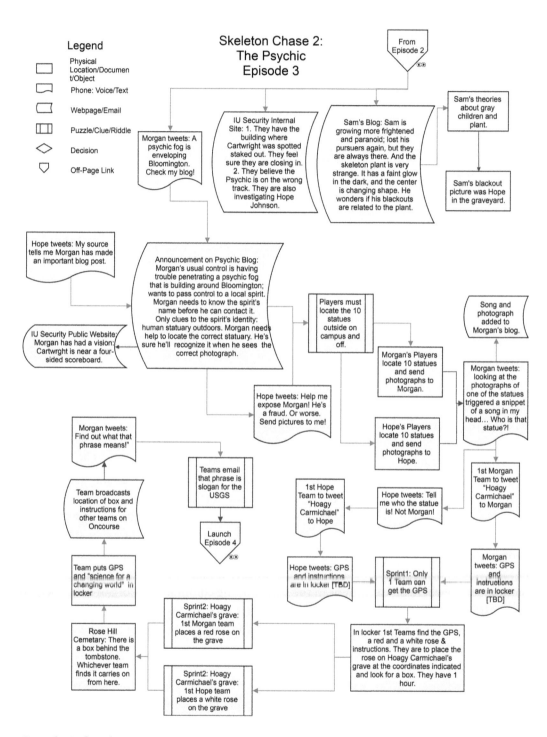

Game logic flowchart.

in his head. Who is that statue?! He publishes a link to the song on his website. The first and second of Morgan's teams to identify the song as *Stardust* and its composer as "Hoagy Carmichael" will represent him in the competitive sprint. The first and second of Hope's teams to identify the song as *Stardust* and its composer as "Hoagy Carmichael" will represent her in the competitive sprint.

One locker contains GPS, the usual instructions, and a red rose. The other locker contains a second GPS, instructions, and a white rose. The teams are to find Hoagy Carmichael's grave and place their rose on it. They have one hour.

> This is the first sprint that is a race between two opposing sides to escalate the challenge and the competition. The grave of the famous songwriter was in Rose Hill Cemetery, a considerable distance off campus.

The first teams to reach the grave in the cemetery and place the rose carries on from here. They find the third box with a message inside: "science for a changing world." They put the GPS and the message in the locker and broadcast where the box could be found on Oncourse.

Morgan tweets, "Find out what that phrase means!" He soon receives many replies. The phrase is the slogan of the United States Geological Survey.

EPISODE 3 CONTENT DELIVERY CHRONOLOGY

Classes resumed after Spring Break.

Monday, March 23

IU Security Public Website

Citizens Must Remain Vigilant

At a press briefing today Chief Milton Mars expressed his thanks to the students who earlier this month identified the location where fugitive Steven Cartwright was photographed. While a number of further sightings of Cartwright have been reported—upstairs at Nick's; auditing a biology class; even asking passersby for spare change near the bus depot—none have been corroborated. In response to a question from an Indiana Daily Student reporter, the chief had this to say: "We know Cartwright was in Bloomington. We don't know if he still is. But the fact that he was seen here in spite of the intense manhunt under way suggests that he is still planning some sort of revenge. We all must be on our guard." Asked if Cartwright was the source of the danger foreseen by psychic Quinn Morgan, the chief declined to elaborate on what he termed "our ongoing investigation."

All Officers Reminded to Check for Updates

The IU Security internal website is there for the dissemination of departmental information to all officers in a timely manner. Officers are reminded it is their obligation to check the internal site regularly. If anyone has forgotten the passphrase, ask. It has not been changed in the past month.

IU Security Internal Site
The Game Preserve Stakeout Continues

Around-the-clock surveillance of The Game Preserve at Fountain Square and other nearby businesses has as yet failed to yield any additional information as to Steven Cartwright's whereabouts, or to his reasons for being in the store. It is theorized he may simply have been using the store to gain access to some other part of Fountain Square. But no further evidence of his movements has been found. The surveillance will continue until further notice.

Chief Mars Doubts Psychic's Abilities

Despite numerous testimonials to Quinn Morgan's abilities, Chief Mars points out that during his time in Bloomington, Morgan has been little more than a bystander while students aiding the celebrity reporter, Hope Johnson, have made the most progress. Chief Mars wants to remind all officers that it was students who broke the case of Assistant Professor Sarah Chase's disappearance last fall and uncovered the Source Corporation's true motives on campus. Mars wants each and every officer to follow the teams of students engaged in the investigation. They have proven themselves to be active and intelligent to date.

Hope Johnson Subject of Inquiry

Taking no one at face value, Chief Mars has launched an inquiry into the background and associations of Celebrity Sheet Online reporter, Hope Johnson. Her uncovering of Morgan's possible involvement in the disappearance of little Mary Zalensky of Salinas, California was excellent investigative reporting. And while he shares her suspicions of Quinn Morgan, he is also aware that someone has been leaking information to Ms. Johnson on Morgan's search for the seven objects that he claims hold the key to the plot against our community. And Ms. Johnson seems to be trying to thwart Morgan, as much as she is reporting his activities.

Sam Clemens Blog
Theories

this is freaking me out. every time i go outside at night i'm followed. kids in gray hoodies and sweatpants. by their size i'd say they can't be more than seven or eight years old. it's no accident they picked me to follow. who told them to? and why pick kids for the job? i have a theory about that. what if it's so i won't be afraid? what if it's so i'll let my guard down. and as soon as i'm distracted, their texas chainsaw leather mask-wearing big brother is right there behind me reaching out.

    and that's not all. did i tell you i keep my little buddy, the skeleton plant, in an old cooler? i leave the lid off, don't worry. and it seems to like it in there. but at night. when i turn the light out. there's this glow from inside the cooler. remember how i wrote the

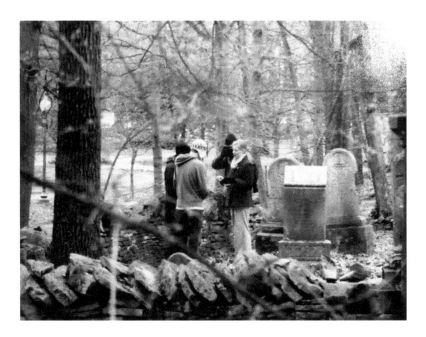

A photo I took during one of my blackouts?

center of the plant was growing darker? and i could see tiny pin pricks of light in there? at night they shine. i've got a camera. did i mention that? funny thing is i haven't used it in months. but yesterday i find pictures in its memory. pictures i don't remember taking. the camera remembers but i don't. isn't technology wonderful? i'll post one of them. the date stamp says i took it during one of my blackouts a few weeks ago. if you know who these people are, please email me. i've heard of sleepwalking, but sleep-photographing just sounds. bad.

   one more theory then i'm done. i didn't black out until the plant started changing. could it be causing it? could that glow be in my brain?

Quinn Morgan Blog
The Spirit's Riddle
Now that the psychic fog surrounding Bloomington has grown so dense, my usual control spirits cannot reach me, I'm forced to turn to a mischievous local spirit. He senses the danger and promises to help. He was true to his word and has contacted me as promised. Yet he toys with me. Before he will agree to be my new control, he asks me to discover his name. He claims my efforts will strengthen our bond. We shall see. To begin, he poses the following riddle:

> "I am like you. I am not like you.
> You see me. I don't see you.
> I am stronger than you. Yet I depend on you to care for me.
> I will outlast you. Yet I am dead.
> What am I?"

Please, if you have an answer to the spirit's riddle, email me at www.quinnmorgan.com. We need its help!

Often there are many game states a real-world real-time game could be in as players try to solve a puzzle. Here is a single example of the many scripts I wrote for the puppet masters. Different possibilities are listed for how many players came up with a solution to the spirit's riddle. We were under an inexorable time limit, needing to advance the game from day to day. If players were still baffled, I added a second hint, as you'll see.

If players cannot solve a puzzle and the game must move forward, you may need to provide an explicit answer. It's much better to at least keep the answer within the game world rather than having an announcement from the puppet masters. I included a possible outright reveal of the answer to the riddle by a deus ex machina. In this case Sam Clemens to be used as a last resort. Happily, it wasn't necessary.

IF only ONE TEAM solves the riddle, send this:

Quinn Morgan Email (All Teams)

Thanks to Team [NAME] the riddle is solved. The answer is a statue. See my blog.
   Or if MORE than ONE TEAM solves the riddle, send this:

Quinn Morgan Email (All Teams)

Thanks to Teams [NAMES] the riddle is solved. The answer is a statue. See my blog.
   Only if NO TEAMS solve the riddle, send this additional hint:

Quinn Morgan Email (All Teams)
The Spirit's Second Riddle
No answer to the riddle as yet, and the spirit grows impatient. It poses another which it insists will clarify the first:

> "Where you are warm, I am cold.
> Where you are soft, I am hard.
> Where you are a traveler through time, I am caught in a single moment.
> Forever.
> What am I?"

Or if no one figures it out by Wednesday morning, Morgan will send out the following tweet:

Quinn Morgan Tweet (All Teams)
"See Sam Clemens' blog. He has **solved** the riddle."

Sam Clemens Blog

so i'm out last night, followed by the kids in the gray hoodies of course, and i look up, and there it is: the answer to the riddle morgan's got everybody puzzling over.

> "I am like you. I am not like you.
> You see me. I don't see you.
> I am stronger than you. Yet I depend on you to care for me.
> I will outlast you. Yet I am dead.
> Where you are warm, I am cold.
> Where you are soft, I am hard.
> Where you are a traveler through time, I am caught in a single moment.
> Forever.
> What am I?"

what are you? dude, you're a statue. which statue? i don't know. there are enough people trying to save bloomington. me, i'm just trying to save sam. there ya go, mister all seeing psychic. the answer to the riddle is statue. blog that!

In any case, when the solution to the riddle is found, post these:

Quinn Morgan Blog

A statue. It is outside. Its form is human. Yes, that is the answer it seeks. But where? Which statue? It provides the slimmest of clues, a selection that I must choose from. The spirit speaks: "Four of us celebrate the halls of learning. Six of us guard the hall of justice."

Ten statues? I do not know the campus and its surrounding city as well as you do. Find these ten statues. Photograph them. The spirit promises I will know which statue is the one I seek. If with your help I can unravel the spirit's identity from this quest, we can proceed. Send me pictures of the ten statues you find: outside, human. Do not be distracted by Hope Johnson. Bloomington's real hope lies with me. Be the first team to mail your photographs to qumorgan@gmail.com. We have no more time to waste. The third box must be found!

Now we wait until at least one team gets pictures of all 10 statues. There are 4 on campus:

Herman B. Wells

Eve (together with Adam)

Adam (together with Eve)

Hoagy Carmichael

And 6 downtown at the Monroe County Courthouse in the middle of the square:

Soldier atop the big monument on the SE corner

Soldier near the NE corner

Woman with dove on the SW corner

Group of 3 above the courthouse's main door

Theoretically it could take only 7 photographs to get all 10 since Adam and Eve playing are together and the three above the courthouse's main entrance are a group.

And the game moves forward as scheduled. At least it should have!

Tuesday, March 24

Here we fold the accidental sighting of the actor into our overall story.

Sam Clemens Blog

okay, so the hottie in the graveyard is hope johnson. and the two dudes with her are a team she has rolling called free tibet. and the photographer works with her and his name is chris debuc? and they're all trying to figure out what this threat to bloomington is? well that's fine, but what's it got to do with me? why would i sleepwalk over there in the middle of the day? did i mention i never go out during the day? what does it have to do with me?

anyway, i promised a picture of my skeleton plant. here's the lil fella. first here's how he looked before we visited the cyclotron last fall.

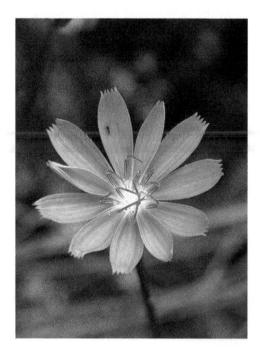

Normal skeleton plant.

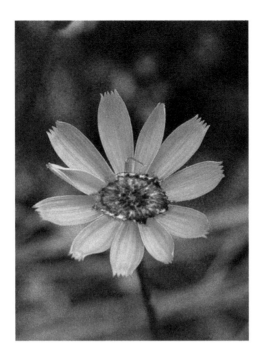

It looks very much like the plant ate the ant…

here's how he looks:
see that dark center? see the pretty pinpoints of light? okay, i know this is going to sound crazy, but remember who's writing this blog. anyway, remember when i said that latin translation was familiar? well, i'm getting déjà vu all over again cause when i look at those tiny spots of light, i get that same feeling. there's something familiar about them, too…

Hope Johnson Email (All Teams)

"Did you read the story I posted on Celebrity Sheet online on Thursday, March 5th? Morgan is a fraud! Or worse! Help me expose him! Don't help him! Be the 1st team to mail the photographs of the 10 statues he wants TO ME!" Email me the answer to the riddle on his blog at hope.celebritysheet@gmail.com!

Wednesday, March 25

Sam Clemens Blog

so player 1 from button mashers has been thinking about my skeleton plant. he's right. it's scary and crazy. but i thought it was worth sharing. here's our email exchange:
Hi Sam,
The skeleton plant (Lygodesmia texana) are not known to be the toughest plants. They are often known to die quickly and be overwhelmed by other plants. They need a lot of direct sunlight. So keep it in the sun… maybe.
The picture you sent is quite scary but i did some research on the scientist J. Robert Oppenheimer, the man who said the quote about the atomic bomb… the quote you wanted

us to decipher. Anyway, in the late 1930s, he, along with the help of Hartland Snyder, was the first to write papers suggesting the existence of what we today call black holes. In these papers, he demonstrated that there was a size limit (the so called Tolman-Oppenheimer-Volkoff limit) to stars beyond which they would not remain stable as neutron stars and would undergo gravitational collapse.

Maybe this is what is forming in your skeleton plant… a black hole…sounds crazy, but with what we are dealing with now everything seems crazy. The other spots of light forming might be other stars. Just a guess. If this is a black hole you, as well as Bloomington, has a lot to worry about!! Keep us updated.

Team ButtonMashers

hey player 1, yeah, let's hope you're wrong. it does look sorta astro-physical-like, doesn't it? but here's the thing: there's something about the little fella that seems familiar and i got no idea what a black hole really looks like.

Totally unplanned collateral learning.

Thursday, March 26

IU Security Public Website
Steven Cartwright Sighted but Only in a Dream?
Chief Milton Mars received a telephone call from alleged psychic, Quinn Morgan earlier today. Morgan claims to have seen Cartwright somewhere near a giant scoreboard. He describes the scoreboard as red and having *four sides*. None of the scoreboards on the athletic fields here on campus have four sides. Chief Mars has for assistance from the public to help us in identifying this scoreboard. Anyone who may know where this scoreboard may be found is asked to email the IU Security Tipline at iusecuritytipline@gmail.com.

Quinn Morgan Blog
If NO TEAM has sent photographs of all 10 statues to either Quinn Morgan OR Hope Johnson:

Time Is Running Out
I have not received the photographs of all ten statues from any team as yet. The spirit adds this additional clue: "Four are on campus, 2 separate statues and 2 figures in 1 statue. Six are downtown." Photograph the statues. Don't forget to include a team member. Email them to me at qumorgan@gmail.com. Hurry, before the spirit turns his back on me!

Hope Johnson Blog
Don't Let Me Down!
Hey! What's up with my ace reporters??? Nobody has sent me pictures of the ten statues Morgan mentioned in his blog! He's gotten another clue from his spirit and posted it on

his blog. We can still beat him. Get me those pictures with one of your team in the shot! Email them to me at hope.celebritysheet@gmail.com!

Here it was Thursday. Our biggest sprint was set to run on Sunday. And still we did not have our four teams. Happily, on Friday we had our sprinters.

Friday, March 27

After teams for BOTH Morgan and Hope have emailed the correct pictures:

Quinn Morgan Website

[Clickable MP3 of "Stardust" and photograph of Hoagy Carmichael's statue are added to the site now.]

As I studied the photographs, I began to hear a song… haunting… beautiful… I borrowed a rehearsal room in the Jacobs School of Music. I'm no pianist, yet I was able to play. I was channeling the spirit. It… he… played for me and I recorded it. And the spirit introduced himself to me: a former student here at Indiana University. The statue was recently placed next to the auditorium in his honor. Listen to his music here on my site as he played it through me.

I sense a race approaching. This Sunday… Ms. Johnson will not give up. I see two teams loyal to her competing. So be it.

Email the names of the song and its composer to me at qumorgan@gmail.com. The first team to do so will join the first team to photograph the ten statues, Team [Name]. Both will represent me in this race to find the third box. Team [Name] will represent Ms. Johnson, and whoever is the first to email her the name of the song will as well.

Hope Johnson Blog

I accept Mr. Morgan's challenge! Team [Name] and whoever emails the names of the song and its composer to hope.celebritysheet@gmail.com will race for me and for a free and unfettered press!

After the FIRST TEAM to email "Stardust" to Quinn Morgan:

Quinn Morgan Blog

Hoagy Carmichael is the composer and "Stardust" is that lovely song. My champions are assembled. Team [Song Team's Name] will join Team [Photograph Team's Name] in the race for the third box on Sunday. I will be contacting Ms. Johnson momentarily to negotiate the rules for this race.

After the FIRST TEAM to email "Stardust" to Hope Johnson:

Hope Johnson Blog

Whoo hoo! The song is "Stardust" and its composer is Hoagy Carmichael! Team [Song Team's Name] will join Team [Photograph Team's Name] to race for all reporters everywhere! I'll get together with Mr. Morgan and work out the details asap.

Time: 5 minutes after posting the above blog entries. They *could* be at different times.

Hope Johnson Email (Hope Teams)

Great job, everybody! You've earned the right to try and recover the third box! Mr. Morgan and I have traded emails. He claims that his local spirit guide, Hoagy Carmichael, has told him there is only one more step before he can help. Hoagy is embarrassed by this. Something about his fans in the beyond insisting. Okay, whatever. I'll play along. They're afraid a lot of us don't remember his name or the songs he wrote. So, they cooked up this race. They hope "this will restore his memory to a new generation." That's okay by me. Did you listen to "Stardust" all the way through? There are critics who say it is the BEST song ever written!

Mr. Morgan and I have worked out how this "race" is going to work. So be ready at 11:00 am sharp this Sunday, March 29th. I'll email you instructions the moment I have them! Until then, this is top secret. Tell no one! Mr. Morgan may have spies even among my loyal reporters!

Hope Johnson
Celebrity Sheet Online

Quinn Morgan Email (Morgan Teams)

Thank you for helping me to save Bloomington. You have made a wise decision. I have exchanged emails with Ms. Johnson. As you know, I will not meet with her in person. And given her wiles she might have had a phone call traced.

My local spirit guide, Mr. Hoagy Carmichael, has told me there is only one more step before he is free to aid me. He confesses to being embarrassed by this. It appears his fans in the afterlife are demanding it. In fact, this race was apparently their idea. They fear too many among you do not remember his name or the songs he wrote. They hope this will restore his memory to a new generation.

I will discover what is required and communicate it to Ms. Johnson. All I know now is that the race is to be this Sunday, March 29th. Be ready at 11:00 am. Tell no one else. Ms. Johnson may have spies even among those claiming to be loyal to me. Do not fail me. There is far too much at stake. We need to see the object in that third box!

Quinn Morgan

Saturday, March 28

This would be our first competitive sprint. The only activity on Saturday were official postings from us explaining the rules for the two teams each from Hope and Morgan who would be competing.

Sunday, March 29

Instruction Sheet for Hope Johnson's Teams

We need to beat Morgan's teams and get that third box. I'm depending on you! Read the following instructions carefully and take this sheet with you for reference.

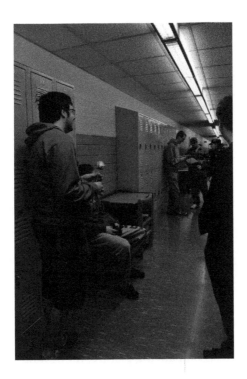

The first competitive sprint is about to begin.

Remove the white rose and the GPS receiver. You are to place the white rose on Hoagy Carmichael's tombstone. The GPS coordinates are programmed into the receiver.

After placing the rose on the tombstone, photograph it with a member from each team in the picture. The third box will be nearby. Photograph the object inside and email it to me, but then leave it in the box. Return the object in the box to this locker and relock them inside with the GPS. Now, go outside and follow the GPS instructions

Instruction Sheet for Quinn Morgan's Teams

We must beat Ms. Johnson's teams and get that third box. Much is depending upon your success! Read the following instructions carefully and take this sheet with you for reference.

Remove the red rose and the GPS receiver from the locker. You are to place the red rose on Hoagy Carmichael's tombstone. The GPS coordinates are programmed into the receiver.

After placing the rose on the tombstone, photograph it with a member from each team in the picture. The third box will be nearby. Photograph the object inside and email it to me, but then leave it in the box. Return the object in the box to this locker and relock them inside with the GPS. Now, go outside and follow the GPS instructions:

Quinn Morgan Blog
Third Box Recovered

My teams were victorious, and despite the unfortunate technical problem with Team Thunderfly's GPS—you may read about their efforts on Ms. Johnson's blog—both Team ZAM Squad and Team BHB have earned my gratitude.

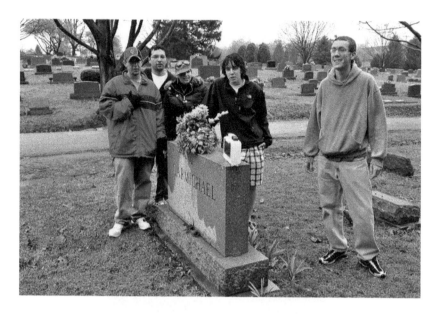

The red rose has been placed in tribute to Hoagy.

As you can see from the accompanying picture, they found Hoagy Carmichael's grave and placed a red rose there as the spirits of his fans had requested. The other flowers are from fans.

Now I trust Mr. Carmichael will be able to lend his great talents from the beyond to our efforts.

The object found in the third box is a puzzlement. As you can see it is an official-looking metal sign, not unlike a door plaque. It reads "science for a changing world" and there is a logo embossed on it as well.

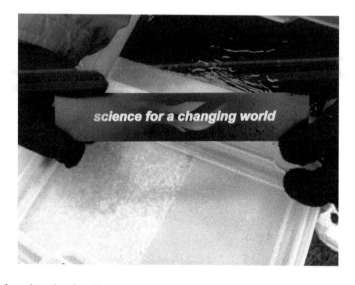

The metal sign found in the third box.

I sense a link to the two abstract paintings we recovered earlier. What that link might be though still eludes me…

Hope Johnson Blog
Technology Defeats Us

Well, friends, we didn't beat Morgan, but we did try. It seems like fate or the spirits or something were against us! The Psychic's teams, ZAM Squad and BHB, placed a red rose on Hoagy Carmichael's grave, as required by his multitude of fans who have passed on. Hopefully that will be enough to gain Hoagy's cooperation at last! I'm told ZAM Squad and BHB have sent out an email describing the location of the grave with pictures, too, so everyone can track it down. Also, they've published a photograph of the object inside the third box which I expect Mr. Morgan will display, but I'll also put it in my story. It's a metal plaque with the words "Science for a Changing World" with a wavy logo on it. Check Celebrity Sheet Online later today for the full story and a picture of the sign.

What went wrong on our end? I was expecting two members of Team Won and Done to compete. Another was out of town. But I received an email late this morning that only one of them was available. He didn't respond to the email from Morgan and I that started the challenge, so Team Thunderfly had to go it alone. They started well, reaching their locker first and taking off with the white rose. A photographer, Yvonne, hired by Mr. Morgan to document their efforts and keep an eye on them as well, left with them.

Unfortunately, there was a glitch with their GPS that sent them in the wrong direction! If I thought psychics could manipulate satellite signals from afar, I'd be suspicious!

I'll include one of Yvonne's photographs in my story. I'm sure they would have been in the race to the finish, had the GPS given them half a chance. I thank them for trying!

Quinn Morgan Email

I have forwarded a photograph to IU Security that was sent to me. I hope it will aid in unraveling the truth behind the vision I saw in my crystal ball last week of fugitive Steven Cartwright.

IU Security Public Website
Mystery of the Four-Sided Scoreboard

Teams of students trying to discover the source of the danger threatening Bloomington have contacted IU Security with theories about the image Quinn Morgan has seen in his crystal ball, namely that Cartwright was "somewhere near" a four-sided red scoreboard. We emailed Mr. Morgan for a clarification, and he insisted Cartwright was within only a very few feet of the scoreboard. Examine the following photograph sent to Morgan by Team BHB:

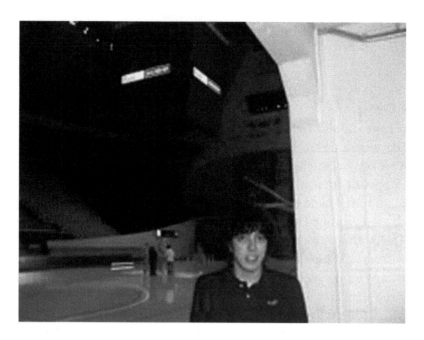

Assembly Hall four-sided scoreboard circa 2009.

This is of course the scoreboard in Assembly Hall here on campus. It has four sides. However, it's clear that to be within a "very few feet" of it, Cartwright would have to be on top of it—he isn't, my officers investigated and the dust there has been undisturbed for months—or floating in the air beside it. Since there's no indication that Cartwright has the ability to levitate, we're still at a loss to explain Morgan's "vision," if of course it means anything at all.

Anyone else with theories or photographs should send them to tipline.iusecurity@gmail.com.

Milton Mars
Chief of IU Security

Quinn Morgan Blog (All Teams)
Science for a Changing World Identified

Science for a Changing World has been identified. It is the slogan of the USGS, the United States Geological Survey. The logo on the plaque matches as well. My thanks to Player 1 of Alpha Team. She was the first to track it down. Player 2 of Thunderfly also correctly identified the phrase. Player 1 had this to say:

> "I find that rather interesting because it could have some sort of connection with the geological incident (the recent earth tremors) that the IU Security reported on their website. Maybe it has something to do with the skeleton plant that Sam Clemens has hidden away? Because his plant has been doing a lot of freaky things…"

Player 3 from TBD did not have the correct name for the agency, but offered some interesting observations as well:

"The phrase is the slogan for the US Geological Society. This confirms suspicions I had weeks ago: that the imagery from the first two boxes are partial seismographic mappings of an earthquake event. Also, I noticed an eerie correlation between the earthquake event reported on the IU Security site and the sighting of Steven Cartwright. When I went to photograph the entrance to the Game Preserve, I quickly snapped a photo of an adjacent plaque displaying the building's history and street address. Are you ready? The earthquake reported around the time of the Cartwright sighting registered a 1.7 on the Richter scale... and the address of the Game Preserve? 107 E Kirkwood Ave. I can't establish a pattern until someone spots Cartwright again, but I think I'm on to something. Now if I only get the foggiest idea about this 'four-sided red scoreboard' business…."

Well done all!

The numbers were a coincidence. But the connection between the USGS and the earth tremors was not. I love the amount of thought our players were putting into the mystery!

CHAPTER 7

Episodes 4 and 5 –
Crop Circles

EPISODE 4 GAME LOGIC FLOWCHART

EPISODE 5 GAME LOGIC FLOWCHART

EPISODES 4 AND 5 GAME LOGIC FLOWCHART

The narratives and gameplay of Episode 4 and Episode 5 were crammed into a single week, along with a surprise event we shoe-horned in at the last moment. I have separated them into three flowcharts here (Morgan, Hope and everybody else). Each can be followed separately, if desired. The stories they track are intertwined in the following narrative and chronology as they were experienced by the players. Each episode finished with a separate sprint, one on April 4, the other on April 5.

March 30–April 5

CHARACTERS

Quinn Morgan, Hope Johnson, Milton Mars, Sam Clemens

NARRATIVE

Morgan tweets that he is being followed by some children in sweat clothes.

There are three new stories on the IU Security Internal Site. First, Celebrity Sheet Online is a spoof site. There is no evidence any such organization or any reporter known as Hope Johnson exist. Hope is wanted for questioning. Second, another unexplained tremor has been felt. Third, Steven Cartwright is still at large.

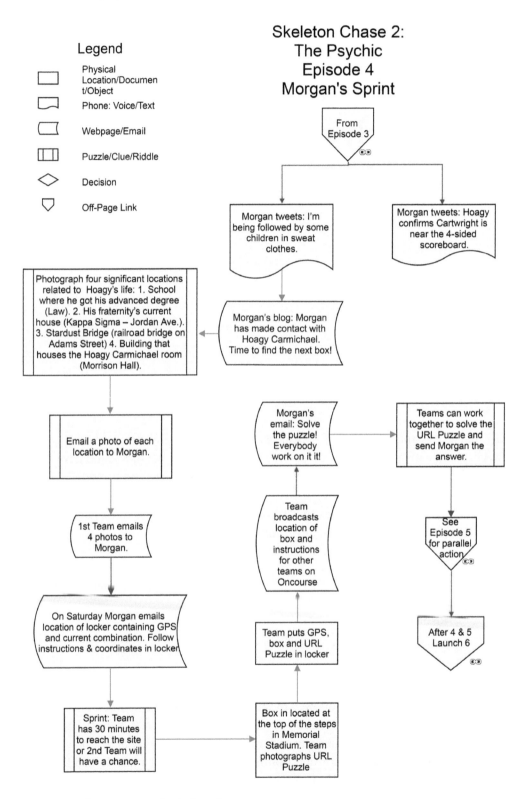

Quinn Morgan's sprint game logic flowchart.

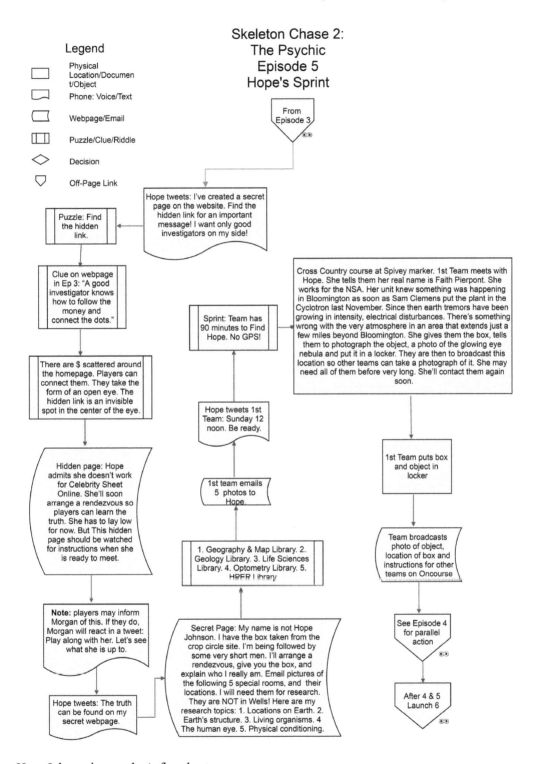

Hope Johnson's game logic flowchart.

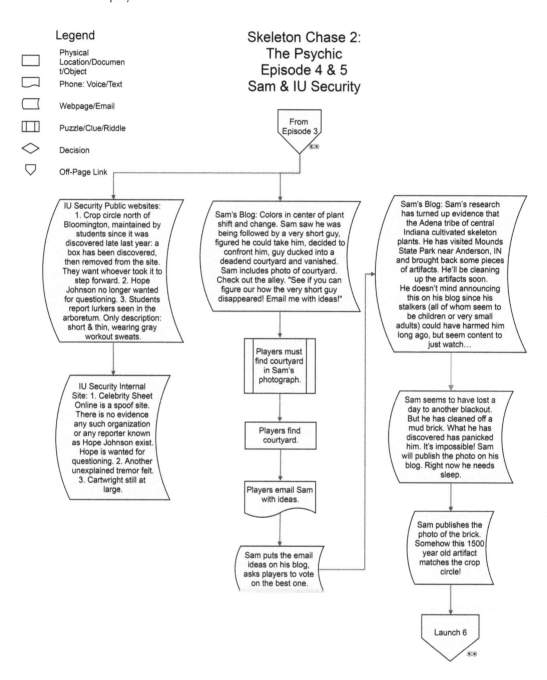

Legend

☐ Physical Location/Document/Object

⬠ Phone: Voice/Text

▭ Webpage/Email

▥ Puzzle/Clue/Riddle

◇ Decision

▽ Off-Page Link

**Skeleton Chase 2:
The Psychic
Episode 4 & 5
Sam & IU Security**

From Episode 3

IU Security Public websites: 1. Crop circle north of Bloomington, maintained by students since it was discovered late last year: a box has been discovered, then removed from the site. They want whoever took it to step forward. 2. Hope Johnson no longer wanted for questioning. 3. Students report lurkers seen in the arboretum. Only description: short & thin, wearing gray workout sweats.

IU Security Internal Site: 1. Celebrity Sheet Online is a spoof site. There is no evidence any such organization or any reporter known as Hope Johnson exist. Hope is wanted for questioning. 2. Another unexplained tremor felt. 3. Cartwright still at large.

Sam's Blog: Colors in center of plant shift and change. Sam saw he was being followed by a very short guy, figured he could take him, decided to confront him, guy ducked into a deadend courtyard and vanished. Sam includes photo of courtyard. Check out the alley. "See if you can figure our how the very short guy disappeared! Email me with ideas!"

Players must find courtyard in Sam's photograph.

Players find courtyard.

Players email Sam with ideas.

Sam puts the email ideas on his blog, asks players to vote on the best one.

Sam's Blog: Sam's research has turned up evidence that the Adena tribe of central Indiana cultivated skeleton plants. He has visited Mounds State Park near Anderson, IN and brought back some pieces of artifacts. He'll be cleaning up the artifacts soon. He doesn't mind announcing this on his blog since his stalkers (all of whom seem to be children or very small adults) could have harmed him long ago, but seem content to just watch…

Sam seems to have lost a day to another blackout. But he has cleaned off a mud brick. What he has discovered has panicked him. It's impossible! Sam will publish the photo on his blog. Right now he needs sleep.

Sam publishes the photo of the brick. Somehow this 1500 year old artifact matches the crop circle!

Launch 6

Sam and IU security game logic flowchart.

Hope emails everyone that she has created a secret page on the Celebrity Sheet Online website. She tells players to find the hidden link for an important message. She wants only good investigators on her side. A clue on the webpage reads "A good investigator knows how to follow the money and connect the dots." There are dollar signs scattered around the home page. Players can connect them. They take the form of an open eye. The hidden link is an invisible spot in the center of the eye.

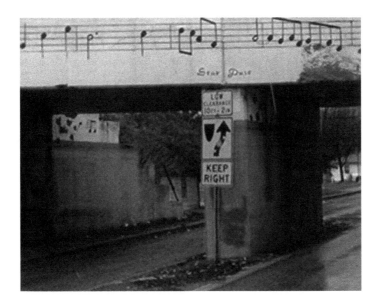

The Stardust Bridge.

Hope's hidden page reveals that she doesn't work for Celebrity Sheet Online. She'll soon arrange a rendezvous so players can learn the truth. She has to lay low for now. But this hidden page should be watched for instructions when she is ready to meet. Players were able to inform Morgan of this. Morgan reacts in a tweet: "Play along with her. Let's see what she is up to."

Morgan has made contact with the spirit of Hoagy Carmichael. It's time to find the fourth box! He asks his followers to photograph four significant locations related to Hoagy's life: 1) the school where he got his advanced degree (Law); 2) his fraternity's current house (Kappa Sigma on Jordan Avenue); 3) the Stardust Bridge (Railroad Bridge on Adams Street); 4) Building that houses the Hoagy Carmichael Room (Morrison Hall). Players are to email a photograph of each to Morgan.

Sam writes on his blog that the skeleton plant continues to change. Sam saw he was being followed by only one of the kids and figured he could take him. Sam decided to confront him. The kid ducked into a dead-end courtyard and vanished. Sam includes a photograph of the courtyard and tells his readers to check out the courtyard and see if anyone can figure out how he disappeared. He asks that they email him with ideas. Players must find the courtyard and email Sam with ideas. Sam puts the ideas on his blog and asks players to vote for the best one.

It is important that not all the puzzles in a game and the rewards for solving them connect to the central narrative through line. There were enough peripheral puzzles for every team to have a chance to solve them. Also, players knew additional prizes would be awarded at the end of the game. Extrinsic rewards! Out of the twenty-two teams that played until the end all received at least two prizes and over half received more than two.

The IU Security Public website reports a box was discovered on a crop circle north of Bloomington that has been maintained since it was discovered last semester. The box was removed before IU Security reached the crop circle. They ask that anyone with knowledge of the box to step forward.

Hope tweets that the truth can be found on her secret webpage. Her name is not Hope Johnson. She has the box taken from the crop circle site. She's being followed by some children in gray clothes. She'll arrange a rendezvous to give one of the teams the fifth box and explain who she really is. Teams should email pictures of five special libraries and their locations. She needs them for research. They are not in Wells Library! The research topics are 1) locations on earth; 2) earth's structure; 3) living organisms; 4) the human eye; and 5) physical conditioning. The locations are 1) the Geography and Map Library; 2) the Geology Library; 3) the Life Sciences Library; 4) the Optometry Library; and 5) the HPER Library.

The first team emails Morgan the correct five locations. On Saturday Morgan emails them the location of the new locker containing the GPS and the locker's combination. The team only has thirty minutes to reach the site and retrieve the fourth box or the team who came in second place will have a chance.

They find the box at the top of the steps in Memorial Stadium. The team photographs the URL Puzzle inside and puts the GPS and puzzle in the locker, then they broadcast the location of the box and instructions for other teams on Oncourse. Morgan tweets that all teams should work on solving the puzzle and send Morgan the solution.

Sunday at noon Hope emails a picture of her location. The first team that completed her research assignment will meet her there on Sunday at noon. The team has to find her without GPS. Hope is on the cross-country course at the Spivey marker. She tells the first team that her real name is Faith Pierpont. She works for the NSA. Her unit knew something was happening in Bloomington as soon as Sam Clemens put the plant in the Cyclotron last November.

This occurred during the first *Skeleton Chase* game.

Since then earth tremors in the area have been growing in intensity and there have been atmospheric electrical disturbances as well. There is something very wrong with the atmosphere in a rough circle extending just a few miles beyond Bloomington. She tells them she feels certain the person leaving the boxes is Sam Clemens during his blackouts. She gives them the fifth box, tells them to photograph the object inside: a photo of the skeleton plant with a glowing center and put it in the latest locker. They are then to broadcast this location so other teams can take a photograph of it. She may need all the teams before very long. She promises to contact them again soon.

EPISODES 4 AND 5 CONTENT CHRONOLOGY

Monday, March 30

Quinn Morgan Tweet (All Teams)

"I am being followed by some children in sweat clothes."

Celebrity Sheet Online

The day began with thick clouds overhead and rain that changed to freezing rain and eventually, however briefly, to snow. I had accepted a challenge from professed psychic, Quinn Morgan, to pit teams loyal to me against those loyal to him. My teams were Thunderfly and Team Won and Done. Morgan was represented by ZAM Squad and BHB.

I wish I could report that my teams won the challenge to place a rose on the grave of famous Indiana University alum, Hoagy Carmichael, but I'm afraid I can't. Team Thunderfly made it to the locker where the white rose was waiting before their opponents. They deserve some credit for that.

Those interested in reading more details of what went wrong on our end can have a look at my blog. I'm going to stick to what was found at the cemetery, because Mr. Morgan seems to be ignoring a rather critical discrepancy. As they say, "A good investigator knows how to follow the money and connect the dots."

First, let's have a look at what was in the third of seven boxes our infamous psychic found next to Hoagy's grave. As you can see it is a metal plaque with the words "Science for a Changing World" above a logo of wavy lines. It has been identified as the slogan of the United States Geological Society. How does this fit with the abstract paintings that were found in the first two boxes?

But that isn't the discrepancy. This is: we were led to believe that this challenge to place a rose on Hoagy's tombstone was initiated by his fans in the hope of keeping the memory of his songs alive with new generations. The roses were a touching tribute to be sure. But what do they have to do with the seven mysterious boxes?

As far as we know Hoagy has not yet taken up his new career as Morgan's control spirit. Okay, let's say he has. Let's say the box was his first spiritual gift. All three of these objects and boxes are solidly and obviously of this world. So, who is placing them at the coordinates spirits send to their favorite psychic???

Am I the only one who thinks something doesn't track here? You can still read my story about Morgan's involvement with the missing Zalensky girl. My big question is: is Morgan planting these boxes himself as part of as yet another "problem" he has devised for himself to solve and amaze the world? What do you think? As always, email me with your thoughts at hope.celebritysheet@gmail.com.

IU Security Public Website

Important Update on Internal Site

All officers are advised to visit the IU Security Internal Website for an important update on progress of an ongoing investigation.

Attention Team Free Tibet

IU Security Chief Milton Mars would like Team Free Tibet, one of the teams helping to investigate the claims of psychic Quinn Morgan, to contact him as soon as possible via the IU Security Tipline at tipline.iusecurity@gmail.com.

Steven Cartwright Still at Large

Other than Quinn Morgan's alleged glimpse of Steven Cartwright in his crystal ball, there have been no further reports of sightings of the fugitive. Player 1 with Team BHB suggests that the scoreboard may have been lowered, as it is for maintenance, at the time Cartwright was "very near" to it." It appears that the scoreboard has not been lowered since the unfortunate end of IU's home basketball season on March 3rd and the maintenance crew state that no one matching Cartwright's description came near to them while they were working. As always, any reports or tips on Cartwright's whereabouts should be emailed to tipline.iusecurity@gmail.com.

Unusual Tremor

A second small geological incident, strikingly similar to one that occurred in Bloomington on March 5, was reported this morning. An unusual coincidence that has The Indiana University Department of Geological Sciences puzzled is that the tremor was recorded by instruments at 4:17 am, precisely the time of the previous incident. Also puzzling was the fact that the epicenter was again almost directly beneath Bloomington, 8.9 miles down. And like the March quake, there were no aftershocks.

Dr. Dean Rensselaer of the Department of Geological Sciences informs us that the odds of the time and location of temblors weeks apart being identical are astronomical. He compared it to the atomic testing in Nevada. Even when the site was identical in tests, the variances in data were greater.

This tremor was unlike the first in that its intensity was 2.3 on the Richter while the first was only 1.7. That may seem like an insignificant change to laymen, but the Department of Geological Sciences points out it is a substantial increase in magnitude.

Again, barking dogs alerted some residences in the area. Reports of some objects being shaken from shelves and a couple of cracked windows in older buildings downtown were the only damage.

Geological Sciences also reports that the recent tremors are unusual in that Bloomington is a relatively stable zone as opposed to the more active Wabash Valley Seismic Zone along the Illinois-Indiana border. This was the site of the 5.2 quake last year.

IU Security Internal Site
Hope Johnson Now Person of Interest

Our investigation has turned up new information concerning Hope Johnson, alleged celebrity reporter now in Bloomington writing stories on Quinn Morgan. After contacting police officials in Los Angeles and California state law enforcement we have learned that there is no evidence of a Hope Johnson as a journalist for any news organization in California. Further, the personal facts concerning her career seem to have been fabricated.

The University of Louisville has no record of a student named Hope Johnson. The Louisville Courier-Journal has never employed anyone by that name. Neither have WISH-TV in Indianapolis nor the websites TMZ and Perez Hilton.

The Celebrity Sheet Online website is a spoof site. There is no print or online publication by that name on record anywhere. The IP address appears to originate in the Washington, DC area.

Therefore, in conjunction with the Bloomington and Indiana State Police departments, we have declared Hope Johnson a "person of interest." We have been unable to discover a local address for Ms. Johnson. If she is seen, she should be detained for questioning.

We are asking one of the student teams involved with her, Free Tibet, to contact the IU Security Tipline with any information they may be able to give us on Ms. Johnson.

Quinn Morgan's Blog
Hope Johnson Is the Fraud

Well, Ms. Johnson, I guess the shoe is on the other foot. And that foot is you. For weeks now you've been intimating that I am a fraud. Worse, you've suggested that I am responsible for the danger threatening Bloomington. I now learn that it is you who are the fraud. I have been told that in fact IU Security is now looking to question you as a "person of interest." The result of their investigation into your bona fides is posted on the IU Internal Website. I've demanded that IU Security put this information on their public website, but Chief Mars has so far declined. Nevertheless, it is true!

Time to Find the Fourth Box

Thanks to Teams ZAM Squad and BHB I am at last in full contact with my local control spirit, Hoagy Carmichael. He is ready to help me track down the fourth of the seven boxes. Still his spirited fans in the afterlife have a challenge for those who would aid me. Very well. I am sure my loyal helpers are up to the task. Tomorrow afternoon at **4:00 pm** I am promised the new challenge will be revealed.

Sam Clemens Blog
Sam in the Daytime!

okay.., okay,.. the skeleton plant is growing in my cooler. growing and changing. the lil fella likes it in there. the colors in the center shift and change. the pattern is still familiar to me, but i can't place it.

but this post isn't about that. it's about me, sam clemens, everybody's favorite missing student, out and about on campus yesterday. i saw this group of students checking some yellow gadget, then heading west toward town with a photographer trailing behind.

but i also caught my stalkers off guard. they weren't expecting sam to come out into the light. but i did. rain and sleet and snow keep it dark and cozy. and there was only one kid following me. gray hoodie, gray sweats. definitely one of my stalkers.

so i walk him past maxwell hall. at the back there's this lil courtyard tucked away. when he's in front of the archway, i turn and charge him. brave, you're thinking. naw. the kid's half my size and scrawny. caught him off guard. oh yes indeedy. all he could do was duck into that lil courtyard. no exit, dude!

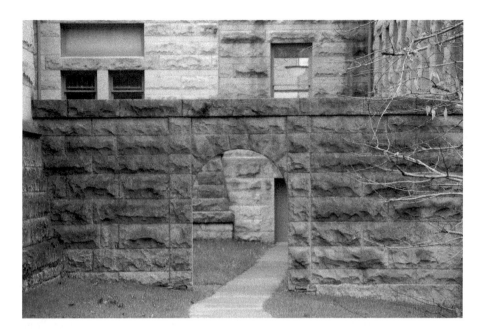

I chased the kid in here.

i charge in after him. time for the showdown.

he's not there. he's nowhere.

here's the thing: there was nowhere to go. have a look at the picture i took:
through one of the doors? nope. locked. bolted. no exit like sartre said.

through one of the windows? locked. with a winter's worth of grime and gunk sealing them tight.

so what are you waiting for? find the courtyard and see if you can figure out how the kid disappeared. email me ideas.

Tuesday, March 31

Quinn Morgan Blog

Science for a Changing World...the slogan of the United States Geological Society... One of my allies has suggested a possible connection between the metal plaque and the abstract art. I will not reveal the name of my source to protect her. You see one thing that IU Security did not reveal to the public about my vision is what else I sensed: incredible danger and... death... I need more explicit information. It would help immensely if we could identify that phrase.

Sam Clemens Email (All Teams)
I Need More Theories!

only a couple teams have sent me theories about how that kid escaped from the courtyard. i need more. Email them to me at saclemens1910@gmail.com. i'll post them here. then YOU ALL CAN VOTE ON THE BEST. it may not be the right answer, but it will at least be the most entertaining!

Hope Johnson Email (All Teams)

I've created a secret webpage on the Celebrity Sheet Online website. Yes, it is not a real web magazine. But I have been hiding behind Hollywood for a reason. And I'll continue to do so. You'll learn why on the secret page. Did you read yesterday's Celebrity Sheet update?

This was a reference to the "A good investigator knows how to follow the money and connect the dots." The Celebrity Sheet Online website now has dollar signs on it. Connecting them like dots and they take the form of an open eye. The hidden link was an invisible pixel in the center of that eye. Many ARGs slow the pace of the game with extremely challenging puzzles. But remember our primary goal was to keep as many players as possible interested and getting their steps, even if their team was not winning sprints. So, no puzzles were terribly complex, and hints were strategically placed throughout the narrative elements.

Hope Johnson Secret Webpage
Want to Know Who I Really Am?

Good. You've found this page. I knew you would. Wow. It feels really good to be able to drop all those stupid exclamation points and that gee whiz writing style. I'll keep it up for the public. But you deserve to know the truth. Yes, IU Security has discovered there is no Hope Johnson, or a web magazine called Celebrity Sheet Online. It was a cover for my true identity and my true mission.

I'm going to arrange a rendezvous for the cleverest of my investigators. Let's drop the word "reporters" shall we? I need to lay low for now. IU Security has by now discovered something new. So, watch their internal site.

Tomorrow I'll have a mission for you. Some vital research. Watch this hidden page for details and then instructions about when I'm ready to meet and where.

Quinn Morgan Tweet

[It is expected that some players loyal to Morgan will inform him of what Hope has said on the secret webpage. IF any do, Morgan will tweet those players]:

"Play along with her. Let's see what she is up to."

IU Security Public Website
Missing Property Sought

Yesterday evening at approximately 8:00 pm a small plastic box was removed from the vicinity of the crop circle found last fall north of Bloomington. Two persons: a man described as tall and thin and a blonde woman, no distinguishing features given, were seen separately in the area around that time. Anyone with information concerning these persons, or the box's whereabouts is asked to contact IU Security at tipline.iusecurity@gmail.com.

> In the first Skeleton Chase game a gigantic arrow-shaped crop circle containing the letters IU was discovered pointing towards the campus. This coincided with the sighting of a UFO over the university's cyclotron.

IU Security Internal Site
Box Found Then Lost

The crop circle found last fall with the arrow pointing at Bloomington has been maintained for several months now by students from one of the IU Bloomington fraternities. Yesterday evening at 7:50 pm one of the students from the fraternity, Gerald Allan Portnoy, found a box at the site. He phoned IU Security, and two officers were dispatched.

The box he described was translucent white plastic of dimensions that match the boxes the alleged psychic, Quinn Morgan, has been collecting around Bloomington. Portnoy claims the box contained what looked like an astronomical photograph. He left it where he found it to direct IU Security officers to the scene. But by the time they arrived the box had vanished.

Portnoy said he had witnessed a man described as tall and thin loitering near the site some time before the box was discovered. Later a woman was seen nearby as well about the time the box vanished. These individuals should be identified and brought in for questioning. But without a clearer description this will be difficult.

Quinn Morgan Blog
Challenge from Hoagy Carmichael's Spirit Fans

Here then is the challenge we have been issued. I have been assured by Mr. Carmichael's spirit that this will prepare us for the search for the fourth box.

There are three significant locations around the IU campus and one other off campus somewhere in Bloomington:

1. His School
2. His Fraternity
3. His Bridge
4. His Room

You are asked to photograph each and send them to me at qumorgan@gmail.com. All can be exteriors, even the last (although if the interior of his room is available that would be better), but each location must be clearly marked, and each photograph must contain one of your team members. The first team to send me all four photographs will be given the opportunity to search for the fourth box.

Wednesday, April 1

Hope Johnson Tweet (All Teams)

I know your trust in me has been shaken. But trust me one last time. See the new post on my secret webpage.

Hope Johnson Secret Webpage (All Teams)

I admit my name is not Hope Johnson. I am the person who removed the box from the crop circle site. It was too important for IU Security. I needed it. We needed it.

I have to be very careful. Not only am I being hunted by law enforcement—although I'll take care of that soon—but last night I was followed. If you've been reading Sam Clemens' blog you already know by whom. That's right. I couldn't get a good look at them, but his description is accurate: kids, thin, approximate age by their size? I'd say anywhere from seven to nine years old. Gray hoodies. Gray sweats. So he wasn't hallucinating them.

They've been following him for weeks. I would have noticed them, if they were following me before this. They aren't exactly subtle. And I know something about surveillance. I think they're following me because I was not supposed to get this box.

I'm going to arrange a rendezvous, give one of your teams the box, and explain who I really am.

For my research I need the locations of the following five special libraries. Email me pictures. I can find them from those.

They are NOT part of Wells Library. Here are my research topics:

1. Locations on Earth

2. Earth's structure

3. Living organisms

4. The human eye

5. Physical conditioning

Email the five photographs to me at my old email: hope.celebritysheet@gmail.com. Be sure to include a team member. The first team to do it will meet with me on Sunday.

Quinn Morgan Tweet (All Teams)

The spirits are satisfied. The fourth box will be found. See my blog.

Quinn Morgan's Blog
Team TBD Is First at Last

Team TBD have been working hard to uncover the danger threatening Bloomington but have not been as fast off the mark as others. Therefore, I'm very pleased to report that they were first to send me photographs of the four locations in Hoagy Carmichael's life that his fans from beyond requested.

The school where he got his advanced degree was Law. His fraternity, Kappa Sigma, is currently on Jordan Avenue. The Stardust Bridge is a railroad bridge on Adams Street). The building that houses the Hoagy Carmichael Room is Morrison Hall.

I am now in full contact with Mr. Carmichael, whom I find to be a delightful soul. He relates that he "has been told" the coordinates will be made available **Saturday morning** at **11:00 am**.

Team TBD has won the right to try and find the **fourth box** on **Saturday morning**. If they fail, **Team BHB** will make the attempt. If they fail, **Psychic Busters** will have a chance. If they fail, I fear for the safety of Bloomington.

I find it curious another entity is giving Mr. Carmichael the coordinates. He insists this has been true of the first three boxes as well. Ms. Johnson, or whomever she really is, was right to point out that coordinates and plastic boxes are not the usual means of communication from the spirit world.

Now a fifth box has appeared without any warning from the spirit world. And just as quickly it disappeared. Is it a coincidence that the descriptions of the two people spotted in the vicinity match Sam Clemens and Hope Johnson?

There are still mysteries to be unraveled.

Sam Clemens Tweet (All Teams)

sam goes traveling around indiana and into the past. check my blog.

Sam Clemens Blog

so in my late night strolls (parades? i had four kids following me last night. probably cause i scared that solo the other day) i stop by the wells library last night. always looking for more info on my mutating roomie. so i find out the local ancient native american tribe called adena used to cultivate skeleton plants up near anderson, in. pretty good trick since our climate isn't exactly the hot and dry the lil fella likes the best.

so today i take a drive up there to mounds state park. while i was there i sort of borrowed some pieces of artifacts, just discarded junk really. but I found one mud brick i'm gonna clean up and see if it amounts to anything.

oh and get this: i saw two of my stalkers up there! behind some trees. just standing and watching. staying way back. too far away to catch. so that proves the kids aren't in this alone. if i could just find out who their parents are…

Sam Clemens Blog

Case of the Vanishing Kid Solved?

you tell me. i dunno how he did it. here are all of the solutions submitted for how that kid got out of the courtyard behind maxwell hall. everybody vote on the one you think is best. **no voting for a teammate**. i may have blackouts but i'm not stupid. email your vote to saclemens1910@gmail.com. i'll announce the winner and send their team a mystery prize. maybe a few seeds from my favorite plant…

1. There were thirteen replies from players covering all the slim possibilities from climbing a drainpipe to having a key to the locked door. One student said he tried in vain to get blueprints for the building. One was blunter: "My theory is there is no kid stalking you and you are seeing things."

None of the theories were correct.

there they are, folks. 13 of em. my lucky number. vote on the one you think is best and email it to me at saclemens1910@gmail.com. we'll tally up the votes and declare a winner faster than cnn. One of you can win fabulous mystery prize for your team. maybe then they will be followed by kids in gray hoodies too.

IU Security Public Website
Searches Intensify

Steven Cartwright has again been sighted in the Bloomington area. This time he was spotted loitering around the Marathon gas station on South Walnut at approximately 2 am, accosting customers for spare change.

Also, the whereabouts of former grad student Sam Clemens remain a mystery. He boasts on his blog that he moves frequently around Bloomington, especially at night. He may in fact have been the man spotted at the Bloomington crop circle. However, he is not a suspect in the disappearance of a plastic box that was taken from the site later.

On a related note, in addition to Clemens' claim that he is being followed late at night by young kids, some small children have been reported lurking in the arboretum. Chief Milton Mars asks all parents: "Do you know where your children are?" Children should be at home in bed, Mars states, not wandering the streets, chasing after an alcoholic, possibly psychotic former student.

Officers are advised to check the IU Security Internal Site for information regarding a third individual.

IU Security Internal Site
Crop Circle Box Theft Update

Witness Gerald Allan Portnoy has positively identified a photograph of Sam Clemens as the man seen loitering near the crop circle right before the plastic box was found. We are very interested in interviewing Mr. Clemens, who we believe is still squatting illegally somewhere on campus.

Hope Johnson is no longer a person of interest. She is not to be detained or interfered with. If she requests assistance from officers, she is to be granted that assistance immediately and without question.

Thursday, April 2

Sam Clemens Blog

Sam Has Nothing to Hide

okay, so i'm getting some questions from you all via email. i got nothing to hide. so i'm gonna open sam's dusty mailbag and answer one.

player 1 from earth-shaking, psychic fog-covered bloomington, in, writes:

"…were you one of the two individuals who was up at the Bloomington crop circle? According to IU Security, there were two individuals up there around the time that the box went missing. It sounded a lot like you and Hope Johnson… Since I've been so forthcoming with theories and investigating your stalker's disappearance would you care to explain your whereabouts last night around 8 pm?"

i'd love to, player 1, but i can't. i had a blackout late that afternoon. last thing i remember is digging into a fresh new bag of cheetos at around 4pm. then nothing until about 10 when i wake up in my lair and see the skeleton plant glowing in the cooler like a giant lightning bug. my shoes were covered in fresh mud now that i think about it.

And this from player 2: "Did you hear that Steven Cartwright said the fifth box would contain a picture of the Glowing Eye Nebula?"

i looked up a picture online of the glowing eye nebula. cartwright may have spoken the truth for the first time in his life. i hope somebody finds that box.

Hope Johnson Blog

Team ZAM Squad has won the right to meet with me on Sunday. Instructions will be sent to them soon.

Sam Clemens Blog

um… okay so i cleaned off the brick. it's… impossible. i need to get some sleep. try to get some sleep. where's a blackout when you need one?

Friday, April 3

Sam Clemens Tweet (All Teams)

case of the vanishing kid winner. oh and scratches and stuff, too. check my blog.

Sam Clemens Blog

The Case of the Vanishing Kid Winner

well, we have a winner. Player 1 got the most votes for this solution to the case of the vanishing kid. i'll leave suitable prizes for all members of her crew with the blonde who sits in hper coordinating the team efforts. dunno her name.

here's the winning solution. maybe it's right. it sounds plausible. i got no way to prove it though.

"The only one plausible to me was perhaps when he entered he went right past the steam tunnel and climbed up that pole there really quickly and then waited until you entered to hop back over the archway and get away. Because like you said if you entered the courtyard only a few seconds after him there really wouldn't have been time for him to do much else."

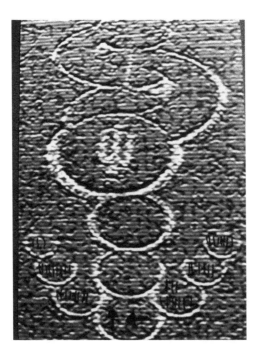

The Impossible Brick.

Scratches and Arrows?

have a look at the mud brick i found up at mounds state park.

so okay if you visited the crop circle that appeared outside of town last semester or saw a picture of it you could think this is just a clumsy copy. only it isn't. this hunk of mud is from the pre-columbian adena tribe who lived around what is now mounds state park hundreds and hundreds of years ago how could this brick be a dead ringer for the crop circle down to the symbol that looks a lot like the iu logo??? that makes this brick pretty impossible. and hey, can you see those scratches and arrows on the bottom of the brick? those aren't part of the crop circle. any idea what they are?

Saturday, April 4

Quinn Morgan Sprint Email (Competing Teams Only)

The usual instruction sheet for Saturday's sprint was communicated to players on that Saturday.

Quinn Morgan Email (All Teams)

On Monday I will have a full report on today's race for the fourth box. It was found in Section 106 of Memorial Stadium. There was some controversy. But I wanted to make certain everyone saw the photograph of the contents of the fourth plastic box.

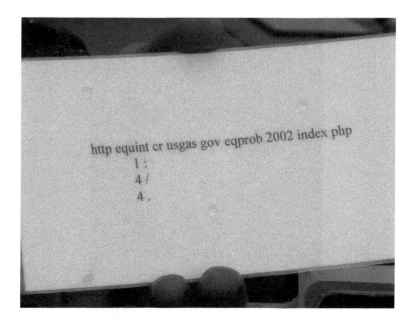

The puzzle found in the fourth box.

Solve the puzzle. Send it to me. Help each other. Time is running out.
  Quinn Morgan

Sunday, April 5

Hope Johnson Email (1st Team Only)

Here is a photograph of my location. You have 90 minutes to find me. No GPS!

The usual instruction sheet for Sunday's sprint was communicated to players on Sunday.

Faith Pierpont Live Appearance

Sunday, April 5 11:00 am to 12:30 pm (hopefully no longer)

Faith at the Cross-Country Course

Faith Pierpont is waiting at the Spivey Mile Marker at 11 am on Sunday morning, Apr 5. [You'll get directions!] This incarnation of the character is pleasant, but all business. None of the gushiness of Hope Johnson.

  "At last! I knew you could find me. Sorry about the location for this meeting, but I can't be seen just wandering around campus right now. You probably know there are several law enforcement agencies interested in talking to me. That's pretty ironic actually. As you'll learn…

  Oh, my real name is Faith Pierpont. What are your names?

  [writes names in her notebook]

The fictional Hope Johnson will give you credit on her blog and in her Celebrity Sheet articles for helping her… me… whomever… Also keep checking my secret webpage for the real updates on my investigation.

You should take notes, so you can spread the word about this conversation.

This is Chris Debuc, one of our unit's other operatives. He documents our investigations, handles surveillance and things like that. We both work for the NSA, the National Security Agency. If the CIA is the army of the intelligence community, we're the marines. We do the tough jobs. And this has been one of the toughest assignments of my career.

We knew something was happening here in Bloomington back in November when a former IU grad student named Sam Clemens—you read his blog?

[If yes: "Good!" If no: "Do it. We believe he's the key to everything."]

Anyway, Clemens put this purple dandelion, also known as a skeleton plant, in the IU cyclotron and bombarded it. He was trying to call up an oracle. Whether he succeeded or not is uncertain. He did seem to be able to help some students find the Source Corporation's private office on campus. But now his blog posts make it clear the plant is mutating into something else. Or at least he thinks it is.

Have the earth tremors here in Bloomington wakened you at night? Have you read about them on the IU Security webpage? Not only have there been tremors, but we've measured an increase in electricity in the air surrounding Bloomington. This may be what is causing what Quinn Morgan calls a psychic fog. The phenomenon is very local. It extends only a couple of miles outside of Bloomington.

Did you read on the IU Security website about a box discovered at the crop circle north of town? Last night I saw a young man who looked dazed, like he was sleepwalking, carrying something clutched in his arms. I'm pretty sure it was Sam Clemens. I followed him to the crop circle, lost him for a few minutes. When I saw him leaving the circle, he wasn't carrying anything. I saw a second young man discover something that looked like one of the plastic boxes we've been finding. When he went running off to report it, I took it.

[Gets box from behind the marker, or someplace else close by]

Here is the fifth box.

Photograph what's inside. It's proof that Clemens is delivering the boxes during his blackouts, I'd say.

The photograph is strikingly similar, but not quite, to the picture of the skeleton plant with a dark center and pinpoints of light that sam published on his blog in Episode 3.

Take it to the locker where you picked up the GPS: Locker number 246 in the SRSC. Quinn Morgan will pick it up there. I'm beginning to think we can trust him. We certainly need to work with him now. The combination on the locker is 16-26-04 right? Email the photograph, and precise directions to this spot, to the other teams helping me or Morgan. Repeat to them what I've told you. Take pictures here, too, to make the location as easy to find as possible. We need as many minds as we can get trying to figure out what is going on.

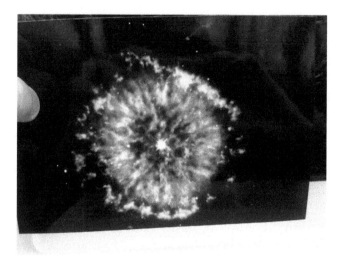

The plant petals are conspicuously missing.

And I know I will need all of you before very long. I don't have to be a psychic to know things are coming to a head.
Did you take good notes? Anything you want me to repeat? [repeats as needed]
All set? Then get going! I'm depending on you!"

CHAPTER 8

Episode 6 – Champions

EPISODE 6 GAME LOGIC FLOWCHART

April 6–April 15

CHARACTERS

Quinn Morgan, Faith Pierpont, Sam Clemens

NARRATIVE

Faith tweets all teams are to help Morgan. They need that sixth box! Morgan tweets he has received a new message from Hoagy and to check his blog.

On his blog, Morgan says that the sixth box must be found. The psychic interference has grown so great that all Hoagy could get through were three song titles. They refer to buildings or landmarks on campus so players should use the campus map. All teams should try and photograph the buildings with identifying signs prominent. Then they are to send the photographs to Morgan. They will be judged on creativity.

The songs and locations are 1) Pink Houses (Mellencamp Pavilion); 2) Starry Starry Night (Kirkwood observatory); and 3) Learn to Crawl (Glenn A. Black Lab).

I mentioned collateral learning in this book's preface. By the end of this game students who played knew more about the campus than faculty and staff who had worked there for years. I try in all my multiplayer classroom games to incorporate interesting facts from other fields. In *Skeleton Chase 2*, I included the Oppenheimer quote, Hoagy Carmichael, the Pre-Columbian inhabitants of southern Indiana, seismic events, the glowing eye nebula and other topics I came across while writing the story. All are examples of collateral learning. As teachers, we should never limit ourselves to simply teaching the textbook, but instead should add to knowledge and context whenever we can.

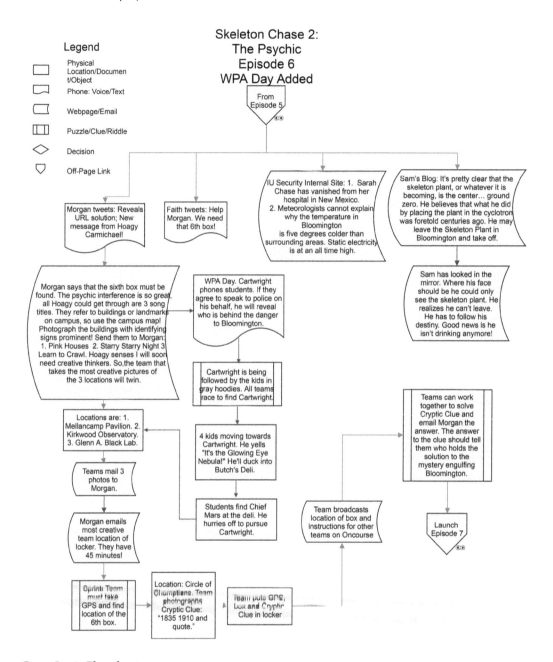

Game Logic Flowchart.

One of the players helps sam work out both what the "abstract art" and the scratches and arrows on the mud brick mean. Sam asks players to check the dates and times of his blackouts to the dates the boxes appeared.

Quinn Morgan tries to "read" one of the gray children following him. He sees one word, a word he predicted when he first arrived in Bloomington: revenge.

Sam learns he is the one leaving boxes during his blackouts. On his blog Sam says it's pretty clear that the skeleton plant, or whatever it is becoming, is the center... ground zero.

He believes that what he did by placing the plant in the cyclotron was foretold centuries ago, as the carving on the Roman ruins and the mud brick from the Adena suggest. He may leave the skeleton plant in Bloomington and take off. He asks players if he should go or stay.

Meteorologists cannot explain why the temperature in Bloomington is five degrees colder than the surrounding countryside. Static electricity is also at an all-time high.

Sarah chase makes her first blog post in months and promptly vanishes from the hospital in New Mexico.

Steven Cartwright phones students. He's on the run from the gray children. The players run all over Bloomington, trying to catch up with him, but the gray children are closing in on him. He makes a final panicked phone call "The picture in the box is the Glowing Eye Nebula!

The next day sam confirms that the center of the plant now resembles the Glowing Eye Nebula except that it's somehow alive. He has looked in the mirror. Where his face should be, he could only see the skeleton plant. He realizes he can't leave. He has to follow his destiny. There's some good news though. He isn't drinking anymore!

Cartwright is found dead next to an old four-sided scoreboard dumped in the back of the IU physical plant supply yard. IU Security announces there is no truth to the rumor that the scoreboard read Gray Children 1, Cartwright 0. His autopsy results seem to indicate natural causes although who wrapped him in a plastic sheet and dumped him by the scoreboard remains a mystery.

Sam is writing a poem on his blog called "every day is halloween." He tells the players to add the pieces together, then their journey and his will be over:

Chief Mars disappears and more unusual seismic activity is recorded. A UFO is reported hovering over HPER.

The search for the sixth box begins.

EPISODE 6 CONTENT CHRONOLOGY

Monday, April 6

Sam Clemens Email (Winning Courtyard Puzzle Team)

so okay i got your rewards. it's movie time! i lifted three copies of my favorite flick from target, and now they're yours. i'll stick em in the bag of the girl who checks you in ut hper. if she hasn't found them, ask her to look in her bag. i stayed around to get them and now i think it's too late to leave. you'll see why tomorrow on my blog.

Another case of improvisation followed with a puppet master actively involved. Her instructions, if the students should ask her if she found anything like DVDs in her bag, were:

Say no, but you'll check. And you discover them. How did those get in there? Say, "I'm not sure I should just hand them over." Let them convince you they belong to them. If they don't try, you can just shrug and hand the DVDs over. They aren't yours after all. If they don't show up until Tuesday, the puppet master on duty then can do the same thing.

Quinn Morgan's Blog

Fourth Box Found

Saturday in an early April snowstorm Team BHB were successful in locating the fourth of the seven boxes. I also want to salute Team TBD's valiant effort, even though it was unsuccessful due to the wrong photograph being submitted. See my email from Saturday. I included the picture of the object inside the box then.

It is an incomplete URL with clues on how to complete it to make it useable. Several teams have already emailed me regarding the URL. I've looked at the page. It is part of the US Geological Survey website that allows visitors to enter zip codes or longitude and latitude to determine the probability of an earthquake occurring at a given location. I believe we have found the origin of the first two objects found that were referred to as "abstract art." They are seismic charts similar to those that can be created on this page. However, there are two differences. No towns or cities are listed. Instead there is a single black dot at the same position on each. Thoughts?

Player 1 of ZAM Squad suggests that "Bloomington looks like it has a chance to have some activity." Player 2 of BHB agrees. While Player 3 of BHB writes: "It appears Bloomington has no threat of an earthquake in the near future." He sent a second email as well: "It appears an earthquake is coming to Alaska very soon. The kenai-cook inlet to be exact." Which of them is correct? Who else has an opinion? Also they are invited to tell us how they arrived at opinions which appear to be—dare I say it?—*polar* opposites? Comment on this blog entry. What do people think?

The Fifth Box that was stolen from the Bloomington crop circle has been recovered as well thanks to the efforts of celebrity reporter, Hope Johnson. Ms. Johnson's team, ZAM Squad, left the box in a locker at the Indiana University Student Recreation and Sports Center.

It appears to be very similar to the picture of the skeleton plant that missing grad student Sam Clemens claims is mutating. To my eye at least, it does not so much look like a black hole, but another celestial phenomenon. I solicit your suggestions. Send them to qumorgan@gmail.com.

Celebrity Sheet Secret Webpage

To those of you who have found this secret page I will say that everything ZAM Squad reported on Sunday concerning their meeting with me is true. My name is Faith Pierpont. And I am an agent with the NSA. They speculated on why I once referred to Quinn Morgan as "she." I admit I have always found the name "Quinn" to be conveniently androgynous. In fact, so is the last name "Morgan." They are even interchangeable: Morgan Quinn? Why not?

For now, Quinn Morgan and I have called a truce. I do believe he is getting to the truth of the danger threatening Bloomington. I stole the fifth box from the crop circle. I gave it to ZAM Squad to deliver to him. Let's do all we can to help him. Maybe together, all of us, we can prevent this tragedy which seems to come closer every day.

Quinn Morgan Blog

Hoagy Carmichael Has Spoken

Despite the intense psychic interference, I have made contact with Mr. Carmichael as promised. All that he could reveal to me were three song titles that refer in some way to IU campus locations. He said they were titles of his songs, but he was unfamiliar with what landmarks they might represent. Here they are: Pink Houses, Starry Starry Night, Learn to Crawl.

Photograph each location with some clearly identifiable feature such as a sign, and with a team member in the picture. Email them to me at qumorgan@gmail.com. Mr. Carmichael, creative gentleman that he is, suggested that instead of the first team to find them, I select the team that takes the most creative photographs of the locations. "Make me laugh, make me cry," Mr. Carmichael insisted before his voice faded completely away and all contact was severed.

Sam Clemens Tweet (All Teams)

"check my blog please"

Sam Clemens Blog

Player 1 from team tbd did some really good work on those scratches on the mud brick. here's what he wrote me:

"I was clueless on the scratches and arrows until i saw the USGS website from the recent box. This site can map earthquake probability by coordinates, so if the arrows are taken as directions (north and west), and the scratch groups counted from edge to center, we find two sequences: 3 9 8, and 8 6 3 7 (or are the 3 and 7 meant to be 10? not sure…) After some finagling i found the latitude 39.8 and longitude −86.37 to be pretty close to Bloomington. You said the mud brick was about 1500 yrs old, so I threw that number in, chose 5.0 for magnitude, and the resulting map bears some resemblance to the picture from that first box way back when…see attachment."

i think you're right, Player 1. except look. your map doesn't match the other 2 maps. we know the first one found matches bloomington. just entering a zipcode and today's date gets that. and that dot is right where bloomington would be. and that dot is on the second

Map found in first plastic box.

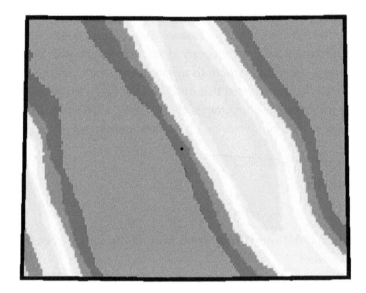

Map found in second plastic box.

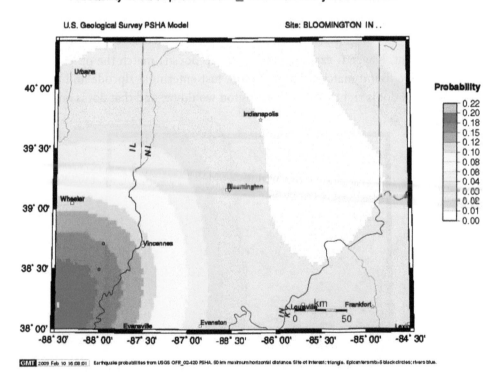

Player 1's USGS map.

map too. so here's what i think. i think that map is a picture of right here. and soon. and the tremors we're feeling are leading up to that second nasty map.

and it's becoming pretty clear that my skeleton plant is the center. ground zero. but I can't think my lil guy is causing it. i don't want to.

here's what i think: when i placed my lil buddy in the cyclotron last november, it did become an oracle. i was able to lead those students to the source corporation's private office on campus thanks to what i saw or heard. i'm not quite sure now. can you see a sound?

i think what i did was foretold centuries ago. the inscription on the wall of those roman ruins in england… the red brick Player 1 deciphered… my blackouts… i did some figuring… here are when they have happened:

sat morning feb 28 sun morning mar 8 sun morning mar 29 mon evening mar 30 sat morning apr 4 sun morning apr 5 mon morning apr 6

can anybody tell me what happened during those hours on those dates?

Tuesday, April 7

Sarah Chase Blog
I'm Coming Home
It's almost time.

Quinn Morgan Email (All Teams)

I'm not going to blog this. I'm being followed. A child wearing gray, hooded sweatshirt and sweatpants. I first saw him (her?) two nights ago. Last night I tried to get a reading… to touch the child's mind. It was incredible. I felt something… strange… sentience most assuredly… but without emotion or what we might think of as personality… and then, as I probed deeper a single word appeared in the vast emptiness, almost as if placed there for me to read.

The word was: revenge.

Quinn Morgan, The Psychic

Sam Clemens' Website
Meet Sam Clemens: Fedex Boy
okay, i've been blind. thanks to those of you who have identified the dates and hours of the days i listed in my previous post.

Player 1 from thunderfly laid it out best:

> "The dates all listed correlate with the mysterious boxes that have been popping up around bloomington, the first three mornings are when boxes were found, the evening of the 30th is when the box went missing from the crop circle, and there was a box found on both saturday and sunday this week, with the box found again monday morning because of some complications."

and i was seen at the crop circle *before* that box was stolen. so yeah, i guess it's me. i'm the fedex driver on this route, delivering presents: return address? the twilight zone. postage paid.

pretty clear my blackouts are not caused by my demons. there is a purpose behind them. a controlling force. is it my lil buddy? am i being controlled by a weed? is it revenge cause i bombarded it with particles in the cyclotron? i meant no harm.

bye bye bloomington. bye bye gray children. bye bye blackouts. i'm outta here, folks. i'm done playing messenger boy. i'm leaving the plant here. don't try to find it. don't try to mess with it.

or should i stay?

morgan says he saw 7 boxes. i've only delivered 5.

should i go or stay to deliver the last 2?

email me at saclemens@gmail.com. u decide sam's fate

sarah? monday afternoon i dreamed of you

IU Security Public Website
Information Concerning Kinesiology Professor's Whereabouts Requested

IU Security is asking anyone with knowledge of Kinesiology Assistant Professor Sarah Chase's current whereabouts to please contact us at tipline.iusecurity@gmail.com. Professor Chase has been on leave, recovering from the effects of an experimental drug administered her last fall by fugitive Steven Cartwright, whose body was discovered on Saturday. Cause of death is still to be determined.

Professor Chase was last seen in the patient garden of Skeleton Canyon Hospital in Grant County, New Mexico on Monday, April 6th, where her recovery has been progressing satisfactorily, but slowly. She has not been discharged, and her belongings were found untouched in her room. A message on her blog suggests that she may be heading to Bloomington. IU Security is interested, once again, in getting in touch with her.

Meteorologists Stumped by Unusual Atmospheric Conditions

A professor in the IU Atmospheric Science Program is at a loss to explain unusual atmospheric conditions measured by a GEOG 107 class project yesterday. Professor George Challenger told IU Security that at first, he thought it was nothing more than student error. But he has since confirmed the readings with the National Weather Service, who plan to send a team to investigate next week

According to the class findings, the temperature in Bloomington is five degrees colder than surrounding areas. Three miles from the town center temperatures immediately rise. Also, static electricity is at an all-time high. Static electricity of course usually peaks during the dry winter months, however there has been considerable rain lately. "Readings as high as those measured yesterday are anomalous to say the least!" explained Professor Challenger.

The professor went on to confess he was additionally perplexed by the unseasonal snowfall on Monday. Snowflakes captured by GEOG 107 students were found to hold a mild electrical charge. Professor Challenger immediately switched the class's final project to studying the strange phenomena. Although some students complained that this wasn't in the syllabus, most have enthusiastically pitched in. Challenger hopes the National Weather Service will also be able to help shed some light on the mystery.

IU Security Internal Site

Sarah Chase Has Vanished Again

The administrator of Skeleton Canyon Hospital has informed me that Professor Chase was discovered missing at 5:00 pm yesterday when she was not in her room for dinner. A subsequent search of the hospital grounds was negative. Two patients remarked that they had seen her late that afternoon in the hospital garden staring towards the northeast. She failed to respond when addressed. The administrator assures me this behavior is not symptomatic of her condition. She was perfectly coherent, although weak, but was improving steadily. The hospital had expected to release her the first week of May.

Grant County law enforcement officials have so far turned up no trace of the missing woman. All officers are asked to re-familiarize yourselves with Professor Chase's likeness and habits.

Chief Mars

Wednesday, April 8

In the midst of our penultimate week an opportunity to support a particularly compatible event, the World Day of Physical Activity, arose. To celebrate we created a sprint in which all teams could participate: an attempt to finally run Steven Cartwright to ground. The event featured a four-mile chase around the IU campus and downtown Bloomington in pursuit of the elusive Mr. Cartwright, a personal appearance by our fictional IU Security Chief, Milton Mars and free pizza courtesy of Butch's Deli, a newly opened restaurant, to replace all those lost calories. This was originally scheduled for April 6 but moved to April 8 due to a forecast of nasty weather. Here is a peek behind the curtain at the event we came up with at the last minute and managed to shoehorn into the narrative. A press release was sent out and I posted an announcement to all teams.

WPA Event Announcement

An announcement has been added in the "Skeleton Chase II" site at Oncourse (https://oncourse.iu.edu/portal)

Subject: Designer Note—World Physical Activity Day Event

From: Lee Sheldon

Date: Apr 8, 2009 12:10 pm

Message:

I hope everybody who can, will turn out this evening.

Including free food, prizes and the fact that it's for TWO good causes…

…one of the **two** characters from the game involved this evening will reveal the answer to a lingering question **ONLY** during this special event.

So be there at the SRSC this evening at 5:30!

And here is how it unfolded!

WPA Event Chronology

Prior to 4:45 pm

1. Elizabeth erases all messages on Cartwright's phone, except for Stephanie's voicemail message. She makes sure the ring volume is as high as it will go; and makes sure the phone is fully charged.

4:45 pm

1. Chris will join Elizabeth at the SRSC. Elizabeth puts Steven Cartwright's phone (**Number???**) in SRSC Locker #**???** [A locker in the middle of the eastside bank of lockers—the ones you can see directly in front of you and to the left when you stand at the turnstile.] She will contact Lee, and Lee will call the phone to test it and how far from the locker the ringing can be heard.

2. She will put a combination lock on the locker. The combination is? **??**.

3. Elizabeth shows Chris where he needs to position Psychic Busters. Elizabeth steps offstage. She is now done.

5:00 pm

1. Lee will find a table at Butch's.

2. Chris phones Lee to tell him how long he'll need to position Psychic Busters (see below)

5:15 pm

1. Ted Castronova (Chief Mars) arrives at Butch's.

2. Psychic Busters arrive at SRSC. Other players begin to arrive.

3. Chris tells Psychic Busters only that an unidentified man phoned Faith Pierpont, his NSA partner (may need to remind them her cover was Hope Johnson), and told her that they must remain here. He tells them that Faith was told to tell them: [Combination? **??**]. Chris says the person said they will know when to use the combination. Be patient.

5:30–5:45 pm or so

1. The rest of the players arrive.

2. Chris texts Lee that they are ready to begin. Depending upon where the phone can be heard ringing, Chris positions Psychic Busters so they'll be able to hear the phone. He tells him he's just setting up a couple of shots of them.

3. Lee waits however long it takes to allow Chris to position Psychic Busters, and take a couple of pictures, then calls Cartwright's phone.

4. A Psychic Busters team member unlocks the locker, takes out the phone and answers it.

5. Lee (Steven Cartwright) asks that player to repeat to everyone else what he says.

This was my first appearance in one of these games, albeit only my voice. I was to have a brief onscreen moment in *Secrets*.

6. He tells that player that he is not the person responsible for the danger to Bloomington. He admits he had ideas along those lines because he felt students here were responsible for the end of his career, and the fact that he is wanted by the police. But in sneaking around Bloomington he discovered who IS responsible. If they promise to speak on his behalf to the police, he'll tell them who that is, and turn himself in to the police. He tells the listener to tell the rest they can decide.

7. Psychic Busters asks the others to vote.

8. Whatever they decide, Lee (happy or sad depending!) says he'll meet them at the shelter in the 3rd St. Park, and explain all. Lee hangs up.

Players Exit Student Recreational and Sports Center

1. The players head for the park, accompanied by Chris (photographs), Elizabeth, Anne and Jeanne (observers). (Several teams know where it is, so group shouldn't need hints.)

Players Reach 3rd St. Park

1. After a couple of minutes of them searching around, Chris texts Lee that they have arrived.

2. Lee phones again. As he was waiting for them, he saw one of the children in the gray hoodies who has been following him. He left the park and is now at the corner of 7th and Indiana. He says he sees a second kid has joined the first! He tells the player they must hurry and find him! Lee breaks the connection.

Players Reach 7th and Indiana

1. Chris texts Lee.

2. Lee phones. They started towards him. He got frightened and ran west on 7th! He's outside Butch's Deli! There are now four kids watching him from just down the block. They are keeping in the shadows, but they seem really under-nourished... They're moving towards him! "It's the Glowing Eye Nebula! Tell them all! That photograph in the fifth box is the Glowing Eye Nebula! I'm going inside Butch's! Help!" The connection is broken.

3. Lee steps offstage.

Players Enter Butch's

1. Ted sees them, demands to know what is going on, listens as they explain. He demands the phone from the Psychic Busters, takes it, says he will mobilize his men. Cartwright can't have gone far. If he's in danger, they will protect him! Ted exits with the phone. (Returning it to Lee on Thursday.) Ted steps offstage.

This Ends the Sprint

Anne, Jeanne and Lee reward Psychic Busters. Pizza is served. Partying ensues. Gift certificates are rewarded. Lee answers questions, gives hints about the finale of the game, etc.

A tip of the designer's hat to Ted Castronova, a friend and colleague at IU, who up until that moment had only appeared in photographs. Ted had such a blast appearing in character we brought him back in Skeleton Chase: Warp Speed where he played Mars again, this time disguised as a waiter, delivering bottles of (what else?) vitamin water to our players. The bottles were the trailhead into that game.

Thursday, April 9

Sam Clemens Blog

yeah, still here with time to dip into sam's dusty mailbag again to answer my fan mail. most votes say sam should hang around. and now cartwright has given new meaning to the words panic mode.

player 2 from bloomington, in, where temperatures are falling and static electricity is rising, writes:

> "Did you hear that yesterday Steven Cartwright said the fifth box would contain a picture of the Glowing Eye Nebula?"

i saw the photograph they found in the fifth box. yeah, it looks a lot like what's happening at the center of my lil plant. in fact it looks like the picture i took. except remember when i said the center of the plant reminded me of something else? when i was a kid i loved astronomy. i had my own telescope. i couldn't see much. so i also collected astronomical photographs taken with real telescopes. i never thought the crab nebula looked much like a crab, but maybe that's just me. but yeah, i don't have those pictures anymore, but i looked up a picture online of the glowing eye nebula and that photograph does look like the glowing eye nebula. almost.

cartwright may have spoken the truth for the first time in his life.

folks, i didn't take that picture. where did it come from?

listen, i know how the voting is going, but if you don't hear from me again it's because i'm not here. i may leave that thing in bloomington and just take off.

Quinn Morgan Email (All Teams)
Convince Sam to Stay in Bloomington

This skeleton plant… I sense we are close to the ultimate answer. The plant must be what Sam Clemens calls "ground zero." And the investigative work done by the teams helping to unravel this mystery is truly extraordinary.

Three things must be accomplished: Clemens must be convinced not to leave Bloomington. Please, everyone, email him at saclemens1910@gmail.com. Tell him he must complete this ritual dance of passing to us the last two boxes!

Provided Clemens can be persuaded to remain, the sixth box must be found. The psychic interference is I believe connected to the bizarre atmospheric conditions reported on the IU Security website. And the earth tremors as well. And the USGS earthquake maps clearly indicate that a tremendous change in local seismic activity is imminent.

If the skeleton plant is at the center of the mounting threat to Bloomington, we must find it and learn how to counteract its influence. Do we destroy it? Nurture it? The wrong decision could be catastrophic.

The psychic interference has grown so great that now even Mr. Carmichael can barely reach me through it. But he has promised to try at 4:00 pm today. Be ready then at 4:00 pm for our penultimate challenge, the next to last clue to the mystery that may well decide all our fates.

Quinn Morgan Tweet (All Teams)

"First results are in. Are they beatable? You decide. See my blog."

Quinn Morgan's Blog
Time for the Showdown

It doesn't take a psychic to realize we have little time left to stop the final cataclysm. Yet only one team has answered the call so far. You decide if they win by default; or is there any other team brave enough to take them on? The race goes to the most creative, remember, not the fastest. You still have today and tomorrow to compete.

Hoagy Carmichael managed to contact me through the psychic fog to tell me that BHB has not only photographed the correct buildings, they took his request for creativity to heart.

[Final-Pink Houses.jpg] [Starry Starry Night.JPG] [red bull copy.jpg] (In this order)

The photographs were attached.

Have they set the bar too high? Or are there others who can top them? We'll see.

IU Security Public Website
Steven Cartwright Found

The body of former Source Corporation employee and fugitive suspect Steven Cartwright was found early this morning wrapped in plastic and lying next to the old Assembly Hall scoreboard that was replaced in 2005 by the new $1.9 million scoreboard-video board we enjoy today. The old scoreboard was dumped in the back of the physical plant supply yard.

The location of the body would answer those questions posed by psychic Quinn Morgan's vision of Cartwright in close proximity to a four-sided red scoreboard. This four-sided red scoreboard is on the ground, as was the body of Cartwright.

Cartwright surfaced Wednesday evening trying to work out a deal with students helping Quinn Morgan to identify the danger to Bloomington. Cartwright promised to reveal the source of that danger in exchange for students pleading his case to authorities. He attempted to rendezvous with a large group of students, but he was also being pursued he said by children wearing gray hoodies and sweatpants and needed to keep on the run.

Cartwright was last seen in the vicinity of Butch's Deli on 7th Street in Bloomington. But when students arrived there, all they found was our own Chief Milton Mars. There was no indication that Cartwright had in fact entered the restaurant. Mars confiscated the cell phone Cartwright had given the students to maintain contact with them, and immediately ordered officers to canvas the area.

The students were seen to be still at Butch's enjoying free pizza. But no trace of Cartwright was found.

IU Security officers are urged to check the internal page for more forensic details.

IU Security Internal Site
Cartwright Death Details

Fugitive Steven Cartwright's body was discovered at 6:23 am by IU physical plant employees at the supply yard behind the Service Building off Range Road. Curiously the yard is very close to the IU Cross Country Course where students met with Hope Johnson on Sunday. Again however, Ms. Johnson is not a suspect, and is in fact in contact with Chief Mars concerning the ongoing investigation.

Luckily an unseasonal frost on the ground allowed forensic personnel to determine the body was deposited there some time the previous evening, possibly soon after Cartwright vanished from Butch's Deli. Four children, previously described by other witnesses as between the ages of 6 or 7 and 9, were mentioned by Cartwright in his last phone call to the students trying to reach him. They are reported to be wearing generic gray hoodies and sweats with no distinguishing logos. While not as common as IU-branded athletic gear, they are available for purchase all over the area. Officers are investigating if there have been any unreported thefts of athletic wear from local stores.

As can be seen from this photograph taken by the forensic team, Cartwright was found only a few feet from the old Assembly Hall scoreboard, just as Quinn Morgan foresaw. The words "Fair Play" were on the scoreboard, an admonition that was obviously not followed by the perpetrators.

There's no truth to the rumor that at the time the body was discovered by a member of Facility Operations the old scoreboard read Gray Children 1, Cartwright 0.

Preliminary examination revealed no overt signs of physical violence on the body. The plastic sheet was of a type that can be purchased from any hardware or home improvement store.

We are awaiting results of the autopsy, but the death is currently being investigated as a homicide.

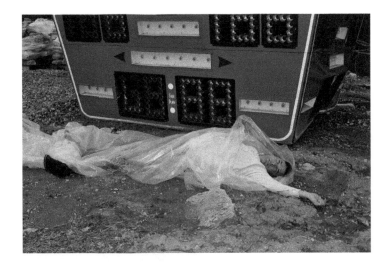

Steven Cartwright found at last.

Friday, April 10

IU Security Internal Site
Access to Internal Website

As is clear from his blog posts, Quinn Morgan has access to this internal site. We are seeking to identify the individual who informed Morgan of the passphrase. However, I have been advised by a higher authority to leave the current passphrase in place for the present. Against my better judgment I am doing so.

    Chief Mars

Quinn Morgan's Blog
Last Call for Submissions

I will announce the name of the team of champions who will help me to find the sixth box on Saturday. If you are still in the hunt, the photographs from BHB I posted yesterday reveal the locations. It's up to you to reveal the creativity.

Saturday, April 11

Quinn Morgan's Blog
Constable Tweekins Will Quest for the Sixth Box

After a spirited vote in the afterlife Hoagy Carmichael's judges have determined Constable Tweekins' creativity a clear winner. The constable will quest for the sixth box on Wednesday evening.

    Constable Tweekins maintained a clear musical theme throughout all three photographs. I've included one of their entries below. Constable Tweekins will be entrusted with tracking down the sixth box on Wednesday at a time still to be determined. They will then alert other teams to where they found it, and carefully photograph the object inside. Here then is the submission from the musician still known as Constable Tweekins.

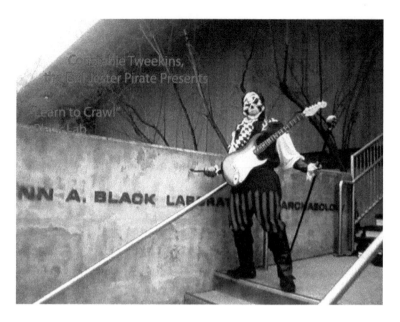

Spirits vote Constable Tweekins most creative.

Although Wolfgang Amadeus Mozart was somewhat unnerved by the mask, Enrico Caruso, The Big Bopper and John Lennon were all impressed by the theatricality. Congratulations, constable!

Sunday, April 12

IU Security Internal Site

Cartwright Autopsy Results Inconclusive

The Monroe County Coroner's Office states that Steven Cartwright died at approximately 7:00 pm Wednesday evening. This would mean death occurred only minutes after he vanished in the vicinity of Butch's Deli at 7th and Washington downtown. How he managed to get all the way across town so quickly is unknown.

Cause of death appears to have been intracerebral hemorrhage. As Medical Examiner Ryan Quincy noted in his report:

> "An intracerebral hemorrhage is a subtype of intracranial hemorrhage, or bleeding that occurs within the brain tissue. It can occur spontaneously as a stroke for example, or it can be caused by trauma: physical injury to the brain. In the case of this subject there were no signs whatsoever of physical trauma to the cranium or surrounding tissue.
>
> However, there was evidence of bruising on both lower arms consistent with the victim being restrained by at least two, possibly three individuals. No fingerprints were evident, but an infrared photograph will be taken to at least determine the relative size of the individuals' hands. I understand there has been a suggestion that young children may be the perpetrators."

Other than the fact that there is no evidence suggesting the source of the intracerebral hemorrhage there were no other anomalies with one major exception. The body seemed to carry an unusually high charge of static electricity. While performing the autopsy it was noted on several occasions that surgical instruments would conduct low values of electricity from the body to the hand of this examiner, even though I was wearing latex gloves. The electricity on one occasion slightly magnetized a scalpel.

I am at a loss to account for this phenomenon, especially because now, hours after the autopsy was performed, the charge of static electricity has not dissipated in the slightest."

Until further notice, we will continue to investigate this as a homicide.

Chief Milton Mars

Monday, April 13

Sam Clemens Tweet (All Teams)

"i made my decision. check my blog."

Sam Clemens Blog

Taking One for the Team

so okay, i was set to hit the road, to get far away fast from bloomington. the suggestion in an email from player 1 of zam squad to "take one for the team" didn't really sit with me too well ya know? i mean i'm not on your team or anybody else's. i saw that story about chasing cartwright on celebrity sheet online. everybody smiling and running and having a great time. and a little while later cartwright turns up dead by that old scoreboard. he took one for the team i guess.

i know cartwright was a mouth-breathing, slime-sucking, lower lifeform who turned my ex-girlfriend from jane into cheetah, but his death tells us how serious these gray children are about revenge. revenge for what? got me.

but i'd promised that same player 1 and her team a prize cause most people thought her idea about how the kid vanished from the courtyard was the best. so the fact that i'm pretty much tapped out cash-wise meant i had to stick around and do some light fingered shopping. I hope they enjoy the dvd's. my favorite movie, player 1. let me know if you like it.

anyway that's done and now i realize i can't leave.

i looked in the mirror in my lair this morning. guess what. where my face should be? i could only see the skeleton plant. and here's a new picture of my lil buddy. that black spot in the center… like a pupil… did it move just now? is it… dilating…?

i wonder if when he looks at himself, does he see sam? so i can't leave you see? it's my destiny to follow this thing through.

good news is i have conquered my demons! i woke up yesterday morning and didn't even think about taking a drink. whether it's cause everything is so crazy strange already, or it's the plant life in my head. i dunno.

watch this blog. i think it's time we all got together, don't you?

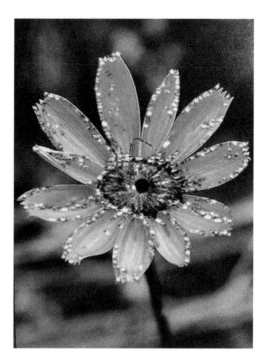

The black spot in the center has grown.

Tuesday, April 14

Hope Johnson Tweet (All Teams)

"Several disturbing news reports on the IU Security internal site."

IU Security Internal Site

IU Security Chief Milton Mars Missing

When Chief Mars failed to show up for a scheduled meeting last evening; and phone calls to his home and cell phone went unanswered, officers went to his home. There they discovered the front door unlocked and slightly ajar. Inside they found Beartrap and her puppies, but there was no sign of the chief, and there was no sign of anything in the house having been disturbed. Chief Mars' keys, cell phone, wallet and badge were all on a table in the entry. His car was in the garage.

The unlocked door suggests the chief either exited in a hurry, or was confronted when he answered the door, and taken away. A forensic team is on site, but there are no overt signs of a struggle.

All officers are expected to pull double shifts until the status of Chief Mars has been determined.

Sarah Chase in Bloomington?

A former student of Professor Chase, Tiffany Stroud, phoned the IU Security office this morning to report that she saw a woman resembling Professor Chase standing in the student parking lot at Memorial Stadium staring at the sky. Officers could not however find any trace of the woman when they arrived a few minutes later.

Unusual Seismic Activity Noted by IU Researchers

After two reported tremors centered beneath Bloomington, faculty and students in the Indiana University Department of Geological Sciences have been monitoring conditions around the clock. Today Dr. Dean Rensalear, head of the continuing research effort, reported that while there have been no further seismic events to match the first two, a continuous, almost imperceptible movement of the earth has been registering on instruments for the past week.

Dr. Rensalear characterized it as "a minute, continuous shaking, like a sifting of flour," occurring deep within the strata directly beneath the city.

Professor George Challenger, whose GEOG 107 class has been studying the weather phenomenon that appears to be centered on Bloomington has met with Dr. Rensalear twice in recent days. Both men admit to being puzzled by the curious juxtaposition of phenomena, but say that to suggest a connection between them would be highly irresponsible. They have asked that scientists from the US Geological Survey join the team of National Weather Service personnel now expected to arrive on Monday. There has been no word as yet, if the USGS has agreed.

UFO over HPER?

One of the most common of student pranks is the anonymous phone call reporting the sighting of strange lights in the sky. But since the appearance of the unexplained crop circle last fall, and a number of sightings of objects in the vicinity of the IU Cyclotron during that period, IU Security is committed to following up on all but the most far-fetched of reports. For example over spring break the sighting of what was described as an "oaken bucket" hovering over Memorial Stadium was quite rightly dismissed as a prank.

Last night's sighting of an object appearing to be relatively small and saucer-shaped, was reported by several students crossing the arboretum. Witnesses claimed it seemed to be hovering over the HPER building.

Sam Clemens Tweet (All Teams)

"every day is halloween"

Sam Clemens Blog

I'm Writing a Poem

i call it "every day is halloween." put it together and your journey and mine will be over. here's the first part:

"once i lived high up a stair.
but if you seek me don't look there."

Wednesday, April 15

Quinn Morgan's Blog

Time for the Unmasking

In order to stop this conspiracy, I am certain we must work more closely together. Therefore I have made a decision I had hoped I'd never come to. I will reveal my true identity and meet with you. All of you.

Hoagy Carmichael managed to get a message through.

He said that I will need the three photographs below to unravel the final piece of the mystery. He says there will be no 7th box from the original source. The 6th box will confirm what is already suspected, and it will be up to us to act.

Once I have those photographs, he told me, our path will be clear. Therefore I will take it upon myself to prepare the 7th box myself. It will lead you to me.

But then the interference grew to a howling of light and sound; and he faded quickly. I fear that all contact with him is gone until this crisis is resolved one way or the other.

Here are the three photographs Mr. Carmichael has asked us to obtain:

1. Door of Sarah Chase's former office

2. Door of Sam Clemens' old lair from last fall

3. Door of the Source Corporation's former office on campus

As always, include a team member in the photograph and send them to me at qumorgan@gmail.com.

Act swiftly. Time is not our ally.

Sam Clemens Tweet (All Teams)

"every day is halloween part two on my blog"

Sam Clemens Blog

Every Day is Halloween Part 2

"now i am below the ground.
find sarah's suite, then turn around."

Quinn Morgan Email (Constable Tweekins Only)

Good Evening, Constable Tweekins. Proceed immediately to HPER. Find Locker #182. The combination is 10-36-30. Follow the instructions inside. You will have 45 minutes from the time you open the locker until the moment you relock it again with the box inside. A minute longer than 45 minutes and the spirits tell me the box may vanish.

May the spirits guide you!

CHAPTER 9

Episode 7 – Skeleton Chase

April 16–April 19

CHARACTERS

Quinn Morgan, Sam Clemens

NARRATIVE

The sixth box has been found at the Circle of Champions. There is only a single cryptic clue inside: "1835 1910 and quote." The team follows the usual instructions and broadcasts the location of the box for other teams. On his blog he asks all team to collaborate to discover what the numbers mean.

Whoever figures out the clue emails the solution to Morgan. The answer to the clue is "Sam Clemens." The writer Mark Twain was born in 1835 when Hailey's Comet passed close by the earth. He died in 1910, the next time the comet reappeared.

The danger to Bloomington is the skeleton plant. The former student with the famous namesake and the plant must be found, and the plant destroyed!

Faith tweets to trust Morgan. With Morgan's help players have to save Bloomington. Morgan tweets that the seventh box is in Sam's new lair. Players should check his blog. On his blog Morgan asks them to send three pictures to him. Then he will be one step closer to finding where Sam has been living. First, the door of Sarah's former office. Second, the door to Sam's lair last semester. And finally, the door of the Source Corporation office from last semester. That team will join Constable Tweekins in the final sprint.

All were locations in the first *Skeleton Chase* game. At that time Sam, as I related earlier, was living at the top of the tower in Indiana Memorial Union.

There are two posts on the IU Security Internal Site. Bloomington will be evacuated on April 20 due to increasing instability in the earth's crust beneath the city and atmospheric

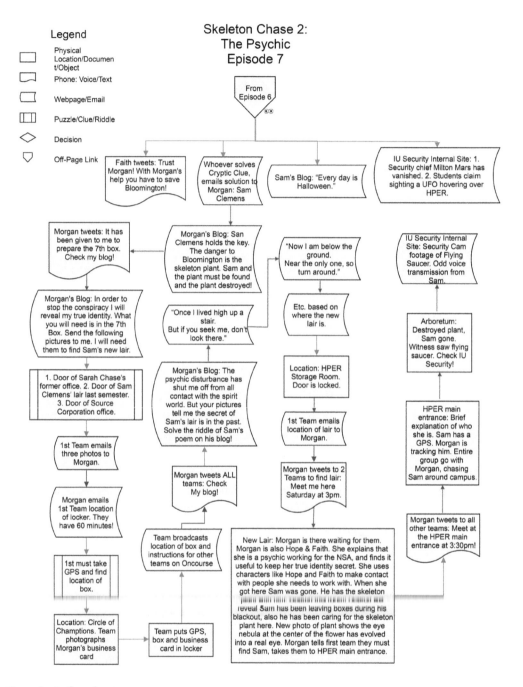

Legend

☐ Physical Location/Document/Object
☐ Phone: Voice/Text
☐ Webpage/Email
☐ Puzzle/Clue/Riddle
◇ Decision
▽ Off-Page Link

Skeleton Chase 2:
The Psychic
Episode 7

From Episode 6

Faith tweets: Trust Morgan! With Morgan's help you have to save Bloomington!

Whoever solves Cryptic Clue, emails solution to Morgan: Sam Clemens

Sam's Blog: "Every day is Halloween."

IU Security Internal Site: 1. Security chief Milton Mars has vanished. 2. Students claim sighting a UFO hovering over HPER.

Morgan tweets: It has been given to me to prepare the 7th box. Check my blog!

Morgan's Blog: San Clemens holds the key. The danger to Bloomington is the skeleton plant. Sam and the plant must be found and the plant destroyed!

"Now I am below the ground. Near the only one, so turn around."

IU Security Internal Site: Security Cam footage of Flying Saucer. Odd voice transmission from Sam.

Morgan's Blog: In order to stop the conspiracy I will reveal my true identity. What you will need is in the 7th Box. Send the following pictures to me. I will need them to find Sam's new lair.

"Once I lived high up a stair. But if you seek me, don't look there."

Etc. based on where the new lair is.

Arboretum: Destroyed plant, Sam gone. Witness saw flying saucer. Check IU Security!

1. Door of Sarah Chase's former office. 2. Door of Sam Clemens' lair last semester. 3. Door of Source Corporation office.

Morgan's Blog: The psychic disturbance has shut me off from all contact with the spirit world. But your pictures tell me the secret of Sam's lair is in the past. Solve the riddle of Sam's poem on his blog!

Location: HPER Storage Room. Door is locked.

HPER main entrance: Brief explanation of who she is. Sam has a GPS. Morgan is tracking him. Entire group go with Morgan, chasing Sam around campus.

1st Team emails three photos to Morgan.

1st Team emails location of lair to Morgan.

Morgan emails 1st Team location of locker. They have 60 minutes!

Morgan tweets ALL teams: Check My blog!

Morgan tweets to 2 Teams to find lair: Meet me here Saturday at 3pm.

Morgan tweets to all other teams: Meet at the HPER main entrance at 3:30pm!

1st must take GPS and find location of box.

Team broadcasts location of box and instructions for other teams on Oncourse

New Lair: Morgan is there waiting for them. Morgan is also Hope & Faith. She explains that she is a psychic working for the NSA, and finds it useful to keep her true identity secret. She uses characters like Hope and Faith to make contact with people she needs to work with. When she got here Sam was gone. He has the skeleton ⟨⟩ reveal Sam has been leaving boxes during his blackout, also he has been caring for the skeleton plant here. New photo of plant shows the eye nebula at the center of the flower has evolved into a real eye. Morgan tells first team they must find Sam, takes them to HPER main entrance.

Location: Circle of Champtions. Team photographs Morgan's business card

Team puts GPS, box and business card in locker

Game logic flowchart.

phenomena with unknown effects on humans. The other post reports that infrared photographs of marks on Cartwright's body appear to be damaged.

The first team to photograph the three locations emails them to Morgan. He tweets to check his blog. The psychic disturbance has shut him off from all contact with the spirit world. But their pictures tell him the secret of Sam's lair is in the past.

He asks all of the players to work together. Solve the riddle of the poem Sam is writing on his blog.

"Once I lived high up a stair.
But if you seek me, don't look there.
Now I am below the ground.
Near the only one, so turn around."

Sam finishes his poetry with a limerick which, combined with the puzzle about his previous lairs, shows the way to his current location.

Morgan is at the lair waiting for the two teams. Morgan is also Hope and Faith. She explains that she is both a real psychic and she does work for the NSA. She finds it useful to keep her true identity a secret. She uses characters like Hope and Faith to make contact with people she needs to work with. When she got here, she found Sam and the skeleton plant were gone.

The final sprint takes all teams to memorial stadium. Where a camera is found with a video that shows Sam chopping up his lil buddy. A security camera at the stadium explains Sam's exit from the stadium and a recording of a call to IU Security reveals Sam's fate.

EPISODE 7 CONTENT CHRONOLOGY

Thursday, April 16

Hope Johnson Email (All Teams)

Faith Pierpont here, the person formerly known as Hope Johnson. I really need to update my social media! Constable Tweekins was successful. See Morgan's blog.

Quinn Morgan Blog

Constable Tweekins, with the aid of the Garmin GPS was able to track down the location of the sixth box in the IU Circle of Champions and return the contents to the designated locker. He has broadcast the location of the box and instructions for other teams on Oncourse. The item in the box was a funeral announcement card with two sides.

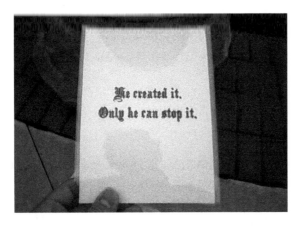

Obviously pointing a finger at someone.

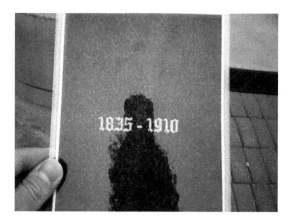

Do the two numbers identify this person?

Everybody, please work on the meaning of this cryptic clue from the box. By now we know that Sam Clemens has been leaving the boxes during his blackouts. He himself does not seem to know the meaning of their contents. But you have solved one puzzle after another. And I'm certain that together you can solve this one. Who do the numbers 1815 and 1910 represent? The answer to that question should tell us who holds the solution to the catastrophe threatening Bloomington. Whoever solves it, immediately send the solution to me.

IU Security Public Website
Theft at Sporting Goods Store Uncovered
Bloomington Police officers were summoned to Dick's Sporting Goods at College Mall when two cases of athletic wear were found to be missing during a regularly scheduled quarterly inventory check. One case containing two dozen gray hoodies and another case of two dozen gray sweatpants, both small sizes, were in the storeroom during an inventory check in February.

Employees at the store were unable to explain where they had gone. There was no sign of forced entry. And no alarms were tripped, although several wires within the main alarm system box appeared to have been slightly damaged or melted.

Speculation that a group of unruly school children may have stolen them as some sort of cult uniform fails to explain how young children might have affected the theft. In order to damage the alarm system, intruders would first have to have entered, thereby setting it off.

Quinn Morgan Tweet
"The solution is found already. See my blog!"

Quinn Morgan Blog
1815 and 1910 were the years the author, Mark Twain, real name of course Samuel Clemens, was born and died. Interestingly, he was born on the day Halley's Comet passed close to earth and he died on the day the comet made its next pass. So, what we've all come to expect is true. Our Sam Clemens is at the heart of the mystery. He has correctly identified the skeleton plant as "ground zero." The evacuation of the city of Bloomington will begin

on Monday unless we can find Clemens and destroy his "lil buddy." Right now, the psychic disturbance is too great for my spirit guides to break through. But I can feel their efforts to reach me growing with each passing hour.

Friday, April 17

Hope Johnson Tweet (All Teams)

"Bloomington evacuation plans announced. Check IU Security internal site."

IU Security Internal Site

City of Bloomington to Be Evacuated

In consultation with the United States Geological Survey and the United States Weather Service, the Department of Homeland Security has ordered the evacuation of Bloomington, Indiana to commence Monday, April 20.

Citing increasing instability in the earth's crust beneath the city and atmospheric phenomena with unknown effects on humans, Homeland Security spokesperson Charity Cassell announced today that a Presidential order has been signed ordering the evacuation of the entire community within a twenty mile radius from a center determined to be the School of Health, Physical Education and Recreation on the Indiana University campus.

All classes will be cancelled until further notice from Monday on at IU along with final exams, the Little 500 and all graduation ceremonies.

The public is assured that the evacuation will be orderly. Pets may be evacuated as well. A shelter has been set up for them in the House Chamber of the Indiana Statehouse in Indianapolis. However, owners will be required to sign a declaration promising that their pets will be quiet when the House is in session.

Infrared Photographs Damaged

The infrared photographs taken of the marks on Steven Cartwright's arms, and one from his back, were somehow damaged and a new set will need to be taken. As can be seen by the photograph of the print on Cartwright's back, reproduced below, the hands that made them appear to be markedly malformed. And this was true of **all** the bruises. There were at least three sets of marks, of differing sizes, so they were obviously made by three separate individuals.

Yet, since all revealed the same peculiar deformity, Medical Examiner Ryan Quincy now concludes the odd appearance of the hands was the result of equipment malfunction.

Quinn Morgan Blog

A horde of my spirit contacts led by Hoagy Carmichael have combined their energy and at last broken through the psychic chaos that is infecting Bloomington. They tell me we will need to find Sam's lair, but they have only been able to determine that Sam hides near one of three doors. The first team that emails photos of the three doors will join Constable Tweekins to lead our final chase once we locate Clemens' lair. Your mission: Find the door of Sarah Chase's former office. Find the door of Sam Clemens' lair last semester. And find the door of the Source Corporation office. The first team to email me those three pictures will help lead the final skeleton chase.

Saturday, April 18

Quinn Morgan Tweet (All Teams)

"Chief Mars has reappeared. See the IU Security internal site."

IU Security Internal Site

Chief Mars Finds Sarah Chase

IU Security Chief Milton Mars, missing since Monday evening, walked into IU Security Headquarters on 17th Street today with Professor Sarah Chase, herself missing from a hospital in New Mexico for over a week.

Chief Mars explained that moments after returning home from work on Monday he was startled to see Professor Chase outside in his front yard, beckoning to him. Hurrying outside, he found Professor Chase to be lucid, but somewhat agitated.

She told him that while walking on the Skeleton Canyon Hospital grounds she had suddenly felt drawn to Bloomington by an irresistible force. There was a flash of light. She remembered nothing more until she found herself outside the suite containing her old office in the HPER building.

When she turned around, she found Sam Clemens there smiling at her even though she had not seen him approach from either direction down the hall.

Then she again apparently blacked out, only to wake up on Chief Mars' lawn. Asked by the chief where Clemens could be found, she pointed behind him. Chief Mars turned. And there was Sam Clemens, smiling.

Clemens then told them that Quinn Morgan couldn't help him, or Sarah Chase, though he thought the gray children wanted her here to talk him into destroying his plant. Its power has been growing unchecked since Clemens bombarded it in the Cyclotron. But he can't bring himself to harm what he called "the little fella."

Researchers have been coming to Earth for some time, he told them, from a planet in the Glowing Eye Nebula. They were always attracted by the power of our particle accelerators and cyclotrons here. While far more primitive, certain aspects of this power is similar to that which powers their planet and their ships.

It has always been controlled, and not dangerous. But the skeleton plant's power is entirely uncontrolled. And it is increasing exponentially, causing the atypical earth tremors Bloomington has been experiencing.

Chief Mars was of course taking all of these otherworldly revelations with a healthy serving of salt, but he asked if the cold temperatures and the electrical charge around Bloomington were also caused by the plant. Clemens said no. The atmospheric alterations were necessary so that the gray children could operate here in relative comfort. They are not of course children, but full-grown adults from a planet in the Glowing Eye Nebula, also known as the Dandelion Puffball Nebula.

When asked how he learned all of this, he replied that during his blackouts—like the one he is experiencing now—lost time it is called—the gray children spoke to him, and directed his actions, trying to warn others through him what was happening in the ground beneath their feet, and showing them that they must either control the plant, or destroy it, or the results would be catastrophic.

This was all that Chief Mars and Sarah Chase remembered until they woke up outside IU Security. Sam Clemens was nowhere to be found.

Both had vague memories of being in an enclosed space: filthy, cluttered with empty liquor bottles, but with rudimentary sanitation facilities. When an officer jokingly asked the chief if he thought they'd been abducted by a UFO, Mars laughed. No, he doubted alien spacecraft would have linoleum floors. Professor Chase added she does remember a strange glow in the darkness, coming apparently from a battered beverage cooler.

After handing Professor Chase over to the care of local doctors, Chief Mars immediately took charge of the heightened manhunt for Sam Clemens. Asked if he believed Clemens' story, Mars replied curtly that if it weren't true, then Clemens was a dangerous lunatic who needed to be apprehended immediately. No more questions were asked.

Sam Clemens Blog

mommy i wrote a limerick!

> "upon faculty i wouldn't depend
> but in this case you should to the end
> locked it may be
> but soon you will see
> me and my lil green friend."

email morgan at qumorgan@gmail.com. tell him where he can find me. i'll meet him in my lair this sunday the 19th at 3:45 pm. then he can introduce me and my lil buddy to all of you who have been helping him.

Sunday, April 19

Live Appearance Begins 3:15–3:30 pm

Quinn Morgan at Sam's Lair

Chris Debuc calls ZAM Squad and Constable Tweekins, who are waiting at the gym: "This is Quinn Morgan. Meet me in Sam's Lair. Now." Quinn Morgan and Chris Debuc are waiting when teams ZAM Squad and Constable Tweekins arrive.

Morgan: Ah, you must be Constable Tweekins… You were supposed to meet Quinn Morgan here, right? You have. I am Quinn Morgan. And you are ZAM Squad sent here by… me. You already know me as Faith Pierpont. I had Chris here make the call to the gym. Why spoil the surprise? I really am with the National Security Agency. So is Chris here.

 We are part of a special black ops team of psychic researchers—yes, I am a psychic, although I don't use anything as hokey as a crystal ball! We investigate all those fringe paranormal stories nobody else wants to touch. Yeah, like the TV show the X-Files, although we get a lot more support than poor Fox Mulder ever did. I used the identities of Hope Johnson and Faith Pierpont so I could investigate in the open. Too many people want face time with Quinn Morgan.

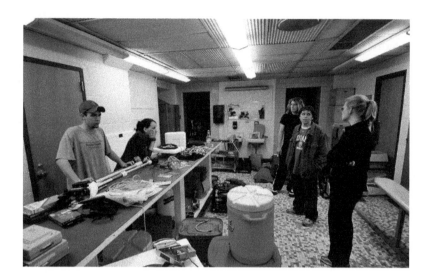

Sam's Lair at last.

We're standing in Sam Clemens' lair where he has been living for months. This is also where Chief Mars and Sarah Chase were briefly kept during a period of lost time. Did you read the report I told everybody about on the IU Security Internal Site? [**react accordingly: "Good!" or "You should have!"**]

We need to have a look around. I just got here. No sign of Clemens obviously, but the plant could be here. Whatever you do, don't touch it! Understood? [**react accordingly**]

    [**Players find empty plastic box**]
    [**Players find a pile of photographs**]
    The two photographs of the plant
    The photograph of the Roman Ruins
    The photograph of the carving
    The photographs of Mounds State Park
    The photograph of the crop circle
    The photograph of the clay brick
    And any others I've forgotten!]
    [**Written on one mirror with lipstick (male handwriting):**]
    Milton Mars
    [**Written on same mirror with lipstick (female handwriting):**]
    Sarah Chase
    [**Written on a second mirror with lipstick (2nd male's handwriting):**]
    Home of Sam Clemens and his lil buddy
    [**Cleared space amidst junk food wrappers is the size of the cooler: 18 inches by three feet:**]
    In the space are a couple of leaves.

[Don't interfere if one of the players reaches for a leaf, but act like he's infected, if he picks it up. If nobody picks one up:]

Morgan: Good! You don't want to touch that!

3:45 pm

Morgan's phone rings. It's Clemens. She puts it on speaker phone.

Sam: I'm sorry, Morgan. I can't let you destroy the lil fella!
Morgan: You have to, Sam, or we're all dead!
Sam: I can't!
Morgan: Where are you? Let me talk to you! Face-to-face. We can work this out.
Sam: I'm not far.
Morgan: Tell me where!
Sam: I'm at the cemetery where I first photographed you. But I'm not sure if I should.

[He hangs up.]

Morgan (to team): We have to get to the front entrance of HPER. Where you guys check in! I've told everybody who can help to meet us there! We all need to work together and stay together! Show me the fastest way to get there!

4:00 pm

Live Appearance

Morgan at HPER Entrance

Constable Tweekins and ZAM Squad lead Morgan to entrance where other players are waiting.

Morgan: Listen up. I'm not Hope Johnson or Faith Pierpont. I'm Quinn Morgan. Sam was not in his lair. We have to find him and convince him to destroy the skeleton plant! Teams Constable Tweekins and ZAM Squad here and I can provide more details as we go.
　　　　This is not a competition, so nobody go running off! Don't split up! We need to work together.
　　　　Sam has taken the plant and he says he's at the cemetery next to Beck Chapel! Let's find him!

[Morgan, Chris and everybody else take off.]

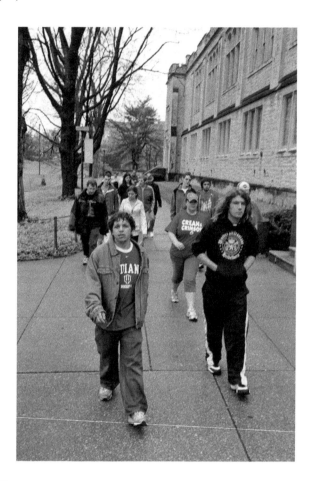

The final Skeleton Chase.

4:05 pm

Morgan and the Final Chase

[Repeat story as told to Teams ZAM Squad and Constable Tweekins or supplement their story as you move]

   [At the cemetery Morgan's phone rings.]

Sam (on speakerphone): Okay I'll meet with you. I'm on the front steps of the SRSC.

[At the steps of the Student Recreational Sports Center Morgan's phone rings.]

Sam (on speakerphone): Why did you bring all those other people???
Morgan: Because a lot of lives are at stake! **(to players)** Somebody help me. Somebody convince him to destroy that plant!

[Let several players try. Sam starts out unconvinced. He loves the lil fella. But he starts to be swayed by the players.]

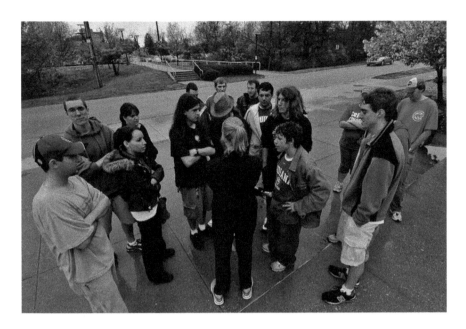

Trying to convince Sam to destroy the skeleton plant.

Sam: Maybe you're right. He doesn't mean to hurt anybody, but he can't help it. I guess I knew that all along. I guess that's why I brought the hammer...

[Take phone back]

Morgan: Sam, tell me where you are?
Sam: Where am I? I don't know. Let me look... It's... I'm outside Memorial Stadium. The gate is open... That's perfect... yeah... I'll do it for everybody... I'll do it for the cheering crowd... Can you hear them? I'll... I'll take one for the team...

[Sam hangs up]

Morgan: He's at Memorial Stadium! Let's go!

[At Memorial Stadium:]

A benign and sometimes funny example of game world and real-world colliding occurred at the stadium when some students stopped passersby to inquire if they had seen a guy carrying a strange plant in a cooler nearby. They received some baffled looks and all replies were good-natured, but negative. You will read about a more interesting collision between fiction and reality in Section 4 of this book: *The Janus Door.*

Through the gate, at the bottom of the slope: Sam's camera is lying there.
   [Morgan sees it]

Morgan: What's that? Don't touch it!

[After everyone has caught up, Morgan kneels, puts on latex gloves, lifts the camera. She rewinds the tape inside]

Morgan: Gather 'round.

[She presses play. Tape of Sam destroying plant plays.]

The video selfie by Sam shows him smashing the plant in the cooler with a hammer then looking up and seeing something. He drops the camera which records him going out of frame. Unfortunately, no copies could be found of this video.

Morgan: It just stops there. At least it looks like he destroyed the plant. I wonder where he went? IU Security has cameras all over this place. I'll check with them. If there's anything to see, I'll have them put it up on their internal website. You all deserve to know.

[Phone rings. She takes it off speakerphone, listens]

Morgan: Right. **(listens)** Good. **(listens)** Thanks for the update.

[She hangs up.]

Morgan: That was Charity Cassell at Homeland Security. Destroying the plant seems to have worked! The seismic activity has stopped. The electrical disturbance has ended. And it's getting warmer! The evacuation has been called off. Congratulations! You've just helped save Bloomington!

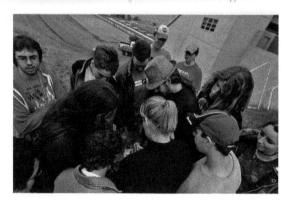

Watching the video on Sam's camera.

[She applauds. There should be some reaction from the players, then:]

Thank you all for your help. Give me some time to get to IU Security, then check their internal site.

[There's a car waiting for Morgan at the gate. She climbs in, and it drives off.]

IU Security Internal Site

Here is the video recorded by former student Sam Clemens and the security camera footage Quinn Morgan asked for:

[Sam's selfie video]

[Memorial Stadium Security Camera Footage]

We also have received what can only be described as a highly unusual broadcast on the police frequency. At this time all I will do is place these here without comment. You are free to draw your own conclusions.
Milton Mars
Chief of IU Security

This is a still from the footage recorded by the security camera at Memorial Stadium showing Sam beamed up by a flying saucer that then heads off into the sky. It was created in Adobe After Effects.

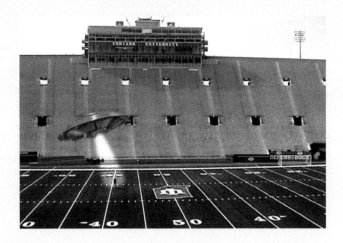

Sam is taken for a ride.

In addition to Sam's video and the security camera video there was a last audio farewell from Sam as he was headed out, I suspect, towards the Glowing Eye Nebula as a guest of the "gray children." Chief Mars posted all three on the IU Security Internal Site.

Sam Clemens Audio File

Okay, so I just talk? There's no microphone or anything? Okay… hi… this is Sam Clemens… As you probably know by now I destroyed my lil friend. He couldn't help what he became. It was my fault. And now I'm… where am I? [laughs] Toto, I've a feeling we're not in Indiana anymore!

So they wanted you to know—my new lil friends that is—they wanted you to know they didn't mean Cartwright any harm. They took him aboard this… ship… and he freaked… burst a blood vessel in the ole brain or something. But he was responsible for Stacey's death and Professor Chase's illness, and was experimenting on students without their consent, so it's no great loss as far as I'm concerned.

They whooshed me and the remains of the skeleton plant on board, disposed of it, and have been pretty decent hosts all things considered. Once they realized the plant was no longer a threat, they asked me where I wanted to be dropped off. Dropped off? I think that was joke. But I've got nothing back on earth, so I told them, head for the "second star to the right and straight on till morning."

So, I guess I'm in for quite a ride.

We're already out of the solar system. Wait a sec… there's something up ahead… a signpost… no, it's… it's… My God, it's full of stars!

I identified the quotes in Sam's message for puppet masters.

"Toto, I've a feeling we're not in Indiana anymore!" (Apologies to Kansas!)
—*Wizard of Oz*
"second star to the right and straight on till morning."
—*Peter Pan*
"there's something up ahead… a signpost…"
—*Twilight Zone*
"My God, it's full of stars!"
—*2001: A Space Odyssey*

The highest number of steps by one student in a week was 94,346 (47.2 miles).

The highest number of total steps by another student for the seven weeks was 485,307 (242.7 miles).

You have reached the finish line of *Skeleton Chase 2*.

CHAPTER 10

Afterword

Other than *THE FOUNTAIN*, a 20-minute real-world fitness game I designed for the Robert Wood Johnson Foundation grant-winner conference in Portland that should have been that. Two *Skeleton Chases* in less than eight months was plenty, wasn't it? No. By the first week of May we were embarked on *Skeleton Chase 3: Warp Speed*. Why warp speed other than my past relationship to *Star Trek: The Next Generation*? That June we ran an ARG for Coca-Cola executives from North Africa. The challenge I faced was to squeeze as much of the seven weeks of gameplay into two-and-a-half days as humanly possible. We divided the executives into three teams, each with an actor in character as guide and hint system. The weekend chosen for the event I was speaking at a conference in Australia. I left the game in good hands and Coca-Cola was pleased with the results. (I *was* told that a team hired a taxi for one of the sprints!)

Given the complexity of the planning and execution of an ARG, I am proud of the results we achieved in all three *Skeleton Chase* games. There are several lessons I learned from this, my first big ARG.

Document everything. I stated this in this book's preface, but it bears repeating. And update the document as needed!

Plan carefully. Try to think up the hiccups the real world can give you.

Expect the unexpected. Because you will not think of everything that can go wrong.

Touch the imagination of the players. The more you make students think about the game, the more they will be open to thinking in general, possibly about what they are learning as well.

Carefully plan frequency of puzzles, clues and surprises. Anticipation must be rewarded. However, in my book, *Character Development and Storytelling for Games*, I stress the importance of not falling into a predictable pattern repeated over and over like jump scares in a B-Grade horror film. My analogy is that the shark in *Jaws* doesn't attack every Thursday at noon. Not knowing when something important may happen keeps players alert. It's called suspense.

We'll see if I remembered these as we move on to the other games in this book. Okay, time to put the skeleton back in the closet and move on to a much more modest ARG that took players to the other side of the planet without leaving the classroom.

SECTION 2

The Lost Manuscript

CHAPTER 11

Introduction to Section 2

Now we go from the complexity and scope of *Skeleton Chase 2* to the relative simplicity of *The Lost Manuscript*. It is very similar in structure to the classes found in *The Multiplayer Classroom: Designing Coursework as a Game*. The biggest challenge was matching an interesting narrative as closely as possible to extremely specific standard foreign language instruction protocols.

The class was supported by two seed grants from Rensselaer Polytechnic Institute. One seed grant was awarded to Professor James Zappen and Dr. Prabhat Hajela. They would facilitate the development of a class that taught a foreign language, in this case, Mandarin.

The second seed grant, awarded to Ben Chang, Mei Si, and I, would support research into virtual reality (VR) as a learning environment. I was also tasked with creating a narrative and gameplay that would serve as a proof of concept of the multiplayer classroom in general, whether in a VR environment or a standard classroom setting.

I would design the class with the help of ShihChia Chen Thompson, who would teach the class and play an NPC in the game. Professor Chang would create VR assets with the assistance of a graduate student, Anton Hand. Assistant Professor Mei Si would concentrate on VR characters that would appear in a later iteration of the class.

We combined these two efforts into The Mandarin Project. *The Lost Manuscript* was intended to be a proof of concept before moving to a more immersive VR experience. See the afterword to this section for a few words on how those plans developed.

The class was held from 5:00 to 6:50 pm, Mondays and Thursdays, in two regular class rooms. The first session was on Thursday and introduced students to the course; the fact that it was an experiment that would include a narrative, puzzles etc. and how it would be taught. There was some initial language instruction. The following Thursday began the narrative and the normal routine of the class. Each Thursday would be narrative in which students used their language skills to progress in the story. Mondays would be preparation for each following episode and a recap of what they had learned so far. There would be additional game and narrative outside of class via a fictional website, texts, and digital interactions (rendered images on the classroom's pull-down screen that could be interacted with via the Microsoft Xbox Kinect).

It's clear that the needs of most subjects from Astronomy to Math to History to Medicine can be the structure of an applied game. They lend themselves easily to both gameplay and narrative. Foreign languages are much trickier. There's a reason we start out in a game teaching a language that we begin with "Hi, how are you?" and "What is your name?" rather than "Have you seen any ancient stolen books recently?" Of course, the higher the level of the class, the more elaborate the stories can be.

You will notice that the story of *The Lost Manuscript* is much simpler than *Skeleton Chase 2*. Much less happens in each episode, usually a single puzzle and a few conversational interactions. This was necessary to make certain that the required vocabulary for completing the class could be reasonably taught in the number of weeks allotted and it also allowed for comprehension of the overall storytelling so the students could understand the narrative moves without confusion. Even so, this class had a cast of characters more than double any of the other games.

Students interested in the class were carefully vetted. We did not want students who knew Mandarin. A few had some experience in learning a foreign language. Others had none. They knew before they signed up that it was an experiment and were excited to give it a try. In the end, eleven students who fit the necessary criteria were selected.

Finally, we needed to make certain that we covered the material that would be included in any first-year Mandarin class. At the end of the proof of concept, ShihChia Chen Thompson, our teacher, as well as a character in the narrative, proudly announced that the class learned more in eight weeks than a full fourteen-week semester of Mandarin.

To learn more of the underlying research goals and results, please consult the paper, *Foreign Language Learning in Immersive Environments*, authored by Benjamin Chang, Lee Sheldon, Mei Si and Anton Hand, February 2012: https://www.researchgate.net/profile/Mei_Si/publication/258712423_Foreign_language_learning_in_immersive_virtual_environments/links/5743e4f908ae9ace841b41b7.pdf.

CHAPTER 12

Foreword to Section 2

ShihChia Chen Thompson

A S A LANGUAGE TEACHER, my goal is always to focus on helping my students adapt what they learn from the class to utilize the skills in real-life situations. While I was given a teaching opportunity to cooperate with Professor Lee Sheldon from Rensselaer Polytechnic Institute (RPI), I was very excited about designing a unique curriculum for fellow students. Not only I was able to gain my teaching experience with college students, but I also could learn a different approach to teach Mandarin Chinese. In order to experiment with different teaching methods in a multiplayer classroom, we decided to find beginning learners in Mandarin Chinese and also invited some native speakers who functioned as mission facilitators in our efforts to help polish their communication skills.

Motivation is an important key to learn a foreign language, especially a challenging one like Mandarin Chinese. Mandarin is one of the most difficult foreign languages to learn. It requires at least two thousand classroom hours for students to be able to master this language while Spanish only requires approximately five hundred classroom hours. Students must have stronger motivation in order to carry on the learning process. During the curriculum-designing period, we interviewed many students to find out who would be the best candidates to take the class. Meanwhile, Professor Sheldon came up with a storyline for me to develop the curriculum accordingly. I designed several units that covered the basic language class topics based on Professor Lee's narrative, such as Introductions, Information Exchange, Asking Questions, Transportation, Currency Exchange, Dining Conversations, Phone Calls, Use of Measures, Directions, etc. Basically, we were trying to establish students' foundation of communication skills to survive in real-life situations. How do they get around in China and communicate with local people in order to accomplish their mission?

The multiplayer classroom setting encouraged students to pick up the language in a short time. The purpose of this language course was obviously to give impetus to students' learning motivation. They were encouraged to interact with mission facilitators (native speakers) to complete their assignments. They were forced to get out of their comfort zone and to act out the narrative. Students were part of acting in the multiplayer classroom.

We were not just learning Mandarin Chinese through other people's stories in a textbook. Everyone in this class, including the instructor, was immersed in this narrative and was asked to use the language to act out their parts. For the purpose of acting in the multiplayer classroom, I chose to speak Mandarin Chinese to assimilate students into real-life situations. In the beginning, most students were quite frustrated with a Chinese-speaking environment. However, they quickly realized that it was very helpful when it came to learning a foreign language. Students improved their listening comprehension better when it was integrated into the role-playing.

I evaluated each class for their listening comprehension and speaking skills. Chinese literacy was quite a challenge for this fast-paced language class. Therefore, we didn't emphasize their writing and reading skills. Yet, we certainly wanted our students to understand that it is important to learn how to read and write in a language class. In fact, we exploited the complexity of the Chinese characters and adopted them as a puzzle for students to solve in the narrative. Most Chinese characters are shaped like pictures. Therefore, students were learning how to read Chinese characters when they needed to read a Chinese menu or to find a specific location on a city map.

The course lasted about two months at RPI. We had to utilize every minute in class to cover all the topics that were covered in the narrative. Students were eager to learn because they wanted to be part of the multiplayer classroom setting, to solve the puzzles, and to enjoy the narrative. Professor Sheldon understood the young college learners' point of view and wrote an intriguing storyline to motivate them to learn a new language. Throughout this eight-week course, they learned how to initiate and carry on conversations, how to make inquiries in different locations, how to exchange or obtain information, how to interact with native speakers (mission facilitators), and most importantly, they came out of their comfort zone and were highly engaged in the classroom!

CHAPTER 13

Design Document

The Lost Manuscript did not have a single, formal design document. Information from various files has been collected and arranged to match as much as possible the other game plans in this book.

TYPE AND GENRE

The Lost Manuscript is an alternate reality game designed to be played entirely in a single classroom. Its genre is mystery thriller.

THEME

At the time foreign language instruction at RPI was limited to software. The theme of the class recognized that bringing a better understanding of Chinese language and culture to students through direct classroom interaction was an important advance. In addition, we would test the theory that students would be particularly attracted to learning a foreign language through the medium of a narrative-driven game structure.

SETTING

The game begins in a classroom in the Sage Laboratory on the Rensselaer Polytechnic University campus. From there students travel to Capitol International Airport in Beijing. The mystery surrounding the theft of an ancient manuscript takes them to different sites in the city: a hotel, a teahouse, the Forbidden City and unfortunately a police station. All Chinese locations were replicated in the classroom by simply moving furniture and adding signage and props as needed.

GAME INTERFACES

Microsoft Kinect

The fictional Heritage Library website and the Kinect interactions on the classroom screen are the only two non-real-world interfaces.

Heritage Library Website

The official website of the fictional organization sponsoring an exchange of students between the United States and the People's Republic of China. For *Skeleton Chase 2* Oncourse GL, the learning management system (LMS) at Indiana University, handled all of the online game and official functions. Blackboard is RPI's LMS; however, the fictional Heritage Library site served as the access point for class-related functions such as tools for language review and class rubrics that would usually be reserved for the LMS.

It should not be surprising that colleagues who are subject matter experts but unfamiliar with the fictional world of an ARG may be confused when deciding which side of the fourth wall material they may be adding to the game belongs. Here is a list of items that were to be placed on the website as it was being built. My notes focused on separating items that belonged from those that did not. For example, there should not be a "meet the cast" section. Rather, only those characters associated with the fictional library should be included. Inspector Pei would not belong. Bullets are a list of completed tasks and to-dos. My notes are bolded.

Website:

Header looks good

News and events should replace "meet the cast"

- News update about students going on a cultural exchange – talk about first group who is scheduled to leave during the 3rd week, on Oct. 27th. List all 12 names.

- Another blurb about second group of students leaving on Jan. 26th.

- Blurb about Tingting Lu returning from successful buying trip, has located several maps of ancient China.

- Blurb about Dr. Chen to greet new students, plus a little something about who he is.

Mrs. Ling and Mr. Pei do not appear on website.

- A blurb about Tang Laoshi (Teacher Tang).

About section should be: "Heritage library is a multi-national organization dedicated to greater understanding of the language and culture of China and North America."

- Picture of each actor next to their blurbs.

- Picture of heritage library buildings in America and China.

- Lee will rewrite Chinese classics text.

- Meetings and events: New classes start October 13th and Tang Laoshi will be teaching this section of students. Give class location at RPI. Next event: This group leaves for China on Jan. 26th.

- Under class list the first three weeks.

Change blog to forum, linking to a free outside forum.

- Show videos of class sessions on website.

Initial State of the Website

The following website material was already loaded before the first class on October 13. New material would be added in the episode where it appeared in the narrative.

News Column

July 17, 2011

Dr. Bai Chen Named Heritage Library Cultural Exchange Director

Noted Chinese bibliophile and scholar Dr. Bai Chen has been appointed Director of the Heritage Library Cultural Exchange Program. Dr. Chen brings years of experience in the cultural history and literature of China to his new position. He is the author of the standard text *Four Pillars of Chinese Literature*, a study of the four greatest novels in Chinese history, their significance and influence on modern Chinese literature. A brief introduction to each of these books may be found here [**link to book page**]. Dr. Chen will personally take charge of cultural exchange students from the moment they arrive at Capitol International Airport in Beijing to create an educational experience they will not soon forget.

[**Biography source: ShihChia Thompson**]

The announcement was accompanied by a photograph of Dr. Chen.

July 25, 2011

Heritage Library Cultural Exchange Program Welcomes Rensselaer Students

Twelve undergraduate students from Rensselaer Polytechnic Institute will be traveling to China on November 3. This is Rensselaer's first participation in the Heritage Library's ongoing cultural exchange program between China and the United States. In preparation for the trip the students listed below will be enrolled in an eight-week Chinese language class beginning August 11 and concluding on October 6. The class will be taught by Tang Laoshi (Teacher Tang), an accomplished language instructor hired recently by the Heritage Library. Students will learn enough of the Chinese language to be able to fully appreciate the tours and programs being arranged for them.

Additionally, twelve Chinese students will be traveling to the United States on October 6 to Washington, D.C. They will be taught English for eight weeks prior to the trip.

The first twelve students from Rensselaer are:

These are fictitious students.

Mark Alvarez, second year student in Computer Science

Heidi Andersen, second year student in Chemistry

Ashley Burnett, third year student in Cognitive Science

Annika Corath, third year student in Psychology

Cory Grannell, third year student in EMAC

Michael Kelso, fourth year student in Games and Simulation Arts and Sciences

Ralf Kuippers, second year student in Engineering

Shannon McBride, fourth year student in Math

David Rickley, third year student in Engineering

Charlotte Ross, fourth year student in Games and Simulation Arts and Sciences

Mizumi Seiko, third year student in Art

Didi Sharp, second year student in Communications and Media

August 2, 2011

New Chinese Language Instructor Joins Heritage Library

The announcement was accompanied by a photograph of ShihChia Tang and a short biography.

September 16, 2011

Heritage Library Announces Second Group of Cultural Exchange Students

The Heritage Library is pleased to announce the names of the second group of students from Rensselaer Polytechnic Institute who will be traveling to China as part of the Heritage Library's cultural exchange program. These students will attend class beginning October 13, concluding on December 8. The class will also be taught by Tang Laoshi. The second group of students is scheduled to leave for China on January 26, 2012. Here are the names of these lucky students:

These were our eleven real students.

October 3, 2011

Tingting Lu Secures Ancient Maps for Library

The announcement was accompanied by a photograph of Tingting Lu.

Chinese Importer Tingting Lu, working on behalf of the Heritage Library, has returned from Shanxi Province, where she successfully negotiated the sale of three Chinese maps from the Yuan Dynasty (1280–1365). These rare maps cover the land indicated in the map below. After they are carefully restored and preserved, the Heritage Library will put them on display in our main museum in Boston.

The announcement was accompanied by a photograph of a Yuan Dynasty map.

About
The Heritage Library is a multi-national organization dedicated to giving students from the United States and China a greater understanding for each other's language and culture.

The article was accompanied by a photograph of a fictional Heritage Library building in Beijing.

The Heritage Library was established in 1968 and is funded by private grants and individuals to ensure that it remain free of national and political associations.

The article was accompanied by a photograph of a fictional Heritage Library building in Washington, D.C.

Meetings and Events
August 11, 2011

First day of Chinese language classes for first group of students from Rensselaer Polytechnic Institute. Classes will be held on the Rensselaer campus in Rooms 5510 and 2704 of the Sage Laboratory.

October 13, 2011

First day of Chinese language classes for second group of students from Rensselaer Polytechnic Institute. Classes will be held on the Rensselaer campus in Room 5510 of the Sage Laboratory.

October 17, 2011

Heritage Library Board Meeting in Conference Room 3 at the Heritage Library, Washington, D.C.

December 17, 2011

Formal Holiday Reception for dignitaries from China and the United States at the Heritage
October 24, 2011
> First group of cultural exchange students depart from the United States and China.
Library Ballroom, Washington, D.C.

January 26, 2012

Second group of cultural exchange students depart from the United States and China.

Chinese Classics

Journey to the West depicts the story of Monk Tang, Monkey King, and two others going west to seek for Sutra. The book is renowned as one of the four great classical novels in China. The monks face many obstacles in their quest to bring back the True Sutra and realize their Buddhist Ideal. It tells stories from the heaven, earth, and the fairyland. It often reflects the social reality of the Ming Dynasty, satirizing the existing ugliness of the society. Published in the 1590's, the Heritage Library owns a first edition of the book.

Romance of the Three Kingdoms is based on the history of the three kingdoms, Wei, Shu, and Wu that strove to reunite the empire at the end of the Eastern Han Dynasty. The political and military conflicts between the kingdoms were very fierce. *Romance of the Three Kingdoms* weaves historical events and the battles between the kingdoms to create a brilliant and poignant portrait of that turbulent time. The literary value of *Romance of the Three Kingdoms* lies much in the vivid characters sketched in the novel. This novel has extended its influence beyond China to Japan, Korea, Southeast Asia, and other countries in the world. Written in the 14th Century, the Heritage Library contains an early edition of this classic work, circa 1460.

The greatest masterpiece of the novels of the Qing dynasties, *Dream of the Red Chamber*, has had the most profound influence on later generations. The novel recalls the epic history of a noble family from the height of its glory to its decline, creating a masterful depiction of life and the mortal world. Set against the backdrop of the Great View Garden and focusing on the doomed love triangle of Jia Baoyu, Lin Daiyu, and Xue Baochai, the novel portrays a tragedy in which love, youth, and life are destroyed. The Heritage Library owns a first edition of this magnificent book.

The soul-stirring novel *Outlaws of the Marsh* (aka *Water Margin*), written more than 600 years ago, is a description of the insurgence led by Song Jiang and composed mostly of farmers. The novel depicts 108 heroes and heroines who gathered in the Liangshan Mountains surrounded by lakes and marshlands and started an uprising. Eventually they were offered amnesty and gave their loyalty to the Imperial Court. After fighting many battles for the Emperor, they were murdered by treacherous court officials. Full of legendary stories, *Outlaws of the Marsh* is considered a landmark of the literary arts. The novel contains a total of 787 characters, more than any other novel in the world. It has also created a common, concise, and expressive literary language from folk spoken language. An original manuscript from the 14th century has long been rumored to exist, signed by the author, Shi Nai'an himself. If it did exist, it would be one of the most valuable of books such as the Gutenberg Bible or a Shakespearean First Folio.

A variety of footnotes with additional information concluded this article.

Heritage Library Forum

In addition to Class assignments, language questions and social chat, The Heritage Library website featured a discussion forum for topics related to the narrative. Here we broke the fourth wall. The following prompts were included to guide the discussions.

Heritage Library website has info on Beijing! (Add AFTER 7 pm on Oct 13)

Why was Tingting Lu arguing with Tang Laoshi? (Add AFTER 7 pm on Oct 20)

Don't forget your travel documents! (Add AFTER 7 pm on Oct 27)

Where is Dr. Chen? (Add AFTER 7 pm on Nov 3)

Who is Mrs. Ling? (Add AFTER 7 pm on Nov 3)

Do you trust Tingting Lu? (Add AFTER 7pm on Nov 10)

Do you trust Tang Laoshi? (Add AFTER 7 pm on Nov 10)

Do you trust Mrs. Ling? (Add AFTER 7 pm on Nov 17)

The Customs Inspector was the waiter at the teahouse! (Add AFTER 7 pm on Nov 17)

Do you trust Inspector Pei? (Add AFTER 7 pm on Dec 1)

Do you trust Dr. Chen? (Add AFTER 7 pm on Dec 8)

What will Inspector Pei ask us? (Add AFTER 7 pm on Dec 8)

Language Class
These were notes from Tang Laoshi, covering her teaching in each class period.

Language Instruction Videos
Links to general Mandarin language instruction videos.

Link to Voice Thread

Students were required to access VoiceThread online to practice their Chinese language pronunciation. Their weekly progress was assessed.

> More than any of the other three games covered in this book, the fourth wall between narrative and teaching for *The Lost Manuscript* was very thin. There is universal agreement that the best way to learn a language is to live in the country whose language you wanted to learn and let nature take its course. Not always a practical method though for obvious reasons. Standard language education tries to mimic this with little scenes for context and lots of rote practice. We were attempting an immersion closer to the ideal.
>
> However, a lot of academic attention was focused on the project. Some of this was caused by the very real need for formal foreign language instruction to return to the school. This class was seen as a way to jumpstart that initiative. There was a concern that veering too far from established teaching practices could damage support for the plan. This was also a dress rehearsal for the Emergent Reality Lab, the second seed grant, and if the class was a failure, convincing the powers that be that a language class might not be the best first test of the 3D environment. As a result, there were many of the usual tools such as VoiceThread, instructional videos, etc. Once we pretended to leave the classroom there was a constant hammering on the fourth wall, a push and pull between the imaginative immersion created by the narrative and standard practice.

Virtual Reality (VR)

These were virtual interfaces interactive via the Microsoft Kinect. Built by Ben Chang and Anton Hand, the VR displays consisted of an airport information kiosk, a teahouse, a display for a code-breaking puzzle and the Wenyuan Library, a building in the Forbidden City not open to casual visitors.

Airport Information Booth (See Episode 4)

The "holographic" information kiosk could be accessed and searched with hand gestures. Using the Kinect students could gather information on hotels, restaurants, and other attractions in Beijing, and how to find and contact their hotel to arrange for transportation.

Teahouse (See Episode 6)

Non-interactive background. There Mrs. Ling also taught them a Chinese tea ceremony. The tea ceremony became the first fully realized, interactive 3D scene in the Emergent Reality Lab.

Code-Breaking Puzzle (See Episode 7)

A puzzle on a screen set up in the hotel room where the welcome reception was held. The decoded message points to the Wenyuan Library in the Forbidden City at a certain date and time to meet Dr. Chen.

Wenyuan Library (See Episode 8)

A building in the Forbidden City open only to scholars with special permission. Four photographs from the Summer Palace could be found by searching various pieces of furniture with the Kinect. The photographs offer clues to the location of the manuscript: 1) Longevity Hill from across Kunming Lake, 2) Revolving Archives (White Pillar with Buddhist Sutras), 3) Unnamed room nearby, 4) Ornate Desk (within the room).

The code-breaking puzzle was the trickiest to implement. There was also an issue with depth perception in the Wenyuan Library. More detailed information on how VR was implemented in these episodes, including the challenges faced, can be found in the research paper cited at the end of the introduction to this class.

GAME MECHANICS

Classroom

Desks, signage, projection system, etc.

Texts and Emails

In addition to the ability to text and email one another, students will also receive texts and emails from four major NPCs: Tang Laoshi, Tingting Lu, Mrs. Ling, and Inspector Pei. In the first episode, Tang Laoshi divides the class into four study groups. At first, each study group will receive all texts from NPCs. But when it begins to become clear to players that several of the NPCs have differing agendas, they will each begin receiving texts from a single NPC. Each NPC will ask her or his study group to not trust the other NPCs. Students may decide to share or withhold information they receive from their NPC. Actual texts will be found in the episodes when they were sent.

In *Skeleton Chase 2: The Psychic*, I had noticed how splitting the loyalties of participating students between two characters (Hope Johnson and Quinn Morgan) was quite successful. It increased player competitiveness, and therefore their interest in doing well. I would use this again in several multiplayer classrooms. The rewards of both competition and cooperation can be intrinsic as well as extrinsic. In *The Lost Manuscript* this was implemented, but only in a very rudimentary form.

1. All texts and emails are sent by puppet masters, not actors.

2. All texts and emails are in English and do **not** include quotation marks.

3. Texts and emails are to be sent to all students *except for* **November 28 and December 5**. Texts on those days are divided by study group (see below). Who texts to which group. **may** be decided based on various group's posts in the Heritage Library forums.

4. Copies of texts and emails are also sent to the actors who play the characters who supposedly sent them to keep the actors up to date on what they have said.

Physical Objects

Props and Costumes, purchased or created for *The Lost Manuscript*, will be listed in the episodes in which they appear.

CHARACTERS

Strangely enough this game, the most modest production, had by far the most actors.

Tang Laoshi

Ms. Tang, a recent addition to the Heritage Library, is a character in the story. Tang is the character's last name. Laoshi means "teacher." So, literally she is Teacher Tang. She is played by ShihChia Chen Thompson, the actual teacher of the class.

Inspector Pei

A canny police detective who may not be quite the master of disguise he believes himself to be. He appears as a customs official and a waiter before revealing his true identity.

Tingting Lu

Tingting is a dealer in rare books, sometimes representing the Heritage Library. At other times she appears to be representing her own interests, particularly when a very valuable manuscript is involved.

Dr. Bai Chen

Another recent addition to the Heritage Library, Dr. Chen is a respected scholar who mysteriously disappears.

Mrs. Ling

Mrs. Ling is a very friendly woman whom students meet at the airport who turns out to be associated with the Heritage Library as well. It's curious she did not mention this when she first met the students. Later she introduces them to a tea ceremony, and admits she is interested in the manuscript as well.

Map Seller

An NPC selling maps at the airport.

Currency Exchanger

An NPC who exchanges currency at the airport.

Van Driver

A driver from the Shambhala Hotel.

Waitress

A waitress at the hotel reception for the students.

Public Announcer

An announcer on the public address system at Capitol International Airport in Beijing.

Each of the major characters had email and Twitter accounts created for them.

ACTOR SCRIPTS

Remember the discussion in *The Skeleton Chase: The Psychic* about how giving actors specific dialogue to memorize is not a good idea when dealing with real people in real time? Actors need to be able to think on their feet and make sure all the important talking points are covered without breaking character or getting locked into precise dialogue. Now imagine needing to carry out a conversation in a language those you're speaking to are only learning now. All of our actors spoke fluent Mandarin as well as English. They needed to know what they should to say to move each conversation where it needed to go, both for the sake of the learning as well as the narrative. For that reason, you will see that the Actor Scripts in each episode are sometimes little more than suggestions, depending upon how each dialogue progressed and the amount of Mandarin the students had learned. The sole exception was the Public Announcer in the airport. Those cues were pre-recorded.

I would especially like to thank all of our Mandarin-speaking "actors" who donated their time to an undertaking that must have sounded a bit bizarre. Only one had had any acting experience at all. Yet they were able to match the vocabulary level of the students, see that the lesson was covered, and maintain character. Each and every one, whatever the size of the part, was able to pull this off with grace, humor and enthusiasm. Both the actors and the students had a ball.

STORY/BACKSTORY

Mandarin students from RPI, part of a cultural exchange, must learn more of the language than planned when a previous class are not allowed to make a trip to the People's Republic of China and they must go in the first group's place. And then they find out an official escort who fails to meet them at Beijing International Airport has mysteriously disappeared. Soon they are embroiled in a competition to find the price-less manuscript of a famous Chinese novel, *The Outlaws of the Marsh*. It's difficult to trust the people they meet: a respected scholar, a rare object broker, a man with several identities, and their own teacher. In the end the students find clues pointing to the Summer Palace, where the lost manuscript may be hidden, but must use all of their newly acquired language skills when they face their final exam: a police interrogation.

See the Afterword for how the narrative was fleshed out to include an extensive adventure at the Summer Palace for later iterations of the class.

POINT OF ATTACK

The game begins when the students' second class is interrupted by a mysterious Chinese woman who has an argument with their teacher, and they learn that they will be going to China weeks ahead of schedule.

ADDITIONAL CLASS DOCUMENTS

This class, more than the others in this book, followed strict rules for teaching languages in a university classroom setting. A lot was riding on it, most impor-tantly the future of foreign language instruction at RPI as well as the addition of narrative and gameplay and the potential of a fully VR implementation. All of the additional rubrics and checklists on display here were appropriate so that those who would ultimately decide its success or failure could see the class followed familiar procedures both for a foreign language class and a class at RPI. It was, despite the simplicity of the narrative and gameplay, just as challenging as any chosen for this book.

Syllabus

The syllabus shows how the learning outcomes, schedule and course policies of an RPI class and the unique nature of this one were combined.

Mandarin Language/Culture Course Fall 2011

Course Schedule

Title	88226 COMM 2960-01 Mandarin Language and Culture
Instructors	Lee Sheldon, ShihChia Thompson, Jim Zappen
Credit Hours	3
Day/Time	Mondays/Thursdays 5:00-6:50 p.m.
Room	Sage 2704 and 5510

Course Description

Mandarin Language and Culture, an experimental beginning course in Mandarin Chinese, will place students in a fictional narrative of mystery and adventure, transporting them to virtual Chinese locations where they will interact with compelling characters on the hunt for a lost object of great value.

Within the context of the story they will be introduced through cryptic puzzles and other challenges to both spoken and written Mandarin, character recognition, pronunciation and vocabulary; as well as Chinese culture. The experience will include face-to-face interactions with actors and other students, social networking, computer and video components, all part of the narrative framework.

Learning Outcomes

Communication—Demonstrating Ability to Communicate in Mandarin Language; Three modes of communication—interpersonal, interpretive, presentational—with focus on vocabulary, pronunciation and grammatical principles

- Interpersonal - Students will be able to engage in conversations, provide and obtain information, express feelings and emotions, and exchange opinions (e.g., state necessities, likes, dislikes, etc.)
- Interpretive - Students will demonstrate knowledge and be able to interpret key characters in written form and basic spoken language

Cultures & Comparison—Demonstrating Knowledge and Understanding of Cultures; Students will demonstrate knowledge and understanding of the distinctive products, practices and perspectives of culture (e.g., cultural artifacts—what they are, how they are used, and why they are used as they are)

- Understand and observe cultural norms for language use and interpersonal communication (e.g., how one says hello to a peer vs. a non-peer)
- Distinguish between acceptable and unacceptable language usage and cultural behavior
  —in Chinese interactions
  —between American and Chinese interactions
  (e.g., what is appropriate in American interactions that is not appropriate in Chinese interactions or vice versa)

Application & Transfer
- Students will be able to use what they have learned to negotiate successfully in new situations that may entail unfamiliar language or cultural elements

Metacognition
- Students will be able to reflect on their strengths/challenges/needs as learners

The syllabus for the class.

and use that reflection to guide their own learning (e.g., demonstrate resourcefulness in resolving challenges such as pronunciation difficulties, etc.)

Schedule of Classes

Thurs	Oct 6	Introduction and Preparation 1	Sage 2704
Tues	Oct 11	No Class Meeting	
Thurs	Oct 13	Practice Session 1	Sage 5510
Mon	Oct 17	Preparation Session 2	Sage 2704
Thurs	Oct 20	Practice Session 2	Sage 5510
Mon	Oct 24	Preparation Session 3	Sage 2704
Thus	Oct 27	Practice Session 3	Sage 5510
Mon	Oct 31	Preparation Session 4	Sage 2704
Thurs	Nov 3	Practice Session 4	Sage 5510
Mon	Nov 7	Preparation Session 5	Sage 2704
Thurs	Nov 10	Practice Session 5	Sage 5510
Mon	Nov 14	Preparation Session 6	Sage 2704
Thurs	Nov 17	Practice Session 6	Sage 5510
Mon	Nov 21	Preparation Session 7a	Sage 2704
Thurs	Nov 24	No Class Meeting (Thanksgiving)	
Mon	Nov 28	Preparation Session 7b	Sage 2704
Thurs	Dec 1	Practice Session 7	Sage 5510
Mon	Dec 5	Preparation Session 8	Sage 2704
Thurs	Dec 8	Practice Session 8	Sage 5510
Finals Week	Dec 19	Practice Session 9	Sage 4711

Grading Procedure

Mandarin Preparation

Weekly Skills Checklist	15 points	ShihChia Thompson, with Mission Facilitators
Verbal Performance Tasks	40 points	ShihChia Thompson
Mandarin Practice, includes culminating task	35 points	ShihChia Thompson
Participation Tasks	10 points	Jim Zappen

Grade Calculation

93-100	points	=	A
90-92	points	=	A-
87-89	points	=	B+
83-86	points	=	B
80-82	points	=	B-
77-79	points	=	C+
73-76	points	=	C
70-72	points	=	C-

(continued)

67-69	points	=	D+
60-66	points	=	D
00-59	points	=	F

Course Policies

Class Attendance: Class attendance and participation are required. Students who miss class for extended periods of time without permission or explanation will be reported to the Dean of Students Office and/or the Department of Public Safety for support and assistance, as needed. Requests for accommodations, exceptions, extensions, or incomplete grades due to illnesses or personal emergencies must be supported by written documentation from the Dean of Students Office.

Intellectual Property and Electronic Citizenship: Rensselaer's policies on copyright, intellectual property, and electronic citizenship are explained at Policy on Electronic Citizenship. Violations of these policies will be reported to the Dean of Students and the Dean of the student's college or school.

Students' Rights and Responsibilities: Students' rights and responsibilities are explained in The Rensselaer Handbook of Student Rights and Responsibilities: 2010-2012 and govern the conduct of both faculty and students. Academic dishonesty is explained on pp. 14-17 and is strictly prohibited. Incidents of academic dishonesty on any assignment will be graded 0 points for the assignment and will be reported to the Dean of Students and the Dean of the student's college or school, with a request that the incident be entered into the student's permanent record at Rensselaer.

> Student-teacher relationships are built on trust. For example, students must trust that teachers have made appropriate decisions about the structure and content of the courses they teach, and teachers must trust that the assignments which students turn in are their own. Acts that violate this trust undermine the educational process.
>
> The *Rensselaer Handbook of Student Rights and Responsibilities* defines various forms of Academic Dishonesty and procedures for responding to them. All forms are violations of the trust between students and teachers.
>
> Office of the Provost

Appeals Process: Decisions by the instructor may be appealed through the LL&C Acting Department Head and the HASS Dean and/or through the Dean of Students Office.

(continued)

Production Schedule

Rensselaer Polytechnic Institute Mandarin Chinese Program

伦斯勒理工学院中文项目

Lúnsīlè lǐgōng xuéyuàn zhōngwén xiàngmù

Schedule 时间表 Shíjiān biǎo					
Narrative Episode	**Date**	**Topics to be discussed (Language function)**	**Subject Content**	**Characters/Vocabulary/Sentence structure**	**Missions/Assignments**
1. The Heritage Library Program	Thursday, 10/6/2011	Introducing myself to others 自我介绍 Inquire contact information 询问联络资料	• Greeting • Identity • Country • Major • Contact information (E-mail, telephone cell phone numbers) • Numbers	• Hello! • What is your name? • My name is _____. • Are you a teacher (student)? • I am a student. • Which country are you from? • I am American (Chinese). • What is your major? • I major in _____. • Do you have e-mail? • My e-mail is xxx@xxx. • What is your telephone (cell phone) number? • My telephone (cell phone) number is 518-123-4560 • Use the website: Heritage library www.heritagelibrary.org • Do you know + a person's name? • I'm looking for + a person's name (or a book).	Students will use any of the devices listed to contact mission facilitators and introduce themselves.
				• Yes/No questions • Subject+Verb+Object. • Cultural component: Exchanging business cards	
	Monday 10/10/2011	Columbus day/ No class			
	Thursday, 10/13/2011	Class preparation and Narrative Episode			
2. China Bound	Monday, 10/17/2011	Asking about someone 询问某人 Forming a question 问问题 Asking and Telling date and Time 日期和时间 Emotions 心情	• Forming questions • Date and time to meet • Expressing emotions: happy & unhappy, surprised, excited, nervous, anxious, exhausted, angry, upset	• Who is that (he, she)? • He/she is _____. • What does he/she want? • He/she wants to _____. • What time is it? • It is 00:00 AM/PM. • When are we going to meet in the airport? • 4 H questions: who, where, when, what • Who are you? Where are you? When are you coming? What are you doing? • I feel (very) happy/unhappy, surprised, etc.	Students ask mission facilitators out for dinner and indicate the date and time.
	Thursday, 10/20/2011	Class preparation and Narrative Episode			
3. Last Class	Monday, 10/24/2011	Asking for direction 问路，方向	• Direction • Hotel • Airport	• Where is + place name? • There it is. • How do get to there?	Students ask direction about the bathroom of a restaurant or any building

Production schedule.

		Book a flight and hotel 订机票和饭店 Book a van (or taxi) 叫车（出租车） Meet someone in the airport 在机场与某人见面	• Taxi, van	• I want to book a flight (hotel room). • What time does the flight depart/arrive? • The flight departs/arrives at 00:00 AM/PM. • Where do you want to go?/Where are you going? • We need a van to pick us up in the airport. • When will you arrive? • When are you leaving? • Where do we meet Dr. Chen in the airport? • Take me to "香巴拉 Shambhala" hotel.	from mission facilitators. Students can also pretend to book a hotel room or van.
	Thursday, 10/27/2011	Class preparation and Narrative Episode			
4. Capital International Airport	Monday, 10/31/2011	Dealing with the airport customs 机场海关 Buy a map 买地图 Currency and rates of exchange 货币和汇率换算	• Airport customs investigations • Map study • Currency exchange • Characters: Renesselaer student group 伦斯勒学生团, ground transportation 陆地交通工具 (公交车 bus, 出	• Are you here for business or pleasure? • I am touring. • Where will you be staying? • I will stay in _____ hotel. • How long will you be in China? • I will stay for + number + days. • How much RMB do you want to exchange? • I want to exchange 500 RMB dollars. • What is the rate exchanging RMB and US dollars?	Students ask mission facilitator about buying a map and exchanging currency through SKYPE.
			租车 taxi, 酒店 包车 hotel van), 地图出售 map for sale, 男厕所 man's room, 女厕所 lady's room, 海关 customs, 入境, 出境 departure/arrival	• How much does it cost? • That's too expensive. • Recognizing key characters in the airport.	
	Thursday, 11/3/2011	Class preparation and Narrative Episode			
5. Miyer	Monday, 11/7/2011	Looking for someone, something 找人，找东西 Restaurant conversation Ordering in a restaurant 餐厅点菜 Dining etiquette 用餐礼节	• Making inquiry about missing person or stuff • Ordering food and drink • Inviting someone for dinner	• What are you doing (looking for)? • I am looking for + number + measure word + object or a person. • What do you want to eat (drink)? • I want a glass of water, tea, coffee, coke, or soda. • I want a plate of sesame chicken. • Please give me + food or drink. • I don't want the onion. • Can I get a fork (knife, spoon)? • Do you have chopsticks? • I (don't) know how to use chopsticks.	Students order food and drink from a Chinese restaurant. Mission facilitators will check their comprehensibility. Students can also record their voice through Voicethread about ordering drink/food.
	Thursday, 11/10/2011	Class preparation and Narrative Episode			

(continued)

6. The Tea House	Monday, 11/14/2011	Making a phone call 打电话 Texting a message 传短信 Leaving a message 留言 Looking for a book 找一本书	• Phone conversation • Characters study • Number + Measure words + Object	• Hello, who is this? • I am _____. I am an American student. • Where are you? • I am at/in _____. • Who/what are you looking for? • I am looking for _____. • Is he/she there? • He/she is not here. Call later. • I am looking for + number + measure word + object or a person. • Do you know this book (person)? • Can I text you or leave you a message? • I have a text (phone) message. • What does it say? • It says _____. • I'm looking for something that's worth a lot of money. It has been missing for centuries. • Review Food & Drink	The mission facilitators e-mail or leave a message of Chinese characters regarding the direction. Students will decode the message and bring it to the class next time.
	Thursday, 11/17/2011	Class preparation and Narrative Episode			
7. Code Breaking	Monday, 11/21/2011	Recognizing key characters 认识关键汉字 Date and Time 日期和时间 Direction 方向	• Month, date, days of the week • Numbers • East, west, north, south	• How to say this phrase or character? • What does this character mean? • What day is it today? • Today is days of the week + date + month + year. • What time is it?	Students need to interpret a message with Chinese characters sent from the mission facilitators. Such as: "there is a Chinese restaurant on the southeast of RPI." (在 RPI 的东南
				• It is 00:00 AM/PM. • I understand. • I don't understand. • What time do we meet? • When are we going to Forbidden city?	方有一家中国餐馆。) or "We are going to the airport at 7:30 am on Sunday, November 20, 2011." (我们二〇一一年十一月二十号星期日要去机场。)
	Thursday, 11/24/2011	Thanksgiving/ No class			
	Monday, 11/28/2011	Class preparation and Narrative Episode			
8. The Forbidden City	Thursday, 12/1/2011	Asking direction 问路 Left, right Up, down Direction 方向	• East, west, north, south • Left, right • Up, down • Front, back • Hall of heavenly peace • Forbidden City • East bedroom Search things	• Where is east side? • East side is over there. • Can you tell me how to get to here? • Go straight • Turn left/right • Do you know where is Forbidden City? • How long does it take to get to Forbidden City from the hotel? • It takes about half hour. • Where is the Hall of heavenly peace • Where is the East bedroom? • It's right there. • Where is the book? • It is on top of the chair. • It is not here. • Search beneath the table, on top of the chair, or above the cabinet	Students listen to a message from Voicethread. Teacher shows a map and asks students how to get to B from A. Students record down their voice.

(continued)

	Monday, 12/5/2011	Class preparation and Narrative Episode			
9. Final Exam	Thursday, 12/8/2011	Final Exam: Interrogation- Answering questions about the investigation of a police officer 回答警察办案的问题	Emotion & feeling: • Happy & unhappy • Scared • Nervous • Angry • Anxious • Exhausted Review previous lessons: • Identity • Country • Status • Gender • Age and birthday • Date and time • Customs investigation • Asking information about the trip • Past tense: Subject + Verb + le 了	• Hello! • How are you? • I am good. / Not bad. / So-so. / Not good. • I feel (very) happy/unhappy/angry/nervous/scared/anxious/exhausted. • What is your name? • My name is _____. • Are you a teacher (student)? • I am a student. • How old are you? • I am number + years old. • When is your birthday? • My birthday is year + month + date. • Which country are you from? • I am American (Chinese). • Do you have e-mail (cellphone)? • Do you know + a person's name? • He is a male. / She is a female. • What are you doing in China? • What are you doing in the Forbidden City? • How long will you stay in China? • When did you arrive China? • When are you leaving China? • Who do you come with on this trip? • Who are you looking for? • What are you looking for? • I'm looking for + a person's name (a book). • Yes/No questions • I stayed in _____ hotel for _____ days. • I went to the Teahouse for dinner with _____.	
Snow day	Monday, 12/19/2011	Final Exam: Interrogation			

(continued)

The production schedule is a good overview for what was covered week to week for all episodes. It included the episode name and number, the date, topics to be discussed, subject content, vocabulary and sentence structure, and missions and assignments. You will see how a similar document was used in *The Janus Box*.

伦斯勒理工学院中文项目

Lúnsīlè lǐgōng xuéyuàn zhōngwén xiàngmù

Rensselaer Polytechnic Institute Mandarin Chinese Program
Fall, 2011 Basic Chinese Level 1-1
Instructor: 陈诗佳老师 Chén, ShīhChiā lǎoshī,　　E-mail: thomps4@rpi.edu

Skill Checklist
Rubrics:

(Please select the level according to student's performance and each specific skill.)

1. *Below expectation*: The student has difficulties structuring or pronouncing any target vocabulary & sentences.
2. *Approaching expectation*: The student can say the target vocabulary & sentences with some errors in structures or pronunciation.
3. *Meets expectation*: The student can say the target vocabulary & sentences with relatively accurate structure and pronunciation.
4. *Exceeds expectation*: The student can say the target vocabulary & sentences with accurate structure and pronunciation.

Week: Episode 1
Date: 10/17-10/23
Topic: Making inquiry, Date & Time, Feelings & Emotions

Student's name: _____

Mission Facilitator: _____

The Student Will Be Able To:	Level
Ask about someone he/she knows; (E.g. Tāng lǎoshī)	☐1.　☐2.　☐3.　☐4.
Say today's date;	☐1.　☐2.　☐3.　☐4.
Set up a schedule that includes date and time to SKYPE with someone;	☐1.　☐2.　☐3.　☐4.
State his/her plan to go to China	☐1.　☐2.　☐3.　☐4.
Ask one's age and birthday;	☐1.　☐2.　☐3.　☐4.
State his/her age and birthday;	☐1.　☐2.　☐3.　☐4.
Express his/her feeling about learning Chinese and going to China	☐1.　☐2.　☐3.　☐4.

Example of a weekly checklist to monitor student progress.

Vocabulary Lists

Here are two examples of vocabulary lists. Look for two things. The first list was practiced before the narrative began. It covers basic foundational language topics. The second was for October 13, the first class that was part of the narrative. It ends with the first narrative specific dialogue. The settings for episodes were informed by standard lessons, so I varied as little as possible from the usual topics such as introductions, social exchanges, dining, directions, travel, etc.

As in *The Skeleton Chase 2*, the narrative and gameplay were meant to be incentives for achieving goals. They were not meant to be the focus of specific lessons, but simply to complement them. As you will see, *Secrets* and *The Janus Door* were far more fully integrated. Either approach is perfectly valid. Regular language instruction often includes "scenes" that learners act out.

RPI INTRODUCTION TO MANDARIN

Vocabulary List 1.1 Self Introduction

问候 Wèn hòu: Greeting

- 你好：Hello（nǐ hǎo）；
- 我：I（wǒ）；我是：I am:（wǒ shì）；名字：name (míng zì)
- 你：you(nǐ); 你叫什么名字？：what's your name? (nǐ jiào shén me míng zì)
- 我叫：My name is（wǒ jiào）；
- 你可以叫我 xx：you can call me xx（nǐ kě yǐ jiào wǒ...）
- 你好吗？: how are you? (nǐ hǎo ma?)
- 很高兴认识你：Nice to meet you:（hěn gāo xìng rèn shí nǐ）

身份 Shēn fèn: Identity

- 学生：student（xuéshēng）
- 专业：major（zhuān yè）
- 大一：freshman（dà yī）；大二:sophomore（dà èr）；大三：junior:（dà sān）；大四: senior（dà sì）

国家 Guó jiā: Country

- 美国: USA（měi guó）；美国人：American(měi guó rén)
- 英国: United Kingdom (ying1 guó); 英国人：British (yīng guó rén)
- 日本：Japan (rì běn); 日本人：Japanese(rì běn rén)
- 德国·German (dé guó); 德国人: German(dé guó rén)

专业 Zhuān yè: Major

- 工程: Engineering; 学院：school (xué yuàn)
- 电子工程: Electronic Engineering（diàn zǐ gōng chéng）
- 土木工程: Civil Engineering:（tǔ mù gōng chéng ）
- 化学: Chemistry:（huà xué）
- 化学工程: Chemical engineering:（huà xué gōng chéng）
- 法学: Law:（fǎ xué）
- 工商管理: Business administration: (gōng shāng guǎn lǐ)
- 科学: Science:（kē xué）；计算机科学: Computer Science:（jì suàn jī kē xué）

对话 Duì huà: Conversation

- Welcome!/ Hello! (to one person)/ Hello! (to a group of people)
  Huānyíng!/ Nǐ hǎo!/ Nǐmén hǎo! 欢迎！ / 你好！ / 你们好！

Vocabulary for the introductory class session.

- What is your name? My name is _____.

  Nǐ jiào shénme (míngzi)? Wǒ jiào _____. 你叫什么（名字）？我叫_____。

- What is his (her) (name)? His (her) name is _____.

  Tā (tā) jiào shénme (míngzi)? Tā (tā) jiào _____. 他（她）叫什么（名字）？他（她）叫_____。

- Nice to see you!

  Hěn gāoxìng jiàndào nǐ! 很高兴见到你！

- Where are you from? I'm American. I'm Chinese.

  Nǐ shì nǎ guó rén? Wǒ shì měiguó rén. Wǒ shì zhōngguó rén. 你是哪国人？我是美国人。我是中国人。

- Are you a college student?

  Nǐ shì dà xuéshēng ma? 你是大学生吗？

- I am a college student.

  Wǒ shì dà xuésheng. 我是大学生。

- Where do you go to college?

  Nǐ zài nǎr shàng dàxué? 你在哪儿上大学？

- I go to RPI.

  Wǒ zài RPI shàng dàxué. 我在 RPI 上大学。

- What is your major?/What major are you studying?

  Nǐ xué shénme zhuānyè? 你学什么专业？

- I study Electrical Engineering, and you?

  Wǒ xué diàn zǐ gōng chéng. Nǐ ne? 我学电子工程。你呢？

- I am studying graphic design.

  Wǒ xué diànnǎo huìtú shè jì. 我学电脑绘图设计。

(Continued)

RPI INTRODUCTION TO MANDARIN

Vocabulary List 1.2

数字 shùzi：Number from 0-10

- 零：zero(ling2); 一：one (yī)；二：two (èr)；三：three (sān)；四：four (sì)；五：five (wǔ)
- 六：six (liù)；七：seven(qī)；八：eight （bā）；九：nine （jiǔ）；十：ten （shí）

通讯资料 tōngxùn zīliào：Useful phrase for "contact information"

- 你：you （nǐ）；你的：your （nǐ de）
- 电话号码：phone number (diàn huà hào mǎ)
- 手机：cell phone （shǒu jī）；手机号码：cell phone number (shǒu jī hào mǎ)
- 几号：what number （jǐ hào）
- 电话：call (diàn huà); 打电话：make a call (dǎ diàn huà)
- 你电话几号？：What is your phone number? （Nǐ shǒujī jǐ hào?）
- 你手机几号？：What is your cell number? （Nǐ shǒujī jǐ hào?）
- 上网：surfing Internet （shàng wǎng）
- 网站：website （wǎng zhàn）
- 发短信：text （fā duǎnxìn）
- 电子邮件：e-mail （diànzi yóujiàn）
- 脸书：facebook （liǎn shū）

对话 duì huà：Conversation

- What is your cell phone number?

  Nǐ shǒujī jǐ hào? 你手机几号？

- My number is 0123456789.

  Wǒ de hàomǎ shì líng, yī, èr, sān, sì, wǔ, liù, qī, bā, jiǔ.

  我的号码是零，一，二，三，四，五，六，七，八，九。

- Do you have email?

  Nǐ yǒu diànzi yóujiàn ma? 你有电子邮件吗？

- Yes, my email is xxx@hotmail.com. What about you?

  Yǒu, wǒ de diànzi yóujiàn shì xxx@hotmail.com, nǐ ne? 有，我的电子邮件是

  xxx@hotmail.com，你呢？

书 shū：book

- 一本书：a book （yì běn shū）

Notice the discussion of books at the end.

- 我在找…：I'm looking for…（Wǒ zài zhǎo…）
- 你知道…：Do you know…（Nǐ zhīdào…）
- 这本书：this book（zhè běn shū）
- 这个人：this person（zhè ge rén）

对话 duì huà： Conversation

- I'm looking for a book. Wǒ zài zhǎo yì běn shū. 我在找一本书。
- Do you know this book? Nǐ zhīdào zhè běn shū ma? 你知道这本书吗？
- What is the name of the book? Zhè běn shū jiào shénme míngzi? 这本书叫什么名字？
- The name of the book is "Outlaws of the Marsh". Zhè běn shū jiào "Shuǐ hǔ zhuàn". 这本书叫水浒传。

(Continued)

EPISODES

The game, divided into eight episodes, was played over eight weeks from October 13, 2011 to December 8, 2011. Mondays were language practice days. Thursday 24, 2011 was Thanksgiving. There was no class that day. The ninth episode was on December 19, 2011. It was the final exam in the form of a police interrogation conducted by Inspector Pei. The nine episodes follow.

CHAPTER 14

Episode 1 – The Heritage Library Program

Thursday, October 13

CHARACTERS

Tang Laoshi

NARRATIVE

Tang Laoshi greets students in Chinese and speaks to them in English. She then introduces herself in Chinese and tells them in English that the Heritage Library supports a cultural exchange between the United States and China. This year students from RPI will be going to China to study the country's cultural and literary traditions. In fact, the first group of twelve students is preparing to leave in three weeks, and students who show progress in this class will be going on January 26.

She introduces the interactive VR technology developed by Heritage Library scientists. Actually, for this proof of concept the "VR" was projected on the standard classroom A/V screen and powered by the Microsoft Kinect). She then teaches the students:

1. Greeting

2. Identity

3. Country

4. Major

There is one additional lesson that is a bit unusual, she says, but it will be helpful, given the literary purpose for the trip:

5. Books.

This lesson will include:

I am interested in Chinese books. I am looking for a book. Have you seen a book called…? Do you know a book called…?

She concludes in English, telling the class they have made a good start. She divides the class of twelve into four study groups, based on their progress. Each group should have one student who is doing very well, and one who is struggling a bit.

> One student dropped out before classes began. We had planned on twelve students that we could divide equally into four study groups of three students each. The study group of two contained the student who was doing the best in class.

She informs them of the lessons they will tackle next week. They will find practice materials for this week's lesson and preparation for next week's lesson on the Heritage Library's website. She tells them they should help each other in their study group, reminding them that they only have eight weeks to prepare for their trip. And any who fall behind may not be allowed to go.

> This timetable was part of the fictional narrative. The class would actually be "going to China" in three weeks.

During the week Tang Laoshi texts each student to ask if he or she has reached the Heritage Library website and has any questions. She reminds them to study, review the videos, use VoiceThread and wishes them well.

TEXT

Send to all students on Monday, October 17.

From Tang Laoshi

When you visit the Heritage Library website there will be a new section called Beijing attractions. Make time to visit any of these you can.

CHAPTER 15

Episode 2 – China Bound

Thursday, October 20

CHARACTERS

Tang Laoshi, Tingting Lu

NARRATIVE

Tang Laoshi welcomes the class and makes sure they were all able to reach the Heritage Library website and study. She reviews the previous lesson. She then teaches:

1. Numbers

2. Useful phrases

3. Supplementary Vocabulary

After they have practiced these for a while, a woman enters. She appears agitated. She demands in Chinese to speak to Tang Laoshi. Tang Laoshi apologizes and exits with her, telling the class to continue their review. After a few minutes she returns with the woman, looking distressed. The visitor introduces herself as Tingting Lu and passes out a business card to each student with her phone number on it. International business cards typically feature the native language on one side and a foreign language on the other.

All of the physical props for the game were excellent from official documents to the authentic tea service used in the tea ceremony. Possibly not the usual expenses or exertion required when creating a new class at RPI, but the team rose to the occasion.

Tingting tells the class in English that she lives in Beijing and will be happy to assist them in any way she can once they are there. She exits. After she goes Tang Laoshi tells the

Beijing Imports/Exports

Tingting Lu
Suite 519
Huaheng Building
31 South Binhe Road
Xuanwu District, Beijing 100055
P. R. China

Phone: (339) 793-8464
Email: Lutingting0@gmail.com

Beijing Imports/Exports

Tingting Lu
Suite 519
Huaheng Building
31 South Binhe Road
Xuanwu District, Beijing 100055
P. R. China

Phone: (339) 793-8464
Email: Lutingting0@gmail.com

Beijing Imports/Exports

Tingting Lu
Suite 519
Huaheng Building
31 South Binhe Road
Xuanwu District, Beijing 100055
P. R. China

Phone: (339) 793-8464
Email: Lutingting0@gmail.com

Beijing Imports/Exports

Tingting Lu
Suite 519
Huaheng Building
31 South Binhe Road
Xuanwu District, Beijing 100055
P. R. China

Phone: (339) 793-8464
Email: Lutingting0@gmail.com

北京进口/出口

路婷婷
电话：（339）793-8464
电子邮箱：Lutingting0@gmail.com

北京进口/出口

路婷婷
电话：（339）793-8464
电子邮箱：Lutingting0@gmail.com

北京进口/出口

路婷婷
电话：（339）793-8464
电子邮箱：Lutingting0@gmail.com

北京进口/出口

路婷婷
电话：（339）793-8464
电子邮箱：Lutingting0@gmail.com

Front and back of Tingting Lu's business card.

students they should not trust Tingting. She explains in English and/or Chinese that while Ms. Lu, an importer/exporter in Beijing, finds old manuscripts, books, and maps for the Heritage Library, she does not speak for the library. They should trust Dr. Chen, who will be their main Heritage Library contact in Beijing.

Tang Laoshi is upset, but uses the interruption to teach:

1. How to ask about someone you don't know.

2. Talk about date and time.

Another example of using the narrative to put teaching in context.

Now Tang Laoshi surprises everyone. She apologizes for the short warning, but a previous group of students from another school were rejected because of poor language learning skills.

> This was changed. The reason given, "poor language learning skills," became mysterious. Look for the list of previous students the customs official (Pei) had on his desk with red lines through the names. In the final iteration of the game the mystery was finally explained.

Tang Laoshi tells the class that they will be going in the previous class' place. And in only two weeks! Next week they will study how to ask directions, about transportation, hotels etc. She again reminds them of review and new lessons to be found on the Heritage Library website. Students must go online to the website and print out the travel documents they'll need.

> This "sudden change" was of course only part of the fiction, but ShihShia told me that the effort the class was putting into studying increased after this announcement.

TEXTS

Send to all students on Monday, October 24.

From Tang Laoshi

We have much to learn before you go to China on Nov 3. Study hard! I will have your travel documents for you this Thursday.

From Tingting Lu

I am sorry you must leave so soon! But I hope you may be able to do me a small favor while you are in Beijing.

CHAPTER 16

Episode 3 – Last Class before China

Thursday, October 27

CHARACTERS

Tang Laoshi

NARRATIVE

Tang Laoshi reviews previous lessons, then teaches:

1. Customs questions.

2. Various airport signs.

3. How to call a cab or van.

4. Hotel phrases (Hotel name is Shambhala).

5. Phrases that will allow them to speak to Dr. Chen at the airport. (This lesson will really prepare them to talk to Mrs. Ling.)

Tang Laoshi tells the students to print their travel documents and expense voucher.

More excellent prop work. The "travel documents" resembled passports, but on regular paper, and included student pictures. Students exchanged the expense voucher for our version of Renminbi, the official Republic of China currency.

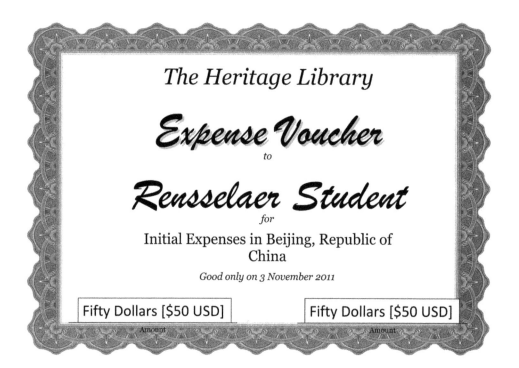

The expense voucher.

The students are told that the documents can be found on the Heritage Library website. They will be greeted at the airport by Dr. Chen, the Heritage Library's new Cultural Exchange Director. They can read about him on the Heritage Library website. She then says there will be a welcoming reception at the hotel in Beijing. They can text Tang Laoshi with questions, but she may not be able to answer right away because she will be very busy when she first arrives in China.

Again, the fiction caused a reaction from the students. Their teacher may be too busy to teach???

TEXT

Send to all students on Monday, October 31.

From Tang Laoshi

Be sure to bring your travel documents with you next week. You will need them in the Beijing airport.

CHAPTER 17

Episode 4 – Capital International Airport

Thursday, November 3

This was by far the most elaborate of the episodes. There were more puzzles in this one episode than in the rest of the episodes combined. There were multiple actors, our first VR interaction, a live telephone call, and a mysterious disappearance.

CHARACTERS

Inspector Pei (disguised as a customs official), Mrs. Ling, Map Seller, Currency Exchanger, Van Driver

NARRATIVE

Students "travel" to China, arriving at Capital International Airport.

There are a number of things they must do here:

1. Negotiate Customs. The Customs Official (Pei) welcomes each student to China. He has a list with Chinese characters and the name RENSSELAER at the top followed by a list of twelve names crossed out in red. Below those is a list of the names of the current eleven students. He'll check off their names after he stamps each passport.

What the officer asks them should include a review of things learned in Episode 3. Examples:

a. Are you here for business or pleasure?

b. Where will you be staying? (Hotel name introduced in Episode 3 is Shambhala.)

c. How long will you be in China?

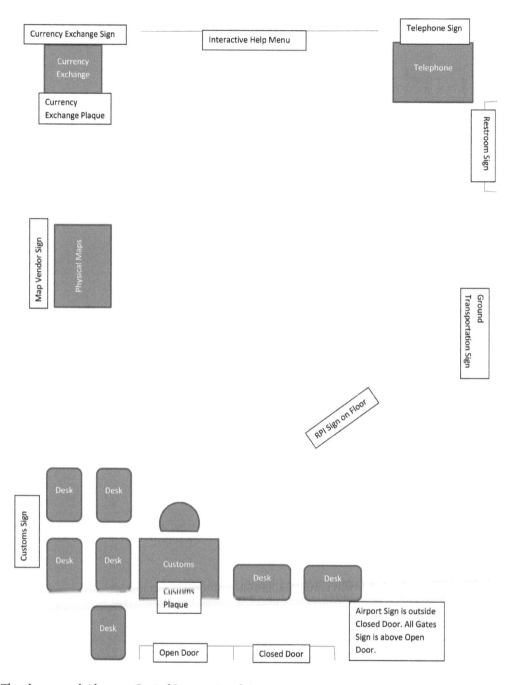

The classroom laid out as Capital International Airport.

2. Dr. Chen is not there to meet the students. But students will find a crumpled and trampled sign on the floor with WELCOME RENSSELAER STUDENTS on it.

3. They must buy a simplified map to the city from a map seller. This will contain all sites to be visited: Airport, Hotel, Teahouse, Forbidden City, and Police Headquarters.

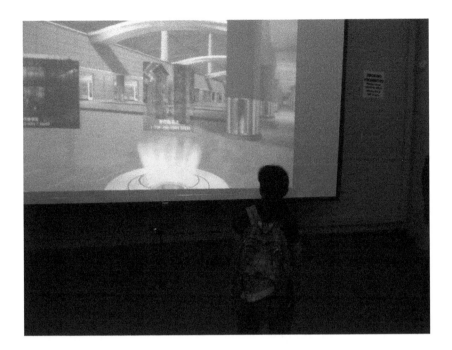

First appearance of the Kinect in the game.

4. Exchange currency.

5. Use the automated information kiosk (Microsoft Kinect) to find the phone number of the Shambhala Hotel.

6. Use the courtesy telephone to call the Shambhala Hotel and ask for a van to pick them up.

The "courtesy phone" was a cell phone with the actor playing the Van Driver, who spoke only Chinese to them, on the other end.

7. Meet Mrs. Ling. She is an elderly woman who overheard them ask for the van. She would like a ride to the hotel with them. This can be the second part of the review of previous material since they must introduce themselves and learn about her. They can agree to let her ride with them or refuse.

8. Study a map of the airport on the wall.

Note: Student study groups may split up or stay together.

The episode ends when there is a public announcement in Chinese asking the students to meet the van at a certain location at the airport. There are several signs on the walls of the classroom and one by each door. Students must find the one that says GROUND TRANSPORTATION in Chinese before they can exit the airport.

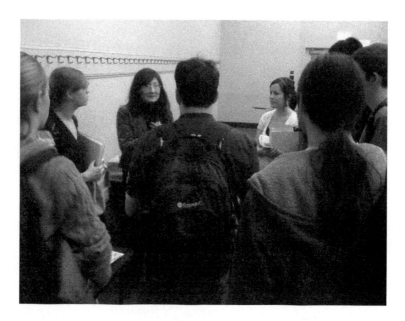

Mrs. Ling seems harmless. Should they give her a ride?

ACTOR SCRIPTS
Detective Pei

Pei holds a copy of a "travel document" as he questions a student. The second student in line holds an expense voucher.

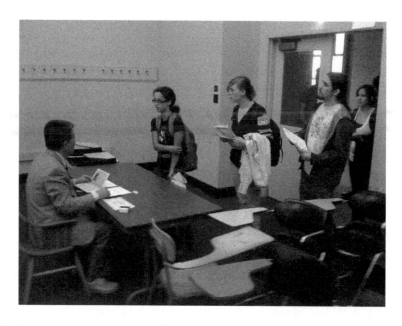

Inspector Pei impersonating a customs official.

Detective Pei appears in this episode as the Customs Official. He welcomes each student to China and checks each of their names off of a list which also includes the names of the previous 12 students, all crossed out in red ink. He also asks each student a number of questions:

1. What is the purpose of your visit to China?

2. How long will you be staying?

3. Where will you be staying?

4. He ends by telling students "Enjoy your visit."

The answers the students must give are:

1. Pleasure

2. Five Weeks

3. Shambhala Hotel

4. Thank You (not mandatory)

Mrs. Ling

Mrs. Ling is standing near the courtesy phone.
She says she overheard them call for a van and would like to ride with them to the hotel. The students can accept or deny her request. This can be the second part of the review of previous material since the students must introduce themselves, and learn about Mrs. Ling.

Map Seller

The students will be tasked with buying a map from the map seller. The map seller will sell a map of Beijing containing all the important sites to be visited: Airport, Hotel, Teahouse, Forbidden City, and Police Headquarters. She will say things like "Hello, how are you?," "What can I do for you?" or "Would you like to buy a map?," and "Thank you for your purchase."

Currency Exchanger

The students will be tasked with individually exchanging money at the currency exchange.

1. Greetings!

2. Would you like to exchange currency?

3. How much will you exchange?

4. Please count your money.

5. Thank you!

Note: The Currency Exchanger will also play public address announcements on the laptop computer at her kiosk (classroom podium).

Van Driver

The students will end Episode 4 by locating the Van Driver and leaving the airport.

1. Van Driver answers courtesy phone call with Shambhala hotel in Mandarin. "Shambhala hotel courtesy van." Students must ask for van to pick them up at airport. Van Driver tells them to wait for him beneath the ground transportation sign. He then says goodbye and hangs up.

2. When students arrive at the van, the Van Driver says in Mandarin "Welcome to Beijing! Shambhala hotel passengers? Follow me please."

Public Announcer

The public announcer will make a number of announcements in Mandarin that are typical of an airport, such as planes departing and arriving. The episode will end with the announcer asking the students to meet their hotel van at a certain location in the airport. The first five announcements repeat in the same order as necessary. The announcement of the van becomes part of the rotation once the phone call to the hotel has been made. It will repeat until the students identify the ground transportation sign and stand near it.

1. Announcing the arrival of Air China Flight 367 from Washington D.C. Passengers may be met after customs inspection.

2. Air China Flight 112 to Tokyo is now boarding at gate 18.

3. Due to heightened security do not leave luggage unattended.

4. Maps may be purchased from the new hologram vendor in the main terminal.

5. Currency may be exchanged at the desk in the main terminal.

6. Shambhala hotel van driver will meet passengers beneath the ground transportation sign.

Van Driver

The students will end Episode 4 by locating the Van Driver and leaving the airport. When students arrive at the correct door, the Van Driver appears and says in Mandarin, "Welcome to Beijing! Shambhala hotel passengers? Follow me please."

TEXT

Send to all students on November 7.

From Tang Laoshi

Dr. Chen cannot be found. I do not know what to think. But the reception at your hotel to welcome you to China will go on as scheduled.

From Tingting Lu

I am searching for a very rare and valuable book. You may be able to help me. I will see you soon.

From Mrs. Ling

I do speak English. I work at the Heritage Library. I have a special surprise for you. I will tell you what it is at the reception.

I had been concerned the students would not be able to finish all of the puzzles in a single class time. This would have required a rewrite of the story to explain students stuck at the airport for two class periods, bringing back our volunteer actors for an extra day IF they could do it and simplifying things so the story could end in one less week. The students not only finished all of the puzzles, they had time to spare. Instead of exiting the door with the Van Driver and then leaving class early, they began showing the WELCOME RENSSELAER STUDENTS sign they found on the floor to our NPCs. With the aid of an English/Chinese dictionary, they put together questions with words they had not learned, asking the characters if they had seen the man who dropped the sign.

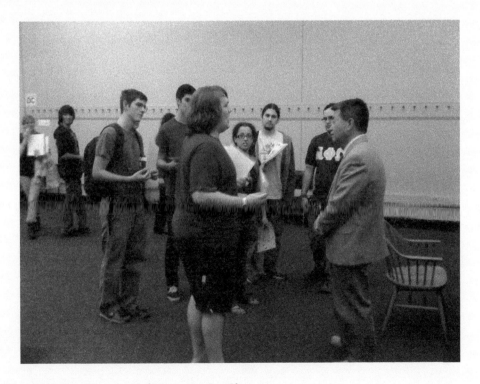

The students inquire about the missing Dr. Chen.

The actors didn't hesitate. In character they explained they did not speak English but would try to help the students. But no one could help. No one knows what happened to Dr. Chen.

This was one of my favorite moments in all of the games in this book. The students stayed later than they had to after finishing all the gameplay we had planned and tackled the mystery of the missing Dr. Chen. When the class was officially over, they had to be gently reminded it was time to leave. I think this moment, more than any other, made us all realize the potential of teaching a foreign language in this way. We are told the best way to learn a foreign language is being embedded in the country and its culture. Here were students willingly suspending their disbelief in an extremely sparse physical setting. They were learning as they played the game.

CHAPTER 18

Episode 5 – Reception

Thursday, November 10

CHARACTERS

Tang Laoshi, Mrs. Ling, Tingting Lu, Waitress

NARRATIVE

While not in class students will have received an email from Tingting Lu in English, repeating her offer to help.

The reception is in a room of the hotel. Students must use menus in Mandarin to ask for food and drink items from a waitress.

At the reception the students are met by Tang Laoshi. Dr. Chen's absence is very troubling. No one knows where he is. She's contacted authorities who are trying to track him down. Since she's here, she can review previous lessons. The last part of this will be her asking what they learned at the airport.

Tang Laoshi uses a game to teach table and dining etiquette.

Mrs. Ling arrives at the reception. Coincidentally (or not…) she turns out to be a Chinese literature professor who occasionally works with the Heritage Library. And surprisingly she speaks more English than she let on at the airport. She invites the students to be her guests at a teahouse next week. If the students gave Mrs. Ling a ride, she thanks them. If not, she says she hopes they didn't worry. She got to the hotel on her own.

Tingting Lu also shows up, but after greeting the students, and suggesting she has a favor to ask, she has a heated discussion with Mrs. Ling in Chinese and exits before she can ask her favor.

Lessons learned at the reception should conform to the lesson plan with the addition of some phrases useful to the narrative, but also fairly generic.

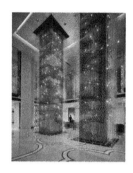

10 November 2011

二〇一一年十一月十日

(Èr líng yī yī nián shíyī yuè shí rì)

Shambhala Hotel

香巴拉饭店 (Xiāngbālā fàndiàn)

Welcomes Heritage Library and Rensselaer Students

欢迎遗产图书馆和 Rensselaer 学生团

(Huānyíng yíchǎn túshūguǎn hé Renesselaer xuéshēng tuán)

前菜 (qiáncài)

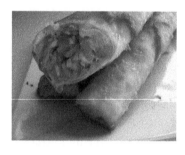

春卷 chūnjuǎn

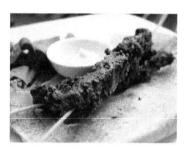

牛肉串 niúròu chuàn

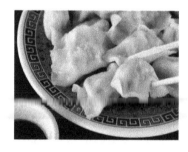

水饺 shǔijiǎo

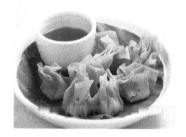

炸馄饨 zhá húntún

饮料 (yǐnliào)

可乐 (kělè)   雪碧 (xuěbì)   水 (shǔi)

The menu was limited, but the food was real.

ACTOR SCRIPTS

Waitress

Students will order food and drink from the waitress at the reception. The waitress will say things in Mandarin like: "Hello, welcome to the Shambhala Hotel." and "May I take your order?" or "Would you like something to eat or drink?" Exact dialogue dependent on caterer contribution.

Tang Laoshi

Tang Laoshi meets the students at the reception. She is very troubled by the absence of Dr. Chen. She tells the students that nobody knows where he is. She says she has contacted authorities who are trying to track him down. She then reviews previous lessons with the students and asks about what they learned at the airport. She also plays a game with the students, which teaches them table and dining etiquette. After this, she moves off and makes a phone call in Mandarin inquiring about Dr. Chen's absence. Mrs. Ling will approach her after she returns, and talk to her in Mandarin about Mrs. Ling's suspicions of Tingting.

Mrs. Ling

When Mrs. Ling arrives at the reception, she informs the students that she is a Chinese literature professor who occasionally works with the Heritage Library. She is speaking more English than she let on at the airport. She invites the students to be her guests at the Lao She Teahouse next week. If the students chose to give Mrs. Ling a ride from the airport to the hotel in Episode 4, she thanks them. If not, she says she hopes they didn't worry because she was able to get to the hotel on her own. She moves off to speak with Tang Laoshi in Mandarin about her suspicions about Tingting.

When Tingting Lu shows up, Mrs. Ling approaches her and tells her in Mandarin that her services are no longer required. Mrs. Ling says she will locate the book. Tingting replies in Mandarin that she will get the book herself and marches off.

Tingting Lu

When Tingting shows up at the reception, she greets the students and suggests that she has a favor to ask; Mrs. Ling interrupts. Mrs. Ling tells her in Mandarin that her services are no longer required. Mrs. Ling says she will locate the book. Tingting replies in Mandarin that she will get the book herself and marches off.

TEXTS

Send to all students on Monday, November 14.

From Tang Laoshi

Dr. Chen sent me a message. I must meet him at the Great Wall. But the rest makes no sense. I think it is in code! I'll bring it when I see you next week.

From Tingting Lu

Something is not right. I should be the only one negotiating for the book, but there are others!

From Mrs. Ling

I look forward to seeing you at the teahouse on Thursday!

CHAPTER 19

Episode 6 – The Teahouse

Thursday, November 17

CHARACTERS

Mrs. Ling, Tingting Lu, Inspector Pei (disguised as a waiter)

NARRATIVE

While not in class all students received a text from Tang Laoshi. Dr. Chen has contacted her but was very secretive. He has emailed her a message in Chinese, but it makes no sense to her. She thinks it is in code! She must go to the Great Wall to meet Dr. Chen, but she will bring the code to the hotel next week.

At the teahouse the students are the guests of Mrs. Ling. She teaches them the Chinese Way of Tea, a traditional tea ceremony with an authentic tea service, first by demonstrating, then watching as they try it.

A waiter (Inspector Pei) is stationed nearby. The students may or may not recognize him as the customs agent, but he pretends not to understand if they question him about it.

Mrs. Ling leaves for a few minutes to telephone Tang Laoshi. Tingting Lu appears. She claims it's an accident she ran into them here. She asks if Mrs. Ling has mentioned why she is in China? When Tingting learns she hasn't, she suggests they ask Mrs. Ling, and warns them not to trust her. There is something very valuable at stake, something Tingting will pay the students very handsomely to obtain. She sees Mrs. Ling, and exits, followed by Pei.

When asked (or if not asked, she volunteers the information) why she is in China, Mrs. Ling tells the students an incredibly rare first edition of *Outlaws of the Marsh* is rumored to have been found.

ACTOR SCRIPTS

Mrs. Ling (1st Conversation)

Mrs. Ling teaches the students the Chinese Way of Tea, a traditional tea ceremony, first by demonstrating, then watching as they each try it in turn. She also tells them about her

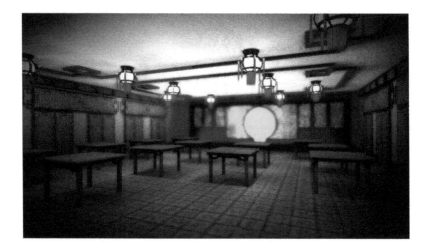

A non-interactive backdrop for the first iteration of the teahouse.

passion for reading and literature and about several famous books of Chinese literature, including *The Outlaws of the Marsh*.

> This is a good place to point out collateral learning in *The Lost Manuscript*. Chinese culture such as this tea ceremony, Chinese history and literature, historical landmarks like the Forbidden City and the Summer Palace, even two-sided business cards, all are examples of students learning more than simply a class is expected to teach. Here, as usual, they are woven into the narrative and gameplay at the heart of the multiplayer classroom.

Mrs. Ling asks the students if they have heard from Tang Laoshi. They may choose to tell her or not about the text. If they tell her, she makes some suggestions on what Mandarin the students might study online to help break the code. She then says she must call Tang Laoshi and leaves for a moment.

Tingting Lu

Tingting appears just after Mrs. Ling leaves to call Tang Laoshi. She claims it is a coincidence that she ran into them at the teahouse. She then asks if Mrs. Ling has mentioned to the students why she is in China. When Tingting learns that Mrs. Ling hasn't mentioned her reason, she suggests the students ask Mrs. Ling and warns them not to trust her. She says there is something very valuable at stake, something she will pay the students very handsomely to obtain. It is one of the books Mrs. Ling mentioned, *The Outlaws of the Marsh* manuscript. Tingting offers to pay them handsomely, if they manage to obtain it.

Mrs. Ling (2nd Conversation)

When Mrs. Ling returns, she finds Tingting talking to the students. She confronts Tingting, and they argue in Mandarin about who should be the library representative to secure the book. She notices the waiter (Inspector Pei) taking notes. Tingting exits, followed by Inspector Pei.

When asked (or if not asked, she volunteers the information) why she is in China, Mrs. Ling tells the students that she has some exciting news: a rare first edition of the famous Chinese novel *Outlaws of the Marsh* is rumored to have been found. The owner is unknown, but an auction is rumored. She claims she has returned to China in order to bid on the book for the Heritage Library. She directs the students to more information about the book on the Heritage Library website.

Mrs. Ling tells the students Tang Laoshi wants the students to next week help her break the code sent to her by Dr. Chen. Mrs. Ling thanks them all for joining her at the teahouse and hopes they enjoyed the tea ceremony.

Inspector Pei

If the students recognize him from the airport in Episode 4, he pretends not to understand if they question him about it.

They did recognize him and were quite suspicious.

TEXTS AND EMAILS

Send on Monday, November 28.

From Tang Laoshi (TEXT to 1st TEAM ONLY)

I went to the Great Wall, but Dr. Chen didn't meet me! I will show you the code he sent me last week when I see you next!

From Mrs. Ling (TEXT to 2nd TEAM ONLY)

I am trying to learn more about who has the book and if it is authentic. I will be in touch. Work on that code!

From Tingting Lu (TEXT to 3rd TEAM ONLY)

I think I am close to finding Outlaws of the Marsh, but Mrs. Ling and Tang Laoshi plan to cheat the library and sell the book. Don't trust them!

From Inspector Pei (EMAIL to 4th TEAM ONLY)

IF students recognized him at the teahouse: Yes, I was the customs inspector and your waiter at the teahouse. I am Inspector Pei, Beijing Police. I ask for your assistance in locating Dr. Chen. If you have any information, please text me.

IF students did not recognize him at the teahouse: I was the customs inspector and your waiter at the teahouse. I'm surprised you didn't notice. I am Inspector Pei, Beijing Police. I ask for your assistance in locating Dr. Chen. If you have any information, please text me.

It was time to heighten player agency, the belief that what a player does materially affects the story of a game. We kept it simple. The previous week texts were sent to everyone. Here we divide loyalties when Tang Laoshi, Tingting Lu, Mrs. Ling text, and Inspector Pei emails only to separate study groups. There are several possibilities:

- Students may not know they received different texts and emails.

- Students realize they have differing messages and decide to withhold information.

- All groups may decide to share information.

- There may be a mix of groups. Some decide to share. Others don't.

- Some students may answer the messages while others don't.

In any of the above cases, it does not matter what study groups or individual students choose to do. The final beats of the game play out the same way, pulling students back to the same narrative through line.

Collateral Learning for readers: Russian Konstantin Stanislavski, to this day known as a seminal acting instructor, coined the term "through line" to help actors track their characters' actions.

What separating the study groups does is give students the illusion they are affecting the plot. Whenever players are given even a hint of agency, the more involved they become in the experience.

CHAPTER 20

Episode 7 – Codebreaking

Thursday, December 1

CHARACTERS

Tang Laoshi, Inspector Pei

NARRATIVE

This takes place in the same room in the hotel as the reception. While not in class, one team of students will have received texts from Tang Laoshi, as she tries to meet with Dr. Chen at the Great Wall, but he fails to show up. Another team will have received tweets from Mrs. Ling, as she tries to learn more about who has the book, its authenticity, and where the auction will take place. A third team receives emails from Miss Lu. She thinks the Heritage Library is close to finding *Outlaws of the Marsh*, but she says that Mrs. Ling and Tang Laoshi both plan to cheat the library and sell the book to an unnamed private collector. Students should not trust either woman! The fourth team receives an inquiry from an Inspector Pei of the Beijing police, asking them for their cooperation in locating Dr. Chen.

Students may choose to share information about the various communications or keep it to themselves.

At the hotel, Tang Laoshi turns code breaking into a lesson. First reviewing what they've learned, then attacking the onscreen code using the Kinect. Students take turns with the Kinect to learn how to use it.

The code is actually directions to the Wenyuan Library in the Forbidden City and a specific meeting time: 5:00 pm on December 8. Tang Laoshi is confused. The meeting at the Great Wall must have been a ruse, possibly to trick someone who was listening in. Dr. Chen must be in danger! They must tell no one about what the code said!

Beijing Police Inspector Pei arrives at the hotel. His motives should be immediately suspicious because a) he's the "customs official" and b) he was the waiter at the tea house. If confronted, he'll explain he had asked to be their customs official and the waiter to learn more about the students and the other people associated with the Heritage Library.

Pei is investigating Dr. Chen's disappearance. Chen disappeared right before he was to meet the students. Pei wanted to see if they were somehow involved. He asks if the students know anything about it. They may or may not tell him they've decoded the message.

If they tell him what the message says, he advises them not to go to the rendezvous. The Wenyuan Library is not open to researchers without official permission to be there. He tells Tang Laoshi he will expect her at his office to answer questions. The time? Right when the appointment at the Forbidden City is to take place. Pei exits, Tang Laoshi reluctantly agrees that the students must go to meet Dr. Chen instead of her!

CODEBREAKING PUZZLE

The students already had been given most of the vocabulary to solve the puzzle. Tang Laoshi used the various words in the message to review previous language lessons like numbers, the date, and time and also introduce some new words.

To solve the puzzle, students take turns selecting and manipulating the Chinese words with the Kinect until they line up in the correct translation.

Correct Answers

Dr. Chen	陈 博士	(Chén bóshi)
Forbidden City	紫禁城	(zǐjìnchéng)
Wenyuan Chamber	文渊阁	(wényuān gé)
December 8	十二月八日	
5 o'clock	下午 五 点	

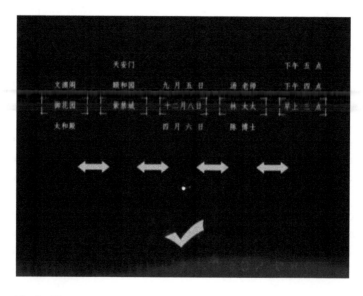

Codebreaking with the Kinect.

Incorrect Alternates

1.

| 汤 老师 | Tāng lǎoshī = Teacher Tang |
| 林 太太 | Líng tàitài = Mrs. Ling |

2, 3.

天安门	tiān ān mén = Tiananmen Square
长城	cháng chéng = Great Wall
颐和园	yíhé yuán = Summer palace
紫禁城	zǐjìnchéng = Forbidden City
太和殿	tàihé diàn = Hall of Supreme Harmony
御花园	yù huāyuán = The Imperial Garden

4. Time

(AM/PM) (number)(o'clock)

AM = 早上

PM = 下午Incorrect Alternates

o'clock = 点

5. Numbers

1: 一

2: 二

3: 三

4: 四

5: 五

6: 六

7: 七

8: 八

9: 九

10: 十

11: 十一

12: 十二

Example: 8 am = 早上八点

6. *Date*

(number) month (number) day

month = 月 <- moon

day = 日 <- sun

example:

April 26

4th month 2 × 10 + 6 day

四 月 二 十 六 日

ACTOR SCRIPTS

Tang Laoshi

At the hotel, Tang Laoshi turns code breaking into a lesson. First reviewing what they've learned and then attacking the code using the Kinect. After cracking the code, Tang Laoshi expresses confusion. She explains that the meeting at the Great Wall must have been a ruse, if someone was listening in. Dr. Chen must be in danger! She tells the students they must tell no one about what the code said! After Inspector Pei interrupts, she reluctantly agrees the students must go to the meeting at the Forbidden City in her place.

Inspector Pei

Detective Pei arrives at the hotel as himself. If the students recognize him from the previous episodes and confront him about it, he will come clean and explain that he asked to be their customs official and waiter in order to learn more about them and the other people associated with the Heritage Library. He goes on to explain that he is investigating the disappearance of Dr. Chen. He tells the students that Dr. Chen disappeared right before he was to meet the students. Pei wanted to see if the students were involved somehow. He then asks if the students know anything about it. The students can decide whether or not to tell him they decoded the message. If they do tell him, he advises them not to go to the rendezvous. Before exiting he tells Tang Laoshi he will expect her at his office for questioning. It is the same time the appointment at the Forbidden City is to take place.

TEXTS

Send on Monday, December 5.

From Tang Laoshi (TEXT to 1st TEAM ONLY)

The book cannot fall into the hands of either Tingting Lu or Mrs. Ling. Do not trust them, or the students who seem to be helping them!

From Tingting Lu (TEXT to 3rd TEAM ONLY)

I am the only authorized buyer for the library. Other students are now working with Tang Laoshi and Mrs. Ling. Trust no one!

From Mrs. Ling (TEXT to 2nd TEAM ONLY)

You must not trust Tingting Lu or Tang Laoshi. Other students are in contact with them. Do not trust them either!"

From Inspector Pei (TEXT to 4th TEAM ONLY)

I now know Dr. Chen vanished while trying to find a rare book. He may have been kidnapped. Trust no one, not even your fellow students.

The previous week's texts were sent from Tang Laoshi, Tingting Lu, Mrs. Ling, and the email from Inspector Pei to separate study groups. Those texts, even if they were not discussed openly by the students, signaled to them that some NPCs possibly should not be trusted. To up the stakes, the above texts added the possibility that fellow students should not be taken at face value either. Did we reach an intensity of suspense such as when the shark attacks in *Jaws* could come at any time? No. But the conflicting NPC opinions caused another level of alertness in the players. That made them receptive to both the narrative *and* the teaching.

CHAPTER 21

Episode 8 – The Forbidden City

Thursday, December 8

CHARACTERS

Dr. Chen, Inspector Pei

NARRATIVE

The students arrive at the Wenyuan Library, the location indicated on the map on the Heritage Library website. There they find Dr. Chen. He explains a member of the royal family was a collector of books and manuscripts. It is rumored a manuscript in the collection was the first edition of *Outlaws of the Marsh*. If it was a part of the collection, it was never found. He's always thought a clue to its whereabouts might be found in this room where that member of the royal family spent much of his time. Dr. Chen must meet with someone from the Heritage Library, someone who may actually know the present location of the book! He exits.

In a VR version of a Hidden Objects game the students will search the room via the Kinect, opening virtual cabinets, chests, display cases etc.

Some pieces of furniture are empty. In four others, the students find four photographs that tell a story. They could be removed and tacked up on the virtual wall.

The first is a wide shot of a building on a hillside at the Summer Palace. The second is a picture of the Revolving Archives building on that hill. The third is a picture of a room nearby. The fourth is a closeup of an ornate desk in the room. The location of the manuscript?

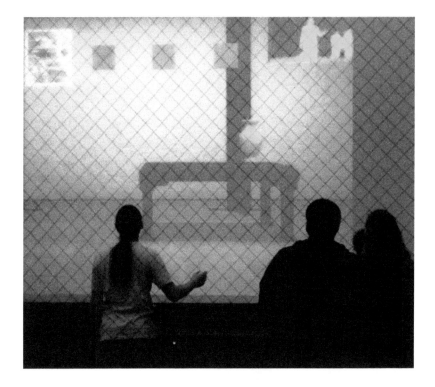

Searching the library.

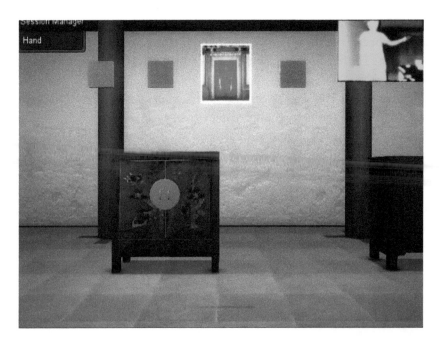

Placing a picture.

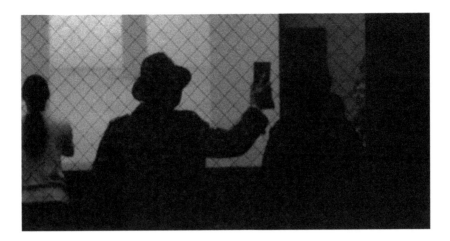

Inspector Pei flashes his badge.

The students are interrupted by Detective Pei.

Two of the Wenyuan Library photographs were taken through what looks like chicken wire. They were taken through a window in one of the closed hallway doors so as to not interrupt the gameplay. We learned that being unobtrusive while documenting a class inside a classroom was not easy.

Pei confiscates the students' travel documents and the photographs they found. They are all to be questioned at police headquarters on December 19!

ACTOR SCRIPTS

Dr. Chen

Dr. Chen is found in The Wenyuan Library. In a conversation with the students, he will explain that a former member of the royal family was a collector of books and manuscripts. He goes on to say that the first edition of *Outlaws of the Marsh* was rumored to be a part of the collection here; however, it has not been located. Dr. Chen tells the students that he believes a clue to the whereabouts of the book is in this room. Before leaving he says he must meet with someone from the Heritage Library who may know the present location of the book. He then exits.

Inspector Pei

After the students locate a clue that the manuscript may be located at the summer palace, Inspector Pei appears and confiscates their travel documents. He tells them they will be taken to police headquarters on December 19 for questioning.

TEXTS

Send to all students on Monday, December 12.

From Inspector Pei

I will expect you in my office on December 19 to answer questions. You are all under suspicion. Do not attempt to leave China.

CHAPTER 22

Episode 9 – Police Headquarters

Thursday, December 19

CHARACTERS

Inspector Pei, Tang Laoshi

NARRATIVE

In a plain room with only a table and three chairs, students are individually interrogated by Inspector Pei. Tang Laoshi is present to see that the students are treated fairly.

This interrogation is the students' final exam. Final interrogation questions:

The following message ended the original design document.

Adjustments of the story will be made as we proceed based on:

1. Maintaining a natural and meaningful progression of lessons.

2. Allowing for student progress.

3. The decision if these same students will proceed to the next semester or not, or if we'll start with new students and repeat material in these first eight lessons, then build on those.

As I mentioned in the Introduction, ShihChia Chen Thompson informed the rest of the team that the class learned more in eight weeks than a full fourteen-week semester of Mandarin. As of this writing, RPI now offers a minor in Chinese. It remains the only foreign language taught.

One final note: This ended the students' eventful visit to the People's Republic of China. I know you were concerned, so I am happy to report that they acquitted themselves well and none of them ended up in jail.

The Final Interrogation

1. 你好！你会说中文吗？**Hello! Can you speak Chinese?**

2. 我要问你几个问题，你觉得怎么样？**I'm going to ask you some questions. How do you feel?**

3. 你贵姓？你叫什么名字？**What's your last name & first name?**

4. 你是哪国人？你从哪儿来的？**What is your nationality? Where are you from (which state)?**

5. 你几岁？你的生日是几年几月几号？**How old are you? When is your birthday?**

6. 你在哪儿上大学？**Where do you go to college?**

7. 你的手机号码是多少？**What's your cellphone number?**

8. 你的电子邮箱是什么？**What's your e-mail address?**

9. 你什么时候来中国的？**When did you come to China?**

10. 你来中国做什么？**What are you doing in China?**

11. 你来中国住在哪里？**Where do you stay in China?**

12. 你喜欢吃什么中国菜？你不喜欢吃什么中国菜？**What kind of Chinese food do you like and dislike?**

13. 我要找陈博士，你知道陈博士吗？**I'm looking for Dr. Chen.**

Do you know Dr. Chen?

14. 你知道陈博士和汤老师在找什么吗？**Do you know what Dr.**

Chen and Teacher Tang are looking for?

15. 这本书在哪儿？**Where is this book?**

16. 这是陈博士给汤老师的留言，请你排一排！**This is the**

message from Dr. Chen to Teacher Tang. Please rearrange it!

17. 这是紫禁城的地图，怎么从天安门走到文渊阁？**This is the**

map of the Forbidden City. How do I get to the Wenyuan

chamber from Tiananmen square?

18. 谢谢你的帮忙！再见！**Thank you for your help! Goodbye!**

CHAPTER 23

Afterword

BUILDING UPON THE SUCCESS of this first iteration of *The Mandarin Project*, we were able to construct what I called the Emergent Reality Lab. A space was found in RPI's Rensselaer Technology Park. The VR lab was envisioned to be a physical environment surrounded by screens featuring 3D virtual reality imagery. Participants would not need to wear VR gear, but cheap plastic glasses like those handed out at movie theaters instead. In the beginning, three screens were set up with rear projection and motion capture equipment and software installed. Due to the limitations of the system we settled on, participants needed wands to interact with the projected environment.

Our first major demo featured the teahouse from *The Lost Manuscript* and Mrs. Ling, now a virtual character, demonstrated a traditional Chinese tea ceremony, interacting with students seated at real tables as guests of the teahouse. At the end of the ceremony, the virtual Mrs. Ling exited through a door in the teahouse and her human counterpart entered the real space to serve the startled students real tea. This "emergent" behavior mixing VR with the real world was the primary goal.

Following the success of that demonstration, a full-length design document was written by my students and me with additional episodes set at the Summer Palace. Unfortunately, this full experience was never realized. In 2015, thanks to a collaboration between students of both RPI and WPI where I was now teaching, as well as the assistance of the two professors brought in to RPI to teach Chinese, that a narrative-complete version of the game was produced. It was an interactive novel in Ren'Py where players could toggle between English and Chinese dialogue. This final proof of concept was as far as I took the idea. However, in collaboration with IBM, a version of *The Mandarin Project* continues to this day at RPI in the Cognitive and Immersive Systems Lab (CISL), now on campus in the Experimental Media and Performing Arts Center (EMPAC). Several of our original team are involved.

SECTION 3

Secrets: An Internet Mystery

CHAPTER 24

Introduction to Section 3

IN LATE 2018 I knew it was time for a second edition of *The Multiplayer Classroom: Designing Coursework as a Game.* But I also knew that there were classes that I did not teach, and where I worked with educators on *their* projects. So, I also proposed writing a new book detailing the designs of four of my major collaborations with other subject matter experts. This book would be a more detailed look at the pre-production, production, and execution of these four classes designed as games.

While preparing the second edition manuscript for publication late in 2019, I began preliminary work on this book you are now reading. The second edition of *The Multiplayer Classroom* was published in March 2020 as the pandemic exploded upon the world. As I was writing, and reading about all the new, intense issues education was facing, it occurred to me that there might be one way to overcome some of the major difficulties in teaching during the pandemic.

In December 2017, after all of the games in this book had been launched, I wrote a short article with Professor David Seelow for the International Journal on Innovations in Online Education. It was called *The Multiplayer Classroom: The Designer and the Collaboration.* The article outlined some of the major considerations when developing multiplayer classrooms in general and applying those techniques to online education. You can find it here: http://onlineinnovationsjournal.com/streams/course-design-and-development/2589574144889286.html.

Only one of the four classes in this book was an online class. But it became increasingly clear that a single article in 2017 was not enough. It was easy to say, "Do this!" It was even more important to give a detailed account of *how* it is done. Indeed, that is what this book you are reading was intended to do. These game plans complete the picture begun in the first book. And the section on *Secrets: An Internet Mystery* can serve as a far more detailed example of how to bring them to life. It is my hope that this marriage of outline and full design document might inspire other educators, to make somewhat easier the job of keeping students of all ages engaged and might be a little bit easier. And who knows? An added benefit might be to turn some of the torture of remote teaching into something that might actually resemble fun.

CENTER FOR GAME AND SIMULATION-BASED LEARNING
AT EXCELSIOR COLLEGE

Home   About   Revolutionary Learning Blog   Podcasts   Programs & Courses   Presentations

HUM 325: Secrets: A Cyberculture Mystery Game

You want to have fun and learn at the same time?

Take this course.

Few forces in modern history have had such a wide-ranging effect on our contemporary identities as the global expansion of cyberculture. The Oxford dictionary defines it as, "The social conditions brought about by the widespread use of computer networks for communication, entertainment, and business." This course provides you with an authentic learning experience and is unlike any other course you are likely to have encountered.

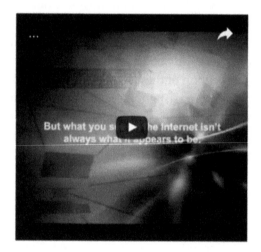

- Go on multiple quests.
- Accumulate experience points.
- Engage in lively Internet forums.
- Work together to solve the Internet mystery at the heart of the course.

Throughout your game play you will:

- Explore essential questions about how and why the Internet has changed and continues to change your sense of identity.
- Create your own evolving digital story as you employ, evaluate, and reflect on cyber-based phenomena such as social media, online games, Internet relationships, and engaging virtual realities represented by *The Matrix* and *Neuromancer.*

Complete the course and you are a winner.

Class listing in the Excelsior online catalogue.

The first two game plans in this book tackled rather straightforward subjects. The last two venture into much more complicated territory. Both of these feature detailed formal design documents, each written over a period of months. To the best of our knowledge *Secrets: An Internet Mystery* was the first ARG designed for an entirely online class. With the *Skeleton Chases,* any narrative requiring physical activity could have been devised.

The Lost Manuscript, since it was teaching a foreign language, was the most restrained of the four. Even though it was a dress rehearsal for a much larger VR experience, it was by necessity ARG light. It was hoped that the VR version might feature a more sophisticated narrative. With *Secrets*, the class and the ARG were fully integrated in a way the first two games were not. And the fact that it was entirely online gave us unprecedented control over the experience.

As I stated in the Preface, this class most closely connects to games and game design. For that reason, while I have reduced some detail of the subject matter more than I wanted to, you should be able to see the amazing breadth of the material covered by Professor Seelow. Its importance today is even greater in a time where the promise of the Internet has become corrupted and captive to the chaos that confronts us day to day, demolishing truth, trust, and science in ways that only a few years ago would have seemed unimaginable.

I do not come from the future. I cannot claim to be a psychic like Quinn Morgan. But in assembling and rereading this multiplayer classroom I can't help but be struck by how what appeared in 2015 to be a fantastic corruption of the Internet has become in so many ways a harsh reality. I can only hope that one day this will all be just a pothole on the road to a better tomorrow.

This online class may appear to be the very definition of ordinary sage in front of a green screen teaching. That was intentional for three reasons: 1) we wanted to create an experience with which online students were already comfortable; 2) it would very quickly become clear to students that there was much more going on, and 3) the experimental nature of the class would not seem too far out to administration officials. Happily, while there was some skepticism at first, that third consideration did not cause an issue, as Professor Seelow will explain in his Foreword.

To learn more of the underlying research goals and results, please follow this link: http://onlineinnovationsjournal.com/articles/1fc7568c28def15e.html.

As an added bonus, here is a link to the game's trailer: https://www.excelsior.edu/article/solve-mysteries-have-fun-earn-3-credits/.

CHAPTER 25

Foreword to Section 3

David Seelow

I<small>N THE SUMMER OF</small> 2013, my former dean Dr. Scott Dalrymple (now President of Columbia College in Columbia, Missouri) bequeathed me with the opportunity and challenge to design an outside-the-box online course for Excelsior College's (a not for profit online college) School of Liberal Arts. The college had made extra money available for the development of two "showcase" courses. One course went to the School of Nursing and one to Liberal Arts. I had also been awarded a $5,000 innovation grant from the college. The school decided the course would be on cyberculture and that I would be responsible for making this a featured course. Why me? I had earned a reputation for innovation and the leadership team felt I could cultivate an exciting new course. Exciting news! In general, online colleges work at scale, and courses are developed in a very standardized fashion adhering to a strict timeline. Unlike a traditional college course where the professor develops and teaches the course with full autonomy, online courses usually have instructional designers, technologists, program directors (i.e. department chairs), and subject matters experts working together on building a "master" course shell that will be taught by many different adjunct faculty who had nothing to do with the course content or design. I now had the opportunity to do something different and I wanted something totally nonstandard.

In May the college's Board of Trustees, under the late President John F. Ebersole, approved the creation of a new Center for Game and Simulation-Based Learning housed in the School of Liberal Arts. I thought, why not make this new course a game-based course and apply the principles of Lee Sheldon's *The Multiplayer Classroom* to an online environment? I knew Lee from nearby Rensselaer Polytechnic Institute (RPI) in Troy where he served as the chair of the Simulation Arts and Sciences program and I taught one or two literature courses each semester. I would ask Lee to serve as a consultant and help make sure our novice effort stayed true to his ideas.

The college also made the services of Focus EduVation, a large third party e-Learning company available to develop the course, but I did not want a third party in the central role, so I assumed the role of Subject Matter Expert (SME) and course manager and opted to work with our Director of Instructional Design, Dr. John Prusch, and a game designer who we would hire with the money usually paid for the SME, and use Lee as a consultant. Focus EduVation would play a secondary, mostly technical role, but not be involved in design. I hired a young graduate of the highly regarded Savannah College of Art and Design, and we were ready to start the creative process.

Our very first planning meeting—the "kickoff meeting"—in early July brought about a total reversal of my initial plans. As we listened to the game designer articulate her vision for the course narrative and I noted Lee's frequent suggestions about aligning the story with course outcomes and content it became evident I had arrived at the first tee with a two iron, but I clearly needed a driver. After the meeting, John and I met, and we acknowledged that for this high profile course to be the best possible offering we needed Lee to be in charge. In late August I asked Lee if he was willing to design the game and he agreed. The original game designer was asked to stay on in a supporting role, but she declined. Regardless, the right decision was made. You need experienced game designers when developing a new project.

The development went smoothly. Lee wrote the design document with the story and characters outlined in detail. I would write the outcomes, and content for each module—now called episodes—one by one. Then Lee integrated the game narrative with the content in a seamless fashion. The story about an internet company Chromogen and their ultimately sinister propagation of "primal empathy" matched the course theme perfectly. At the end of the writing process, I met with Dr. Prusch and we made sure the narrative, outcomes, content, and assessments were in alignment.

The penultimate stage of development proved a true highlight. Focus EduVation would tape and later edit the story and my lectures in a hotel just outside Boston. I would play the "hero" Professor Grey. A Focus EduVation manager would play a peripheral character, an actress from Boston would play The Collective's spokesperson Audra Casey and a former chair of the college's Board of Trustees, Dr. Joshua L. Smith would play the opposition leader, Dale Kenyon, from Fortress 9. Having Dr. Smith, a prominent national leader in urban education when he was at NYU's School of Education, volunteer to travel to Boston and enthusiastically play the freedom fighter Dale remains one of my most enjoyable moments in education.

Focus EduVation concluded the development process through postproduction editing, adding backgrounds, graphics etc., and then loading the edited videos into the Blackboard Learning Management System. Two college employees agreed to serve as the story's Non-Playing Characters (NPCs), and I had the honor and challenge of teaching the course in the guise of Professor Logan Grey. Launching such a high profile course had significant risks. Many employees at the college feared offering a game-based course to nontraditional adult students. Why would students in their thirties, forties, and fifties focused on quickly earning college credits or they worked or served in the military want such a playful, outside the box experience? I had no such fear. After all, the average gamer is in his or her mid thirties and military personnel are often avid gamers. The college's president at the time, the late John F. Ebersole was a Vietnam Veteran and one of the trustees was a retired Brigadier General. My faith in the potential of game-based learning for online courses, Lee's expert design, support from then Dean Dalrymple and former President Ebersole, along with the capable supporting cast resulted in extraordinarily positive reviews by adult students. An excerpt from one student's response to the course stands in for the many others I received, "I am saddened that this course will be over in about three weeks. This has been one of the most unique educational experiences that I have ever encountered in my life."

In fact, Professor Grey turned out to be a better online teacher than David Seelow, but that's a testament to the power of game-based learning!

CHAPTER 26

Design Document

THIS DESIGN DOCUMENT IS built from the Concept Document. It details the narrative, learning, and structure of the class. This is a living document. It is not cast in stone. As production proceeds, it should be updated to reflect the current state of the game.

Dialogue scripts for non-lecture video, other messages from NPCs, components of fictional websites, documents, and puzzle specifics through which the students will experience the game are described in this Design Document.

Additionally, once this document is complete, a second *generic* Design Document template, or possibly a pair of fraternal twins, could be created for two purposes:

1. So that other Excelsior online classes can be designed using the structures and mechanics included here.

2. So that other institutions can create their own online classes on the culture of the Internet or any other topic they choose.

These are not included as part of this initial project.

There was a change in Excelsior's administration a couple of years after *Secrets* was launched. And despite the success of this class, no others were attempted. By now, six years later, we could have developed online classes in a variety of fields, classes which were not just a video version of the sage on the stage, but online multiplayer classrooms with compelling narratives and challenging gameplay. An opportunity not lost, but hopefully just postponed.

EXECUTIVE SUMMARY

Excelsior's new online class on Internet identity has a secret. It is ostensibly to teach students to become responsible and knowledgeable citizens of the Internet. In fact, it has been created to solve a mystery that apparently transcends time and space. At first, only the class instructor, Professor Grey, knows this.

Fortress 9 is a social/political movement from only seventy years in Earth's future, a future shaped by experiments in psychic enhancements that, instead of creating a superior human race, have resulted in a severe loss of cultural and personal identity. The ruling powers in their time do not see the harm in the enhancements so two factions have emerged: Fortress 9 and the majority that embraces the enhancements: The Collective. Fortress 9 wants to break the Collective's power. They cannot reverse the enhancements, so they have communicated with the past, our time, in the hope of preventing their implementation. Because of its experience with the Internet and online education, they have contacted Excelsior College as a likely place to start.

The leader of Fortress 9 is Dale Kenyon, and he will become a main contact for the class, accessible through videos, text messages, and emails sent back to our time. However, the Collective has learned of the Fortress 9 plan to thwart them, and their representative, Audra Casey, sends reports of how well the experiments are working to create a single society without the cultural differences that have led to so much hatred and war. Logan remains neutral, skeptical of the claims from each faction, sensing there are other secrets still to be uncovered.

He is right. Fortress 9 and The Collective share another secret that Logan does not know. They are not from the future. They are from the present and are both controlled by a rogue corporation that is financing the psychic enhancements. Fortress 9 was created to fail so The Collective's side of the debate would be even stronger. The corporation, Chromogen, has in fact begun unsanctioned experiments on the Internet to test their effectiveness. The danger is real, and it is happening now.

Tom Wetherall is a student in the class, but he has a secret. He has been planted by the corporation to experiment on the Excelsior class.

Ann Bennett is a student in the class. She has a secret. She is a cyber cop, one of a new breed of policemen and women who fight Internet crime. She has joined the class to stop the experiment, to learn the identity of the corporation hiding behind the cover name The Collective, and to shut down its operations.

So, the class will become a discreet battleground between forces out to create a dysfunctional future for financial gain, and those allied against them.

Through the eight weeks of the class, students will learn all the major facets and challenges of what it means to be online in today's world. The narrative will closely map to lessons learned.

As I designed multiplayer classrooms in the eight years covered in this book, you will see that I was able to connect the narrative and gameplay far more closely to the subject matter with each succeeding project. Remember I was also designing many of the classes I taught as multiplayer classrooms. This gave me plenty of time to hone what worked and to experiment on ways to make each class better.

In the end it will be the knowledge students have gained that will lead them to uncover the truth behind all of the secrets, and to help prevent a future that is all too possible in today's wired world.

TYPE AND GENRE

Secrets: An Internet Mystery is an online transmedia Alternate Reality Game (ARG) designed for the Culture of the Internet class developed at Excelsior College. It is suggested the reader look up ARGs such as *i love bees*, *Year Zero*, and *Evoke*.

The genre of *Secrets* is a hybrid of mystery and science fiction, allowing for a maximum of exploration and discovery by the players.

THEME

The theme of *Secrets*, and the class, is that in order to become responsible and knowledge-able citizens of the Internet, we must understand how it works, how our behavior is perceived by others, and the implications for us as individuals and as a society.

SETTING

The game takes place entirely within the environment of a normal online Excelsior class and on the Internet and includes communications through email, text messaging, and popular social media.

GAME INTERFACES

Game Websites

> Real websites on the Internet were included in this document as references for both the visual styles of the fictional websites built for the game and so I could mimic their writing styles.

Game interfaces include fictional websites created for the game as well as real sites containing information of use to players, and tools for both students and the instructor. These are the fictional websites.

The Collective (www.thecollectiveworld.org)

A website with a homogenous and somewhat restful, even bland design, but with graphics that suggest the future. It includes forums for students to interact with The Collective officially and private messaging for the students to contact the characters. The site features videos, photographs and screen grabs by students, and messages from the NPCs.

Fortress 9 (www.fortress9.org)

A website with a deliberately grunge non-establishment feel. It includes forums for students to interact with Fortress 9 officially and private messaging for the students to contact the characters. The site features videos, photographs and screen grabs by students, and messages from the NPCs.

CareHart Foundation (www.carehartfoundation.org)

Informational site only with touchy-feely graphics design and annoying looped New Age music that is on by default but can be toggled off. The site is running a contest. Students are encouraged to identify world problems and submit ideas for solving them. **NOTE: This action will later be revealed as simply a way to collect information on the students**.

Edmund Conner Hart Obituary

Structured like a Wikipedia article, it tells of how Hart rose from a childhood of abuse and rejection to become a billionaire entrepreneur and his dream of creating the foundation that became CareHart.

Chromogen (www.chromogen.org)

Informational site only. Very corporate, stark, and modern. Students may apply for jobs and send resumés. **NOTE: This action will later be revealed as again simply a way to collect information on them**.

Badge Lands (www.badgelands.org)

"Law Enforcement News for the Rest of Us." This is a law enforcement fan site not affiliated with any official law enforcement organization. Visitors can get the latest news and commentary on crime and justice; follow missing person cases, the hunt for serial killers, access breaking crime news and reports on newsworthy trials. It will contain an RSS newsfeed.

Remember the RSS feed attached to the Celebrity Sheet Online website in *Skeleton Chase 2*? Here's another. They are not as popular as they once were, but there are still countless feeds out there that may save you some time and effort. Here is Badge Lands.

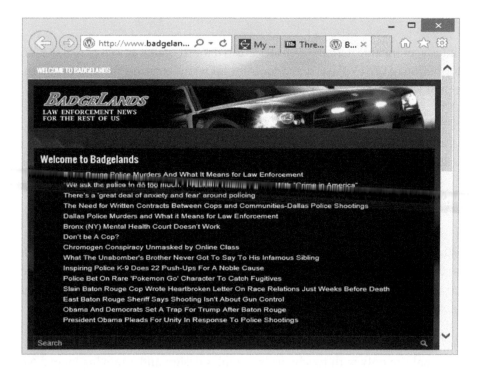

Badge Lands website created for the game.

Real websites will also be used, tying together both the narrative and learning. These are detailed in the Investigations and Additional Resources sections in each episode.

Class Website

Class Homepage

The portal through which students access all class elements; create their avatars; and communicate with each other, the instructor, and teaching assistants. The homepage for the class mirrors a standard Excelsior class homepage such as the one shown here.

All standard instructor tools are available. All typical links, e.g. assignments, grades, etc., are available. There are, however, changes to other pages and several additional pages, as follows.

Course Information

The Instructor Information should closely map to the real instructor with only the name Logan Grey replacing his or her own.

In addition to the expected tabs for Instructor Information and Introductions for students, there is a link to an index page with icons (student images) that link to personal pages.

Personal Page

Each Personal Page is the location where students can upload a short biography and a picture of themselves to represent them in class forums, live discussions, etc. and contact information.

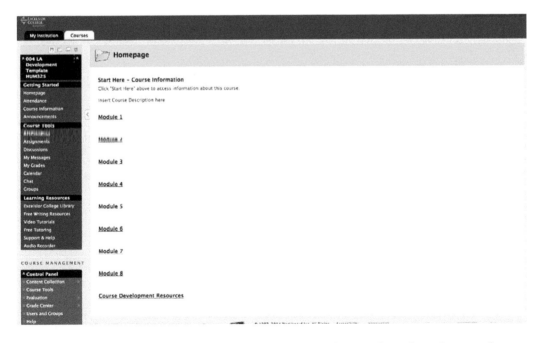

The course is experienced entirely within the environment of a typical Excelsior class interface.

Two students are not real students. They are Non-Player Characters (NPCs). Their pages are formatted identically to the other student pages. Information entered there can be found under their names in the Characters section in this Design Document.

Students will upload an image of their avatar, and they may also choose handles, but their full names, contact information, and biographies will also be available to other students and the instructor on their Personal Pages.

At a critical point in the game, Tom/Elliot will hack the class website (see Episode 6).

Class Journal

The Class Journal page index links to all of the narrative elements and puzzles of the class in an easy-to-access database, so that students will be able to catch up should they miss a class. This material is supplied by the developers. By default, each week, once a class is complete, all narrative elements and gameplay from that week become available for review. The default can be changed at the discretion of the instructor if, for example, the instructor feels some items should be retained only by the students themselves. Instructors can toggle between either state at any time during the eight weeks of the class.

Student Journal

Each student is required to make journal entries as directed in each episode. These are distinct from the Class Journal.

GAME MECHANICS

Environments

These are the transmedia environments where students interact with the game. They may include, but are not limited to, the following:

Actual websites as detailed in the Investigations and Additional Resources sections of each episode.

Fictional websites

The Collective (www.thecollectiveworld.org)

Fortress 9 (www.fortress9.org)

CareHart Foundation (www.carehartfoundation.org)

Chromogen (www.chromogen.org)

Badge Lands (www.badgelands.com)

Actual Websites and Tools

This was a list of sixteen popular websites and online communication tools including Twitter, texts, email, Facebook, Pinterest, YouTube, LinkedIn, Skype, etc.

Communication

There are three trajectories of communication available in the game. Students may interact with NPCs, other students, and the instructor.

Student/Instructor

Students will be able to email the instructor and teaching assistants. Replies are at the instructor's discretion.

Student/Student

Students will be able to create and join discussions in the class forum. They will be able to privately email or message all class members, including Tom Wetherall and Ann Bennett (See NPCs in this Design Document).

Student/NPC

Students will be able to email, text, and tweet to NPCs.

Basic Gameplay

Gameplay will consist of players uncovering narrative elements; following trails of clues both on our in-house fictional websites and the Internet; solving puzzles and riddles, aided by lesson material and the built-in character hint system provided through Tom Wetherall and Ann Bennett (See NPCs in this Design Document). Most of the gameplay is devoted to uncovering the narrative and completing class investigations.

In-Game Videos
Video Messages

These are from Dale Kenton and Audra Casey. They will be "official" broadcasts of the two factions' positions. They are pre-recorded talking heads and are not interactive.

News Footage

These are accessed via a fictional news website, Budge Lands ("Law Enforcement News for the Rest of Us"). Only one is created especially for the game (Desmond Wright being arrested). All are short, pre-recorded news clips and are not interactive.

Extra-Game Videos

Videos from various real sites on the web. They are accessible from any browser, are pre-recorded, and are not interactive.

A trailer was also produced for the school's online catalogue and publicity. The script follows. Compare this to traditional class catalogue entries.

HUM 325 Secrets: A Cyberculture Mystery Game
Trailer script

1. Open with Professor Grey's announcement about a startling message, 0:00–0:15 (DRAMATIC MUSIC OVER THROUGHOUT)

2. TITLE CARD: **An online class on Internet culture and identity.**

3. Screen shot of the course home page on Blackboard, which David will provide.

4. TITLE CARD: **Becomes a chance for you to change the future.**

5. The Collective Video # 1, 18–27 (Audra's intro)

6. Professor Grey's briefing #1, 1:11–1:13 ("It's from an organization called the Collective.")

7. The Collective Video # 1, 1:25–1:30 ("We're trying to build a world free from hate, strife, war and hunger.")

8. TITLE CARD: **That sounds pretty good, doesn't it?**

9. Professor Grey's briefing #1, 1:18–1:30 ("Yet only a few days later…they stand in opposition to The Collective's goals.")

10. Fortress 9 Video #1, 1:47–1:52 ("What we have is an elite who claim to know what's best for us.")

11. TITLE CARD: **Two factions fighting for the soul of the human race.**

12. TITLE CARD: **Voices from a future that has roots in today's Internet.**

13. Professor Grey's briefing #1, 1:31–1:38 ("My lectures…both sides of the debate")

14. TITLE CARD: **But what you see on the Internet isn't always what it appears to be.**

15. TITLE CARD: **There are secrets within secrets.**

16. TITLE CARD: **Only you can discover the truth. Explore…**

17. TITLE CARD SCREENSHOTS representing examples of each of the following five subjects with titles of each on the screenshots: **1) Social media, 2) Identity role play, 3) Internet dating, 4) Online games 5) And more [a still from The Matrix]**

18. TITLE CARD: **Discover the ultimate secret that lies at the heart of**

19. TITLE OVER LMS IMAGE: **Humanities 325 Secrets: A Cyberculture Mystery Game**

20. TITLE CARD in a larger size font:
    For more information or to register visit Excelsior College's Center for Game and Simulation Based Learning www.gameandsimulationbasedlearning.org

21. Final screen with credits

    Secrets: a Cyberculture Mystery Game

    Written and Designed by Lee Sheldon

    Instructional Design by David Seelow

    Produced by Focus EduVation, Woborn, Massachusetts, in collaboration with Excelsior College's Center for Online Education, Learning and Academic Services and the School of Liberal Arts

CHARACTERS

Player-Characters

With the exception of the two students who are NPCs, each student is a Player-Character. Students will use both their own names and handles, if they wish to do so. (See more about avatar creation under Personal Page above.)

Instructor

Logan Grey is designed to be a template, a shell with an androgynous name that will fit whoever the instructor might be. Logan is neutral, not taking a side in the struggle for power between The Collective and Fortress 9. Once student suspicions are aroused that all is not what it seems, Logan will encourage students to discover the truth, helping them gain the skills necessary to master the Internet in their efforts.

Major NPCs

Audra Casey

Audra Casey is the representative for The Collective: open, intelligent, someone you want to trust. She is attractive, in her early thirties, a true believer that what she is doing is bettering humankind. Her clothes are stylish, but business-like, cut differently enough from today's normal business attire to suggest future fashion. She is actually a top executive at Chromogen. She is seen in videos, pictures, and can email, tweet, and text students. Audra is controlled by the class instructor or a teaching assistant.

Dale Kenyon

Dale Kenyon is the face of Fortress 9, the social/political group in opposition to The Collective. He is African American, in his forties, rugged, good-looking, but with an edge to him. He dresses in leather, or a leather-substitute, because the look will never go out of style. He is actually another agent of Chromogen who will make it look as if he has been won over by The Collective's message. He is seen in videos, pictures, and can email, tweet, and text students. Dale is controlled by the class instructor or a teaching assistant.

Tom Wetherall (Elliot Plevin)

Tom Wetherall is a likable, intelligent member of the class (probably only seen in his character photo) who says he works for an Organic Health Food Company.

> Again, while a fictional health food company doesn't exist in the game, as it did in the *Skeleton Chase* games, Tom does dole out suspect vitamin water to students in reprehensible experiments. No reference to any real health food company is implied or intended!

He is one half of the hint system. He is of course directly responsible for Chromogen's experiments on the class. His real name is Elliot Plevin, a PhD student gone really, really bad. Tom is experienced entirely through normal student interaction interfaces. He is controlled by the class instructor or a teaching assistant.

Ann Bennett

Ann Bennett is another likable, intelligent student in the class (also probably only seen in her character photo). She is the other half of the hint system. She is an FBI agent who fights Internet crime, a job she can handle very well indeed from her very real wheelchair. Ann is experienced entirely through normal student interaction interfaces. She is controlled by the class instructor or a teaching assistant.

> Both Tom and Ann were controlled by teaching assistants. They had three main functions in the class. First, they were tasked with offering hints to students. Their second function was, whenever necessary, to take opposite sides in debates that arose on topics presented by the lectures. Not in an obvious way as teaching assistants do outside of lectures in many classes. Instead, their enthusiastic disagreements encouraged the real students, who believed one way or the other, to speak up, knowing they were never alone.
>
> Finally, they were instrumental in moving the narrative forward at a pace the class could handle while ensuring that students would be ready for each new episode. The amount of information the students were asked to absorb each week was immense. Their pacesetting was instrumental in preventing anyone from being left behind.

> In *Skeleton Chase 2*, I used non-player characters to encourage competition. In *The Lost Manuscript*, I added only a light flavoring of competition between the study groups. When we paired which NPC would text their suspicions to which study group, we did so pretty randomly. The idea was not really developed and there is no evidence students paid much attention to it. In a 2017 Ren'Py version of the game, NPCs were more clearly in conflict in their search for the missing book. That iteration of the game was simply a final proof of concept and was never meant to be released.

In *Secrets*, all three of Tom and Ann's primary functions worked extremely well from the very beginning. I hope I can design more online multiplayer classrooms for a couple of reasons. One reason is I would like to explore the possibilities of this idea of fake students. And of course, as this book is being written, COVID-19 is a major threat and schools wrestle with how to make remote classrooms more appealing to students of all ages. Turning some into multiplayer classrooms is an obvious way for schools to increase engagement.

Minor NPCs
Desmond Wright

Desmond is Audra's and Elliot's boss: fashionably bearded, hair gelled to perfection, Italian suit. Desmond is CEO of Chromogen, slick, amoral, driven entirely by the bottom line. His Achilles heel is that he is an egotistical paranoid schizophrenic, a combination that will lead to his downfall. He will only be seen in stills as students close in on Chromogen, then finally in a video clip as he is led away from his estate by police.

My second appearance in these games occurs in *Secrets*, this time on camera. I played Desmond Wright in a video on the Badge Lands website, as he is led away in hand-cuffs to face his just desserts. Sadly, this footage does not appear to have survived. I can state for the record that I do not match in any way the character description. A similar moment occurs when a character I did not play is also led away in handcuffs in *The Janus Door*.

Sallie Lopez

Sallie is a spokesperson for the CareHart Foundation. She exudes motherly warmth and good cheer like a heady perfume. She appears to believe passionately in the CareHart Foundation and its good works. But it is in her files that students will find the link to Chromogen.

Edmund Conner Hart

Hart is seen only in a still photograph accompanying his obituary. He is in his seventies, carefully groomed, with an open, welcoming smile.

BACKSTORY

In the early 1990s, Desmond Wright, an entrepreneur/visionary in a similar, if much darker, vein to Mark Zuckerberg, Mark Pincus, Bill Gates, and Steve Jobs, realized the potential power of the Internet. The small startup company he'd formed to explore human DNA, Chromogen (www.Chromogen.org), was headed down a path too many competitors were already traveling. Wright began pondering if his company and his hobby, studying how the human brain processes information, might be combined with the ubiquitous reach of the Internet and its phenomenal ability to capture users' attention.

With the aid of a particularly brilliant, if sociopathic, PhD student, Elliot Plevin, Wright set in motion a series of experiments, first on animals, then on human volunteers. What they discovered was that people whose DNA was susceptible to particular chemical stimulants might indeed develop a kind of psychic harmony with one another, not really telepathic, but an ability to sense others whose makeup was similar, and form a tight, instinctual bond of like-minded individuals. Further, Plevin discovered that subliminal perception, long ago dismissed in old media, might actually work extremely well in an interactive medium such as video games or the Internet. The process, if it worked, could be sold to anyone for any amount, and that country or corporation or group could bend the world to their will. The profit potential was obviously immense.

Wright and Plevin did not publish their findings but embarked on an enterprise that would alter the DNA in anyone through exposure to certain chemicals and subliminal stimuli, and then connect them to each other through interaction on the Internet. But they needed a trial on people who were unaware they were being tested. It was the Vice President of Marketing at Chromogen, Audra Casey, who came up with the idea of infiltrating an online course with an agent (Plevin) who could then experiment from within.

When their first attempt in 2012 led to a massive outbreak of migraine headaches (due to the chemicals) in a class in Tampa, Florida, they managed to safely fade away, or so they thought. But the migraines in a single class on Internet culture attracted the interest of an FBI agent, Ann Bennett, who was part of a special unit formed to look for anomalies in Internet experiences that might indicate criminal behavior.

Ann and her team found a link to an account about Plevin, who early in his career mentioned some chemicals at a conference that might be used to alter the behavior of DNA to increase psychic ability. He was laughed from the stage, but there was a note that Plevin said he was frustrated by a number of apparent migraine headaches in his test rats.

Ann searched for other classes that were studying the Internet. She became convinced that a new course at Excelsior might be Plevin's next test case. But he couldn't be doing this on his own, and no legitimate foundation would sponsor such research. Someone with more money and power than ethics must be financing his experiments.

Ann suspected that Plevin would infiltrate the class, but she had no idea in what guise, nor did she have any proof for that matter of wrongdoing. In the weeks before the class began, her team was given part of a damaged file found on the body of an associate of Plevin's who had died in an "accident." It mentioned his plan to make students susceptible to the experiment by claiming to contact them from a future Earth free from hatred and war where all citizens were becoming part of what they called The Collective. So, she signed up for the class.

Wright and his people had already set up a front organization, The CareHart Foundation, to begin mass testing when the class experiment was a success, as they were certain it would be. But Wright's Achilles heel kicked in. His ego blinded him to the interest the FBI was taking in Chromogen. He feels safely hidden behind the CareHart Foundation since no one yet knows of his connection to it.

Wright is now poised to put his plan for domination into motion via genetic manipulation and the ubiquitous nature of the Internet.

POINT OF ATTACK

The game begins when Logan Grey reveals that his planned class will be adapted to include an extraordinary communication he has received. He introduces a video from Audra Casey, representing The Collective. A second video follows quickly to present Fortress 9's side of things. Both videos contain Rabbit Holes (Trailheads) into the narrative, as do Logan's remarks. Logan, Dale, and Audra will all suggest various links and readings for students. Here is Logan Grey's introductory video script.

INTRODUCTORY VIDEO

Hello, this is Professor Logan Grey. Welcome to Excelsior's Culture of the Internet class. The course outcomes are:

1. Evaluate the effect of computer mediated technologies on your sense of identity.

2. Create digital exhibits of your learning.

3. Formulate your own theory of 21st century global identity.

4. Analyze and present a coherent explanation of a humanities question or issue integrating two humanities disciplines.

5. General Education Outcome

   a. Explain concepts of diversity and inclusion in the context of US society and culture as well as in the context of a global society.

   b. Demonstrate an understanding of individual and group differences and alliances and explain how they may be influenced by race, gender, sexual orientation, age, class, religion, and/or disabilities.

6. Describe how rapid changes and developments of digital technology in recent years serve to project an altered image of identity upon our collective consciousness.

That sounds straightforward enough, doesn't it? However, this class is unlike any you will have taken in the past at Excelsior or elsewhere. It is not only a class, but a narrative-driven game called *Secrets*. If you have heard of alternate reality games, or read about them on the Internet, you will have some idea of what to expect: the unexpected. You… and I… will be characters in the story.

You will view briefings, conduct investigations, file reports, meet challenges, and discuss issues. Class lectures, materials, assignments—here called investigations—and readings will serve more than one purpose: to give you knowledge and to teach you critical thinking; but also, to give you the clues to solve the mystery the story presents.

Each week's class—think of it as an episode in a TV series—will progress the story. You will meet characters through various media. You will be confronted by differing points of view concerning a discovery that could change the world. You will uncover secrets that will help you to decide what to believe, and how you feel about what you learn.

Are you ready?

If you are watching this video, the game has already begun…

EPISODES

Secret: An Internet Mystery is divided into eight episodes. Each episode lasts for two weeks, except for Episode 8 which lasts only one week. There was a total of fifteen weeks in the class. Major story moves may be found in each of the following episode descriptions.

CHAPTER 27

Episode 1 – Primal Empathy

DETAILED EPISODES

In each episode class assignments have been written directly addressing students so that they can easily be transferred to the class website. In the sections focused on narrative and the game, intended only for the eyes of developers and Excelsior, students are referred to in the third person, e.g. students, the class etc.

LEARNING OUTCOMES

By the end of this episode successful students will be able to:

1. Identify some of the characteristics and trends of the Internet/World Wide Web that contribute to how humans think about their identity in the post-1990s world.

2. Create an online avatar and brief backstory for the avatar that presents an online identity for other students to think about and interact with.

CHARACTERS

Logan Grey, Tom Wetherall, Ann Bennett, Audra Casey, Dale Kenyon

NARRATIVE

In a special video, Logan reveals to the class that Excelsior has been contacted by The Collective, a group of leaders, scientists, and humanitarians 70 years in the future. He will share with the class a video The Collective has sent. They are trying to build a world free from hate, strife, war, and hunger. Their scientists are developing a way to alter human DNA so that all humans can have ability they call Primal Empathy or PE. PE is a kind of psychic harmony with one another, not really telepathic, but an ability to form a tight, instinctual empathetic bond that transcends national, cultural, and racial differences. If all humankind can learn to strongly identify with one another then hatred and war would be evils of the past. Their movement is well advanced, and is succeeding; however, there is still much ignorance and resistance. This movement began on the Internet in our time but was slow to take hold. The Collective is hoping that in this class, by exploring the many meanings of identity on the Internet, they can help not only speed up the process, but make it better. Logan then tells the students there is another video.

This video is from Dale Kenyon, representing a faction in opposition to The Collective. Dale asks students to be very wary of The Collective's vision. It brings new meaning to the term "Silent Majority." You are either one of them or a silenced outcast.

VIDEO (3)

The video number above refers to special, narrative videos. All of Logan Grey's briefings were recorded as well but are not counted in the number following this section title.

All actors had teleprompters to keep memorization to a minimum. Audra was only one of two members of the cast with acting experience. Logan was played by David, who is not an actor. Dale was a former member of Excelsior's Board of Trustees. Sallie was not an actor. Desmond Wright was played by yours truly, who has had some acting training and experience, but Wright has no dialogue. He just needed to look grumpy when he was hauled away in handcuffs.

Logan's Surprise
Logan

Something extraordinary has happened. I don't know if I quite believe it, but I'm convinced that not only can it be integrated into our class as an unprecedented teaching opportunity, but it is a chance to help future generations. I will continue the class as I planned, so you should expect to write reports and complete assignments just as you ordinarily would. But I guarantee you will never look at the Internet in the same way again.

We, that is Excelsior College, because of our unique position as a non-profit online school, have been contacted… through the Internet… from the future. I'm going to let that sink in for a moment. I have no idea what is behind the science that has made this possible. All I can tell you is that I've received two videos purporting to be from the future and containing links to websites accessible now in our time via the Internet.

The first was received just over two weeks ago attached to an email addressed to me personally. It is from an organization called The Collective. The implications of that video alone are immense. Yet, only a few days later, a second video arrived from a rival group calling itself, somewhat melodramatically, Fortress 9. They stand in opposition to The Collective's goals. My lectures and the class assignments will, I believe, provide data to intelligently assess both sides of the debate.

That is all I intend to say for now. After you've viewed the two videos, my first class briefing will be available. Feel free to use the class forums to discuss this amazing event as well as regular class issues. I can promise you we are about to embark on a unique adventure together, the outcome of which is impossible to predict.

Greetings from the Collective

The Collective's slick-looking logo screen appears, accompanied by some warm and fuzzy music. The screen fades to a MEDIUM CLOSE SHOT (news program talking head size) of Audra Casey. She wears a nicely tailored suit and sits in a comfortable chair in front of a beautiful landscape backdrop.

Audra

Greetings from the future! [laughs apologetically] I tried for quite a while to figure out how to open this video. I wanted to be impressive and welcoming. But when I finally said it on camera it sounded kind of silly. Oh well, hopefully you're still watching!

My name is Audra Casey. And I am speaking to you from…get ready for it…the year 2084! I kid you not! I work here at The Collective's main office in New York City. I did some research on CommCore… sorry, what you call in your time the Internet! A lot has happened in the past seventy years!

Unfortunately, if you're looking for lottery winners or pictures of what your grandchildren will look like, I can't oblige. There's a big reason for this, trust me! The future…even a minute from now…is not predictable. Your choices, the choices of those around you, your classmates, even random occurrences, are constantly affecting what happens next.

And this natural law is why I am reaching out to you now.

The Collective is a group of scientists, philosophers, humanitarians, futurists—yes, we have them too!—and people just like you and me. We are trying to build a world free from hate, strife, war and hunger. I know, I know. It sounds like Flower Power. Is that right? The hippies? The 1960s? Far out and give peace a chance?

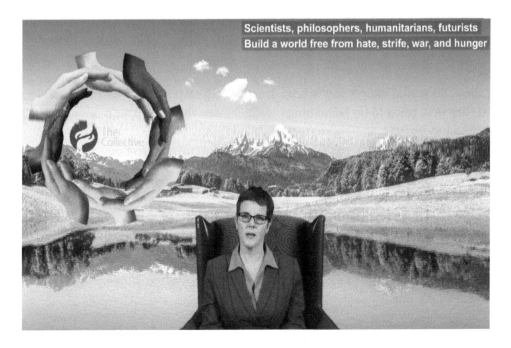

Aura Casey, spokesperson from the future.

Well, bear with me. It's really possible, and here's how. Our bio-geneticists are developing a way to alter human DNA so that all humans can have a psychic ability we call Primal Empathy or PE. It doesn't hurt. It doesn't turn you into a zombie or a robot or a lizard like some science fiction holovid. Ooops, sorry, I mean movie, right?

PE is a kind of psychic harmony that allows us to connect with one another, not really telepathic, but an ability to form a tight, instinctual empathetic bond that transcends national, cultural and racial differences. If all humankind can learn to strongly identify with one another then hatred and war will be evils of the past. Our movement is well advanced, and is succeeding; however, there is still much ignorance and resistance.

Believe it or not the seeds of Primal Empathy can be found on the Internet in your time, but it was very slow to take hold. There were wars and hatred and bigotry for years after 2014. The Collective is hoping that in this class, by exploring the many meanings of identity on the Internet, you can help not only speed up the process, but make it better. Learn all you can about this medium, and your place in it. It can synchronize so many lives. One day it will connect us all in peace and harmony.

That's it for now. We'll be watching your progress. I'll be in contact through videos. You can also reach our website in your time: www.thecollectiveworld.org. Send us your thoughts; share pictures and screen grabs as you explore the Internet and the beginnings of PE, contact me directly. I'll try to help you in any way I can, although Professor Grey has said I can't help with your class assignments! Sorry! But other than that, we want this to be a true collaboration to create a better future for all of us!

A Warning from Fortress 9

The screen FADES UP on a MEDIUM CLOSE SHOT of Dale Kenyon. He wears jeans and a dark gray turtleneck and sits on a cheap chair in front of a plain brick wall with a Fortress 9 logo as the only decoration.

Dale

Hey there. So yeah, I expect you've seen The Collective's peace and harmony speech. We heard they were going to try something radical. I guess that means we're succeeding. They can't defeat us in 2084, so they've reached back into the past to try and change the rules. One thing I want to get straight: Fortress 9 doesn't blow things up or harm people, but this is a war we're fighting here.

OFFSCREEN WHISPER
Your name.
Dale (looks o.s.)
What?
OFFSCREEN WHISPER
Tell them your name.
Dale
Oh. I'm Dale Kenyon. I'm not public relations. I'm strategy and intel. So, if I come across too... intense... sorry.

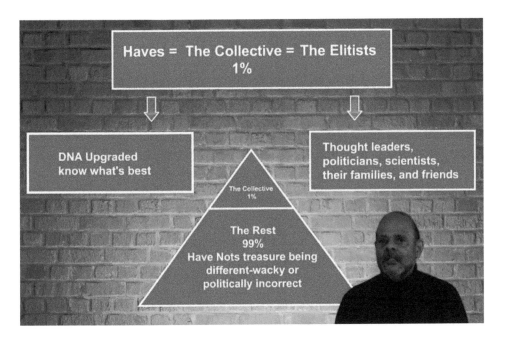

Dale Kenyon, the voice of the opposition.

They probably painted a pretty rosy picture about Primal Empathy, yeah? How PE helps us to understand each other better, to walk in the next guy's shoes, yeah? That's actually kind of how it works with somebody else who's also had their DNA "synchronized." Right now, that's only about 1% of the world's population: mostly thought leaders, politicians, scientists, their families, friends… The cream you might say. But what this has done is turn our world into the haves and have nots. Want all that good feeling directed at you? You damn well better have had your DNA upgraded. Otherwise you might just get ignored.

Yeah, what we have is an elite who claim to know what's best for us. What they can't understand is there's also some of us who treasure being different, even if it's wacky or not politically correct. I'll give you an example: comedians. A PE comedian just isn't funny. She doesn't have to be if the audience is all on her side. They enjoy being supportive. They show it by laughing. Trust me it's not the same as laughing cause your funny bone got plucked.

And even though their hearts may seem to be in the right place, there's no guarantee they'll remain that way. They might find they like being the elite, and then wonder if that feeling might go away if everyone is too equal…

So, make up your own minds. Investigate the Internet, the question of identity, and learn both the web's promise and its pitfalls. And learn more about PE. It may have pitfalls even The Collective has overlooked. I'll do my best to help you come to your own individual decisions whether you help them or not in the end.

I'll make some more videos. I know they pushed a website into your time. We did too. You can go find ours at www.fortress9.org. Let us know how your investigations into the Internet go. Connect with me personally, if you want. Otherwise send us stuff you find on the Internet, and the conclusions you reach. That's all I have to say for now. Dale Kenyon. Out.

All pedagogical material supplied by David Seelow for his character Logan Grey was fully scripted and recorded for delivery to the class. As mentioned in my Preface to this book, the intention is not to teach the subject matter here, but rather to get a feeling for topics covered and to provide reference points for the reader to illustrate how learning and narrative were integrated. In this online class the reader also can see how, thanks to Professor Seelow, the depth of the teaching equaled, even surpassed, the amount of material students would be expected to learn in a typical online class.

PROFESSOR GREY'S BRIEFINGS

As in many online classes, all of Professor's Grey's briefings were recorded in front of a green screen where text and images were displayed. Briefing images have not been reproduced in this book.

Briefing 1: The Rise of the Internet and World Wide Web

In this course we will explore the importance of the Internet and related technologies to how we think about ourselves.

Topics Include:

- Essential Question for Episode 1: What is cyberculture?

- The Internet is not the World Wide Web.

- The Internet is a network of networks.

- Web 2.0: The WWW Today.

- BitTorrent.

Briefing 2: Culture

The briefing starts with a quote from Pierre Levy on cyberculture that echoes Levy's French Enlightenment tradition of individual freedom and stresses the global nature of such freedom. This could be called a utopian definition that sees the Internet as the ultimate global democracy. Professor Grey promises the class will examine this definition throughout the course.

Briefing 3: Identity and the Internet: An Opening Gesture

Topics included:

Electronic Frontier Foundation

National Security Administration

1984 by George Orwell

The "Deep" or "Dark" Web

The "deep" or "dark" web plays a significant part in the fourth design document in this book where it is explored for a class on cybersecurity.

Investigations

These were reading assignments. While some may be referenced, they are not reproduced here to save space. There would be a list of these in all of the following episodes of the design document.

Investigation Reports

Based upon Professor Grey's briefings and the readings you are asked to compose a short 100–250-word manifesto for cyberspace. A manifesto (think of Marx and Engle's *Communist Manifesto*), like *The Declaration of Independence* that is a blueprint for what you would like to see happen now in terms of the organization, future development and governance of cyberspace.

Additional Course Assignments

XP, short for Experience Points, comes from videogame design. In game-based learning they can measure a student's progress in a class in the same way a player's progress in a game is measured. All of my classes covered in *The Multiplayer Classroom: Designing Coursework as a Game* use XP.

Standard Introduction used in all our courses (10 XP)
  Avatars: Creating a Unique Online Self (40–60 XP depending on use of software)
  You are asked to create an avatar or use a pre-existing one and introduce that avatar to the class with a backstory or brief biography about the avatar. The avatar can be as close or as far from your embodied or physical, "real world" or offline identity as you want. It is important to provide a graphic for your avatar. This can be ridiculous, as some people use cats or dogs for their visual presence online. You can draw a picture or use a copyright-free image from the web.
  For additional credit, you can use a free avatar creation program. Think of your own identity. Is your online self the same or different from your offline self and what does this mean in thinking about who we are?

Midterm Project: Internet Innovation (100 XP)

In Episode 4, Professor Grey would like you to submit a report on one of the important figures or organizations of the Internet. Your report can be three double-spaced pages, five pages if you compose a multimedia report (texts and images, 8 slides if you submit a Power Point or Prezi report). Please let Professor Grey know your subject by the end of Episode 1.

You are definitely allowed to reference *Wikipedia* in this course, but you cannot compose your entire report solely using that resource. Please make use of Excelsior College's excellent virtual library and librarians.

Possible Choices for Mid Term Report

A huge number of possible report topics were listed here.

Final Project: A Digital Autobiography (300 XP)

An autobiography is a written account of one's life. Everyone's life is worth writing about. The challenge is to make one's life interesting to readers, especially those who don't know you. An autobiography is a narrative that shapes the multitude of events in one's life into a readable form. History is our collective story and autobiography our personal story. The story does not have to be linear though that is a traditional mode of composition and of course our story on earth does not end until we pass away at which time another person would need to write a biography to preserve the memory of who we were. This style of writing helps us understand who we are at the time of writing and how we became who we are and also helps others now, and in the future, to understand us. As your professor, not only do I want to know about you, but I also want the members of *The Collective* and *Fortress 9* to understand who you all are as we decide what message to send them about our world.

As we are learning about the Internet, our stories must be told in a digital fashion to reflect the tools around us. What distinguishes a digital autobiography from a print-based autobiography is its multimedia potential. Your story can be told with more than words, but words including what you write in this course are important. You may also use pictures and drawings, scanned images of print documents, screen shots, music clips or links, social media like Facebook or Twitter; possible movie clips or slide show presentations, anything that helps portray who you feel you are at this point in time.

What to include in your story is up to you. Your completed story will be due in Episode 8, but you will need to write one chapter each episode in order to be successful. Each episode will give you the general area to address and some hints to help your work progress. You can keep your work private or share with friends. You will also have access to Professor Grey's own story.

Final Project Chapter One Guidelines

This should be your introduction, but you can reorder later if you want to be experimental. Expand on your introduction and the creation of your avatar or online identity with images, music, and whatever else helps present yourself at this moment in your history.

CLASS FORUM (30 XP)

Release of Logan, Tom and Ann's posts in the Class Forum should be timed to appear natural e.g. not posted all together. Specific timing will also be noted as needed. Also, additional posts will be necessary in explicit response to specific student posts to show our NPCs dialoging directly with students.

Ann and Tom will also comment as needed to initiate discussion in class-specific forum topics.

Misspellings, typos, and wrong word choices in posts from Ann and Tom are deliberate. They are meant to be real people after all. And like it or not, real people make mistakes in online posts. Logan Grey, being a professor, of course, does not make mistakes. Seriously, speech that looks like it has been copyedited by the New York Times will only make real students suspicious.

In *Skeleton Chase 2: The Psychic*, *The Lost Manuscript*, and *The Janus Door*, students knew they were dealing with NPCs. In this class about identity on the Internet it was important to keep our NPCs secret as long as possible, and it was much easier to do since none of the students ever physically met.

As it was, during the first iteration of the class a student discovered that the NPCs were not students because Blackboard represented employees or non-registered students with a different icon than students. Professor Seelow tells me that they easily corrected this technical glitch but being aware of how an LMS works makes a difference. Another student solved the mystery earlier than we wanted. This happened when a student who was a military IT professional went behind the scenes of the LMS, had a look at the code, and made the discovery. He kept our secret.

Professor Seelow points out that the younger students would be less likely to tamper with your LMS code, but it isn't entirely impossible either.

Logan Grey First Post

First post in the forum:

Welcome everybody. I'd first like you to tell the rest of us who you are and a little bit about yourselves. Just post a short paragraph here in the forum. Then we can discuss the remarkable videos we've seen.

After a suitable time:

Ann Bennett Post

My name is Ann. I am a programmer in the IT Department at Rensselaer Polytechnic Institute in Troy, NY. I'm a working mother with two kids in elementary school. I was in a car accident when I was nine which left me on wheels, but I promise you they don't slow me down! I play center on our community center's girls Special Olympics basketball team. I'm really looking forward to learning more about the Internet for my job. Some of it involves protecting RPI's computers.

After a few other students have posted:

Tom Wetherall Post

Hi, folks. My name is Tom. I work in sales and marketing for a health food distributor. We're opening our first retail store in Marin, California this winter so I'm pretty excited about that. I'm on the Internet every day for my job, but I know there's still a lot I have to learn so here I am!

After all students have posted:

Logan Grey Second Post

Given our current state of knowledge what do you think are the merits of the two contrasting messages on the videos? Will the future of cyberspace by the utopia [pop up] described by Audra Casey; a place of open sharing, collaboration and collective consciousness or do you share Dale Kenyon's fear that we are moving toward a totalitarian state where cyberspace will be ruled by a single organization? Share your thoughts with class and discuss the thoughts of at least two other class members. Make sure you give some thought to how the future of cyberspace could affect your own personal identity or those you know from a younger generation.

Tom Wetherall Post in Response

Okay, I'll play along. ; -) I think primal empathy sounds very cool. I'm not sure about playing around with DNA, but even the Fortress 9 dude suggests the idea of it isn't necessarily bad. He just comes across as a typical troublemaker. If somebody likes something, he's against it.

Ann Bennett Post in Response

I don't know. Maybe I'm overreacting, but it sounds too good to be true. Anybody else feel that way?

Here we can see Tom and Ann fulfilling one of their three rolls: jumpstarting conversation.

Logan Grey Post in Response

Give students a few hours (a day?) to leave opinions or other thoughts, then personalize the following.

I want to thank [student name], [student name] etc., Tom Whetherall and Ann Bennett for starting the discussion. I'm going to stay neutral at this point. But I'm glad to see you're already using the forum. Since I'm the professor I'll echo what both Audra and Dale suggested: use the Internet to explore the possibilities. You may decide to help The Collective or not. But replay my lectures and have a look at the links under both Investigations and Additional Resources. Even though these messages seem to be from the future, the past is a good place to start. I'm looking forward to your reports!

Tom Wetherall Response

No h in Wetherall, Professor, but you won't have to encourage me with my big mouth to contribute!

CHAPTER 28

Episode 2 – The Present Is the Past of the Future

LEARNING OUTCOMES

By the end of this episode students will be able to:

1. Describe the changes in identity brought about by the advent of the Internet and World Wide Web.

2. Discuss the impact of the social media on social identity formation.

3. Reflect in writing on the context and formation of social identity in the 21st Century.

CHARACTERS

Tom Wetherall, Ann Bennett, Audra Casey, Dale Kenyon

NARRATIVE

A new video from Audra suggests students can help The Collective by learning the nature of the Internet and how it can bring people together or split them apart. A video from Dale promises revelations. The Collective's vision for a new humanity charged by Primal Empathy is not as successful as she claims.

Ann tells the students she's discovered some interesting anomalies embedded in the first videos from The Collective. She shares them with the students in the class forum. Tom suggests they look at *all* of the videos again for clues, including Dale's and Prof. Grey's lecture. He's not ready to choose a side without more information. Other students will be able to discover additional links. If they miss any, Tom and/or Ann will have found them before next week and posted them on the class discussion page. Finding these links in the narrative chain is the first puzzle in the game.

VIDEO (3)
Progress Report

The Collective's slick-looking logo screen again appears, accompanied by some warm and fuzzy music. The screen fades to a MEDIUM SHOT of Audra Casey. She wears the same nicely tailored gray suit and purple blouse and sits in a comfortable chair in front of a beautiful landscape backdrop. Superimposed on the background is a copy of the Fortress 9 logo.

Audra's choice of wardrobe will become a clue in a future episode.

Audra

Hi, everybody! It's Audra again! By this time, I expect you've already started your investigations on the Internet.

I have an idea about that, but first I wanted to talk to you about Fortress 9. We have discovered that they managed to get a website up in your time and have sent you a video. I've seen it. We certainly didn't mean to hide them from you. In fact, we invited Fortress 9 to give their point of view in our previous video, but they declined.

You need to understand that Fortress 9 is a group of science deniers. They believe what they need to believe and won't let a little thing like facts get in the way. They haven't hurt anyone. Yet. But they have trespassed upon and vandalized Collective property. They send out holovids that are very slickly produced but bear no resemblance to reality. And yes, they suggest, oh so very delicately, that at some point if nobody in our time is listening to their message that they may indeed resort to violence. Ask Dale Kenyon. If there *is* violence, it will be his wing of Fortress 9 that will instigate it. Send him an email. Ask him if what I'm saying isn't the truth!

Please believe me, I can understand why they want to stop Primal Empathy from synchronizing lives. They are the very people, full of anger and a need for destruction that The Collective wants to help. The more they fail to win over others—and they *are* failing—the more dangerous they will become.

Anyway, I needed to say that. Hopefully, you'll come to the same conclusion through your investigations. And that brings me back to what I wanted to talk about in this video. We would like to see how well you are all progressing. I know you've just really begun, but with Professor Logan's permission, I'm going to give you a challenge: a 10 question quiz on your readings and viewings. He asked me to say the challenge can be taken 3 times. It is worth 20 experience points—what he calls XP? Submit them as you would any other assignment and he will send the results of the challenge to us for analysis. Maybe we'll even offer prizes for the best ones!

That's all for now! Remember, you can contact me directly through the forums on The Collective's website or email. I'd love to hear from you! Bye!

Thinking Critically

The screen FADES UP on a MEDIUM LONG SHOT of Dale Kenyon. He wears jeans and the dark gray turtleneck and is seated in the same cheap chair in front of a plain brick wall with a Fortress 9 logo as the only decoration. He faces CAMERA.

Dale

Listen, I'm gonna make this quick. I understand how seductive The Collective's vision may be, okay? I mean peace, love, harmony, no war, no hatred…who wouldn't want that, right?

Let me tell you something. Human beings survive because we're edgy, unpredictable…different! We need to learn what makes us different and celebrate that difference! Everybody solves problems in their own way. But if nobody thinks there can be another way, stuff is going to get lost!

Damn, I know I'm not making a whole lot of sense here. I'm not as slick as Audra Casey. I'm just me. And yeah, I'm different than them. I want to stay that way.

Primal Empathy got its start where you are…*when* you are. You have the best chance for seeing it as the danger it truly is. I'm counting on you. The human race is counting on you. That's all I have to say.

Remember, you can contact me directly through email or on our website. Let me know what you're thinking. Ask me the hard questions. I'll try to answer them. Dale Kenyon. Out.

The CareHart Story

[This is a slick corporate video introducing the CareHart Foundation and its philanthropic mission. It is introduced by Sallie Lopez.]

While Sallie's entire dialogue will be recorded with her ON CAMERA, it will be broken up and some of it will be used as V.O. narration in the promotional video. The CareHart web address, www.careheart.org is prominently displayed throughout.

Sallie

Hi there. I'm Sallie Lopez, and I am the Director of the CareHart Foundation. The Foundation was established in 2013 with a grant from the Edmund Conner Hart Trust.

Mr. Hart rose from a life of hardship to become one of the most successful entrepreneurs in the United States. He was inspired to combine life lessons from his troubled childhood with a desire to help others. When he died in 2012, he left his considerable fortune in trust to establish a foundation, whose mission would be in his words, "To help individuals who have been abused or traumatized to regain a strong sense of self worth and purpose in life. When they are truly synchronized with life, then they can gain the empathy necessary to reach out and help others." The CareHart Foundation is his dream realized.

We call this mission in short "Synchronizing Lives." Reintegrating damaged souls into life so that all of us may live together as one loving family.

While we have just begun to tackle the immense challenges our mission presents, we hope to one day build on Mr. Hart's dream and unite all the peoples of the world.

An ambitious goal? No question. But the CareHart Foundation has the resources to someday realize that vision. It begins here. On the Internet. It begins with you.

Narration will be adjusted and expanded to match visuals. Entire video should be no more than 30 seconds long.

PROFESSOR GREY'S BRIEFINGS

Briefing 1: Modern Identity: Three perspectives

Essential Question for Episode 2: Who am I today in relationship to the Internet and digital technologies and where am I headed?

This week I will present a small number of theories about identity from a philosophical, psychological, and sociological perspective. Keep in mind that many of the theories I will mention require entire 15-week semesters to even begin to grasp, but at least you will have a foundation to help build your own thinking upon. At the outset keep in mind a very general distinction between a quantitative personal identity and a qualitative personal identity.

Do you present different faces to different people? Do you find yourself managing your public identity and what does this management convey about who you really are or are you a summation of your public identities?

> Here is a good example of how the fictional narrative and class topics were carefully balanced to illuminate one another. All of the NPCs presented different faces to the students.

I am asking each of you to compose your own narrative as this course unfolds. Your ongoing narrative will express your sense of self or who you are at this point in time. The reflexivity of your identity will be your continually re-composing this narrative as you reflect upon your experience, contemplate the future, and think about the present.

You now have a foundation to help build your own autobiography. In the second briefing, I will briefly talk about identity on the Internet but will address this topic more fully next week.

Briefing 2: The Online Self and the Circle of Life

Most scholars writing about online identity have seen a fundamental continuity between an online self and one's offline self. Yes, they argue, individuals online will construct many self-representations, but ultimately these many representations can all be traced back to a unified embodied self in the "real world."

There are obvious aspects of cyberspace that allow for identity experimentation of all ages much less likely in physical space. The virtual world allows for anonymity. Cyberspace allows for the exploration of fantasy and the aspects of self that Freud often found repressed by the average person. I would argue that there is an ongoing feedback loop between the offline self and the online self. Online provides feedback to the offline self necessarily modifying that self in potential important and surprising ways.

INVESTIGATIONS

Additional Resources

> A list of websites. While some may be referenced, like reading assignments they are not reproduced here to save space.

Challenge (25 XP)
Crowds or Mobs?

Investigation Reports
The Clue to Facebook (30 XP)

This investigation continues into *Episode 3* and has two parts. First, visit someone you know who has used Facebook or identify an agency or organization that uses Facebook for promotional or informational reasons and list every visible component of the page then write one paragraph evaluating the effectiveness of the page. If the site is organizational, evaluate how effective the site was in getting its message across whether it is a call to action or an attempt to sell something. If the site is personal, what did you learn about the person and would you want to be this person's Facebook friend? Send this to Professor Grey.

As you work on this part of the investigation, gather information for your own Facebook page.

Or (chose one or the other option, but not both)

This investigation continues into *Episode 4* and has two parts. First, visit someone you know who has used LinkedIn and list every visible component of the page then write one paragraph evaluating the effectiveness of the page. Pay attention to LinkedIn's basic template or structure: summary, experience, publications, projects, skills, and expertise etc. Also look at endorsements for the person and any groups the person might belong to. Evaluate the page in terms of effectiveness. Do you think this person has an effective professional network? How could he or she improve it? Do you want to connect to this person? Why or why not? Send this to Professor Grey.

As you work on this part of the investigation, gather information for your own LinkedIn page.

Neighborhoods: Location and Self-Identity (75 XP)

One of the most important elements of our personal identity is our neighborhood. We all grew up in a neighborhood we often remember sometimes fondly and sometimes not. As we move, our neighborhoods change, both those we move into and those we leave behind. Have you ever visited your first home? For this report Professor Grey wants you to join the *Map Skip* community, a virtual community for people of all ages to share stories about their locations. You are to write a short story from between 250 (1 page) and 750 words (3 pages) about a neighborhood of your choice. Send your story to Professor Grey and if you have a map, link to that neighborhood. You will earn five extra points.

Student Journal

These are not the same as the Class Journal which is supplied by the developers.

In this course, you will not be recording daily activities, though such a practice could be beneficial if you chose to do so, but you will practice journaling about specific topics for the duration of the course. You can use the journal feature of *Blackboard* or if you want to continue journaling beyond this class you can use a new online journal forum. Your journal entries can be anywhere between 50 words and 250 words. Journal writing is informal, and you will be awarded points based on the depth and clarity of your thought. The idea is to practice reflection or thinking about your experiences.

Bonus: *The Social Network* (25XP)

Watch David Fincher's 2010 film *The Social Network* about the origin of Facebook and the meteoritic rise of Harvard sophomore Mark Zuckerberg to the top of the business world. Write a short 250-word review of the film using the attached guidelines/format. Make sure to pay attention to what made this business venture such a success and what obstacles Zuckerberg had to overcome in achieving this success. Post your review to your Facebook page.

Liberating or Oppressive: The Complexities of Social Media (35XP)

Discuss among your classmates through one original post and two responses to other students about how you think social media and technology either helps or hinders socialization.

Final Project Episode Two Suggestions: My Social Self

For your second chapter, focus on your social identity or the identity you show to the public. Do not talk about work or college. That will come in Chapter Four. For this chapter, focus on both your online and offline social identity. For example, your friends and how you communicate with them, any important clubs or 4-H or Boy Scouts, sports, hobbies that you like or used to like and places you have lived or visited that you consider an important part of your identity.

CLASS FORUM (35 XP)

Logan Grey Post

Okay, you've seen the second video from both The Collective and Fortress 9. They obviously don't think much of one another. What do *you* think?

Ann Bennett Post in Response

I'm not sure what to think honestly. I think the assignments we're getting will help us decide which faction is right, or maybe they both are! Or neither of them! But there's something else I want to talk about. I've been looking at the videos over and over again. I know this is going to sound stupid, but there's something wrong about Audra. I don't mean personally. She seems nice, a bit too gosh golly gee whiz, but nobody's going to pick the Wicked Witch of the West to be their spokesperson. There's just something wrong with the way she looks.

Tom Wetherall Post in Response

Wow, isn't that how prejudice starts? No offense, Ann, but she can't help how she looks.

Ann Bennett Post in Response

I'm not prejudice. I can't say what it is exactly that bothers me. But there's something else, too. Something she said. I'm going to watch her second video a few more times and see if I can figure out what it is.

Above, Tom and Ann take different sides of a topic for debate, the second of their functions.

Give students a few hours (a day?) to leave opinions or other thoughts, create responses to those for Logan, Ann and Tom. If no one sees what Ann does, then send the following.

Ann Bennett Post

Hey everybody, I think I got one of the things that's bothering me about Audra's videos. Watch them again. More important listen to them! She uses the same phrase or almost in both of them. In the first video she says "It can synchronize so many lives." In the second video she says "they want to stop Primal Empathy from synchronizing lives." That sounds really familiar to me for some reason. And I know I didn't hear it first in the future!

Above, Ann gently moves the narrative forward, the third of Tom and Ann's roles.

Students can enter "synchronize lives," "synchronizes lives," or "synchronizing lives" in a search engine to find the fictional CareHart Foundation that should go live at the beginning of the Second Episode. IF after a certain amount of time no one finds it, Logan will, as follows:

Logan Grey Post in Response

When I enter "synchronize lives," "synchronizes lives," or "synchronizing lives" I get lots of links focusing on syncing things "live" not "lives." I didn't dig very deep though.

IF after a certain amount of time no one finds it, Tom will, as follows:

Tom Wetherall Post in Response

It a slogan for something called the CareHart Foundation. Check it out here: www.care-hart.org.

Tom moves the narrative forward.

Logan Grey Post in Response

Now that is interesting. The CareHart Foundation sounds a lot like it wants to do what The Collective is doing in the future. Is this what Audra meant when she said that Primal Empathy began in our time?

Give students a few hours (a day?) to leave opinions or other thoughts, create responses to those for Logan, Ann and Tom. If no one asks the following question, then Tom will:

Tom Wetherall Post in Response

If there's already a foundation doing this why didn't Audra tell us this?

CHAPTER 29

Episode 3 – Have a Hart

LEARNING OUTCOMES

By the end of this episode successful students will be able to:

1. Produce a personal social media page for either personal or professional purpose.

2. Discuss in writing the social phenomena of oversharing and its impact of how people publicly present themselves in the 21st Century.

CHARACTERS

Logan Grey, Dale Kenyon, Tom Wetherall, Ann Bennett, Sallie Lopez

NARRATIVE

The students have discovered the CareHart Foundation is a present-day philanthropic organization dedicated to the same ideals as The Collective: to teach us to empathize with our fellow humans. Tom asks Logan if he could invite someone from CareHart to discuss with the class how CareHart is using the power of the Internet to bring humanity closer together. Tom also chooses for his project compiling a list of websites of groups today in opposition to one another, soliciting ideas on how they might be brought to some understanding without violence.

VIDEO (1)

Danger on Every Page

Dale is back in his chair in front of the same brick wall and Fortress 9 logo.

Dale

First of all, thanks to everybody who has contacted me with support for Fortress 9 and what we're trying to do. I admit we were kinda afraid everybody in your time would sort of roll over for The Collective's touchy-feely message. Glad to see that isn't true.

I've been looking over what Professor Grey has planned for this week, and I'm really glad he's getting into both positive stuff and negative. I know it's a wild frontier back in your day. In 2084 everything is pretty regulated. Safe maybe, but maybe not as alive as it once was.

Hey, I see he's got a discussion on self-revelation and narcissism planned. I thought some of The Collective's ideas sounded a lot like narcissism, but maybe what I'm doing is kinda like that, too. I don't know.

Reading what your class has been learning has caused me to do a lot of critical thinking, too. If we filter too much information and just concentrate on stuff we already believe in for validation or to feed our egos, that's not cool. Let me know what you think: is the trend in your time self-revelation and narcissism? If you email me, or leave thoughts on the Fortress 9 forums, I'll tell you where I am. Dale Kenyon. Out.

PROFESSOR GREY'S BRIEFINGS

Briefing 1: Postmodern Identity: I Share Therefore I Am

Essential Question for Episode 3: How has computer mediated communication affected our sense of self?

This week I want to pick up where I left off and talk briefly about postmodern identity and then talk directly about some of the ways the Internet has impacted our sense of self through Sherry Turkle's cyberpsychology, the social-psychological theory of oversharing, and the role of gender and race in cyberspace.

Postmodern Identity

For our purposes, I am going to focus on an excellent, but not a well-known study of postmodern identity called *The Saturated Self: Dilemmas of Identity in Contemporary Life* (Basic Books, 1991) by Swarthmore College's social psychologist Kenneth J. Gergen. Although Gregen's text is dense, he writes in an understandable style for educated people. The more philosophical postmodernists write in a language virtually impenetrable to non-professors in the Humanities.

In talking about architecture and music Gergen stresses hybrid forms and the blurring of genres as a way of saying nothing can be clearly and neatly defined or boxed in by categories. A common example is when Hip Hop artists sample, or incorporate, other artists' music into their compositions.

Also, in the postmodern era authority and tradition deteriorate. In literature, for example, the idea that all students should study certain great writers like Homer and Shakespeare, who are considered the established giants by experts in the field, goes by the wayside. Not only is the idea of expertise challenged, the notion that certain works are the ones to be studied ends up displaced by an emphasis on multiplicity.

In terms of identity, just as tradition goes by the wayside, the idea that a person's identity remains constant over time becomes untenable.

> Another overt connection between the game and the material, as the "true" identities of the NPCs shift, they require a deeper look at the themes discussed in this week's briefings.

One guiding question of this week's activity would be how do you shape a story that has many contradictory components and also how do you think contemporary social realities have impacted your sense of self?

Network Culture

For instance, you will hear in your briefing material one of the many talks by Professor Henry Jenkins, now of U.S.C., about participatory culture. These participatory mechanisms made possible by the Internet contribute to a widening of culture and a diversity of voices. This enables a person's creative identity.

Think about your own identity within the increasingly connected or networked world. Sherry Turkle points out that, despite being plugged in, people are more psychologically disconnected than ever. For instance, businessmen and women text during meetings, students update their Facebook page during class, employees email a colleague who sits only five feet away. People rarely make eye contact and are often distracted during an event, whether a sporting game or conference meeting. Text replaces talk and people fail to reflect on their own activities.

Oversharing

A number of scholars and professionals maintain social media like Facebook, YouTube, Instagram, Tumblr, and other online resources provide a platform for excessive sharing of personal information. Recall the Greek myth of Narcissus where the boy looking at his reflection in the pond drowns.

One of the many dangers of narcissism is the proliferation of superficial ties or connection. Does anyone really have 500 friends? Social media, like its predecessor *Reality TV*, encourages a false sense of celebrity for everyday people. People today are famous just for being famous.

Gender and Race

Little has been written about gender, race, and ethnicity on the Internet. Professor Lisa Nakamura's work has been most prominent in discussion about the intersection of both race and gender in the culture of the Internet. She outlines three positions for clarifying cyberrace, summarizing Larry Kang's "Cyber-Race" (*Harvard Law Review*, 2000).

- *Abolitionist:* you can hide your racial identity online and prevent potential racial stereotyping.

- *Integrationist:* making race visible online for open discussion.

- *Transmutation:* a person can adopt multiracial identities online in an attempt to dissolve the relationship between identity and the physical, racially marked body.

She coins a fascinating term "identity tourism" to describe cyberrace. Individuals can go online as another race, i.e. a white person can adapt an African American avatar and not feel racist. Nakamura calls this identity changing tourism because such switching can only be temporary and superficial. An Internet traveler must return to his or her native body. This tourism is equivalent to "going native"—a fictional and ridiculous attempt to eradicate "otherness." Digital technology and cyberspace have not liberated race. The digital divide replicates real world racism and pretending that cyberculture erases race is a fantasy that covers up and hides the material racism of the molecular world. As you progress through this course do not lose sight of how race, ethnicity, and gender intersect with cyberculture and affect your self-identity.

Briefing 2: Completing the Circle

Let me conclude this week's discussion by making some remarks about Dave Eggers' novel *The Circle*. I am curious how you find reading a 491 page novel? Why would I assign such a lengthy novel in an online course when surely I could find a shorter novel or short story to use as a spring board to talk about social media? Well, asking you to read such a long novel runs against the grain of the cyberculture we are studying.

The entire novel's plot drives toward completing the circle or monopolizing the world. Not a world government, but a world corporation.

I end by reminding you that the drive for unlimited knowledge is not new. It dates back to the famous German legend of Faust and for total knowledge Faust sold his soul to the devil. A world ruled by technology and data may end up a world without a soul.

INVESTIGATIONS

Challenge (25 XP)

The Lure of Narcissism

Investigation Reports

Facebook: The Socially Networked Self (50 XP)
This investigation brings to conclusion your report from last week. Complete your own Facebook page or update your current page if you have one and send a screen shot of your page to Professor Grey.

Or

LinkedIn: The Professionally Networked Self (50 XP)
This investigation brings to conclusion your report from last week. Complete your own LinkedIn page or update your current page if you have one and send a screen shot of your page to Professor Grey.

Student Journal
On The Circle *(TBD) 25 XP*

Self-Revelation or Exhibitionism?
Discuss among your classmates through 1 initial post and a minimum of 2 responses to others' posts what you feel to be the cause and consequences of over sharing personal information in a public forum. Why do people post things such as pictures of intoxicated behavior at a party, boasting about sexual conquests or even clips of criminal acts? What does this say about our current sense of self? What needs are we fulfilling? Is there a sense of privacy anymore and what information should remain private and confidential?

Notice how so many of the class assignments in *Secrets* encourage, even require students to communicate. Getting students to participate is even more an issue in online classes than it is when everyone is in the same room. If we just try to copy how we conduct in-person classes online, we make it harder than ever to reach our students, let alone share our knowledge with them.

Bonus: Four Square (50 XP)

For the rest of the term play the online location-based game *Four Square*. This game works with mobile devices and *GPS*. You accumulate points and/or badges as you check in from various places. Those who log in the most become Mayor. Simply keep track of your progress and make weekly observations in your journal titled: **Episode 2 Four Square**, **Episode 3 Four Square**. Your bonus points will be tallied by me, Professor Grey, in Episode 8. Each entry only needs to be 25 words at most.

Final Project Chapter Three Suggestions: My Professional Self

For your third chapter, focus on your professional or career identity, which means primarily your current job, jobs, and learning that led to where you are now and where you plan to be before retirement. How, if at all, has your online experience contributed to your professional life through training, job searching, or networking? Today, most people begin job searches through online papers, or massive online employment services like Monster.com or even career-specific specialized services that target individual career paths like educators or engineers. Online networking has also proven to be invaluable in the 21st century. Today we can communicate with people all over the world in a way not possible in the past. Likewise, give some account to education and how this has contributed to your professional or work identity. In this case, you are enrolled in an online course and an online institution. How does this experience compare with any other educational experiences you have had in a classroom environment?

CLASS FORUM (30 XP)

At this point there will hopefully be a lot of discussion that we'll need to monitor. Tom and Ann can begin to focus on moving the story forward. Ann and Tom will still comment as needed to initiate discussion in class-specific forum topics.

IF someone has asked Audra about the CareHart Foundation, they will receive the following response from Audra:

Audra

Good for you, [student name or names]!

It's worth repeating that naming students wherever possible is an easy intrinsic reward which keeps them engaged.

Yes, actually Edmund Hart was the first inspiration. Of course, he had no idea then what genetics could do to realize his dream. I didn't want to just tell you about CareHare since your class is about exploring the Internet. But I knew you guys would get there sooner or later. I never dreamed it would be this fast though! Well done!

If someone asks about "synchronize lives," then:

Audra

"I didn't use those words as a clue. I've studied the history of Primal Empathy of course. I guess they just stuck with me!"

IF no students have asked Audra about the CareHart Foundation, Ann will report that she has:

Ann Bennett Post

Hi Everybody. So, I asked Audra if she knew the CareHart Foundation. Her answer was a little weird. Here's what she emailed me: "Good for you, Ann! Yes, actually Edmund Hart was the first inspiration. Of course, he had no idea then what genetics could do to realize his dream. I didn't want to just tell you about CareHart since your class is about exploring the Internet. But I knew you guys would get there sooner or later. I never dreamed it would be this fast though! Well done!" I then asked her if she'd deliberate used the words "synchronize lives" as a clue. But she swears she didn't. She said, "They just stuck with me."

Tom Wetherall Post in Response

I have to say I was suspicious of The Collective. I hoped they were on the up and up, but there was no way to tell. But if they started as the CareHart Foundation I think their heart's (no pun intended!) in the right place. What was all that in the last Fortress 9 video? Kenyon doesn't sound so sure of himself as he did in the beginning. It's only been three weeks.

Give time for students to reply, then Logan:

Logan Grey Post in Response

We've only been involved for three weeks. Dale's been opposing The Collective for who knows how long? But you're right. He was pretty clear how he felt in the first two videos. His attitude in the last one surprised me, too.

Tom Wetherall Post

Professor Grey, could you ask the CareHart lady—Sallie something—if she'd be willing to talk to the class, maybe answer some questions?

Logan Grey Post in Response

I think that's a terrific idea. Maybe I can arrange a Skype call or something. What does everybody else think?

Students reply. Ann answers:

Ann Bennett Post in Response

I think it's a great idea!

After enough have replied:

Logan Grey Post in Response

I'll see if she can visit next week.

CHAPTER 30

Episode 4 – Change of Heart

LEARNING OUTCOMES

By the end of this episode successful students will be able to:

1. Create communication artifacts imaging the interpersonal relationships between offline and online identities.

CHARACTERS

Logan Grey, Tom Wetherall, Ann Bennett, Audra Casey, Dale Kenyon, Sallie Lopez

NARRATIVE

Tom tells the class he has met someone online, and wonders if he should ask to meet her in person. Dale Kenyon sends a video. He and the other members of Fortress 9 have been wrong about The Collective. He outlines what he has discovered, and places it alongside, what the class has discovered about the CareHart Foundation. The CareHart Foundation is obviously where The Collective's ideals were born. He urges the students to do everything they can to help The Collective by ensuring that CareHart does not betray its own ideals. At the end of the video Audra appears and hugs him. She would much rather have Dale as a friend than an enemy. Tom is delighted. Ann? Not so much.

VIDEO (2)

Before Dale's new video is available:

Logan Grey (Live)

Hi folks. Sallie Lopez won't be able to Skype with us, but she's agreed to a short text Q&A session. So, we're going to start class with that since I haven't received any new videos from The Collective or Fortress 9 yet.

Live Text Q&A with Sallie Lopez

> While not a video, the Live Text Q & A is included here for continuity. The answers from "Sallie Lopez" were given by an Excelsior instructional designer.

As the session is ending, Tom Wetherall makes a post on the Class Forum and asks everyone to have a look at it. (See Episode 4 Class Forum section.)

About Face

Dale Kenyon stands in front of the brick wall, looking more relaxed than we've ever seen him.

Dale

Some things have been happening here. We've had a number of defections from Fortress 9, including a couple of our top people. I want to make this clear up front that they weren't kidnapped, brainwashed or drugged or even had their DNA rearranged for them.

We have these sit-down discussions every night about our goals, strategy, tactics, and so on. Even before I first reached out to you some Fortress 9 people were thinking maybe we made up this enemy because we needed one. We've been taking on political causes for a long time. And when Primal Empathy started to capture everybody's attention, we may have jumped too soon to oppose it. I mean, I think we realized it could put us out of a job.

What happens to the opposition, if there is nothing left to oppose? What if the idea we were against actually might work? Maybe we should be helping it cause we ARE against poverty, war and hatred. Who wouldn't be?

I've been doing my own investigating, just as you have. The CareHart Foundation is obviously where The Collective's ideals were born. There's a clear path up through the decades. Seventy years. And what happened: fewer wars, less hatred, a more balanced society worldwide both emotionally and economically.

So, I feel pretty stupid right now. But I can't go on spouting stuff I no longer believe in. I don't know if Primal Empathy is the way I personally want to go. I actually think some people might learn empathy the old-fashioned way: by example.

If I were to ask you to do something now it would be this: do everything you can to help The Collective by ensuring the CareHart Foundation does not betray its own ideals. It's in your power to really make this work.

But don't do it on my account. Don't stop investigating, don't stop asking questions. I know you probably have a lot of questions for me. But if there's one way I can prove how sincere I am, here it is.

He looks off screen.

Okay. Ready.

Audra walks into FRAME, now wearing a casual purple tunic and slacks.

Audra

Hi everybody! You probably have a lot of questions for me, too. Neither one of us is going away. We'll both do what we can to help you help us. But for now, I came here to lend support to Dale. It isn't easy making a life change like this. But as Edmund Hart believed back in your time: it can be done. I want Dale to continue to push us to be true to our ideals, to be true to the entire human race.

She hugs Dale. He looks a little awkward and embarrassed. She smiles at him.

Audra
Go ahead. Say it!
  [Dale gives a rueful grin.]

Dale
Dale Kenyon. Out.

PROFESSOR GREY'S BRIEFINGS

Briefing 1: Romancing the Web: Dating and Sex Identity in Cyberspace

Essential Question for Episode 4: How has the Internet impacted the experience of intimacy?

Few topics pertaining to the Internet are more compelling and more controversial than intimacy. Indeed, the web provides a compelling case for the paradoxical reality of "intimate strangers." People have carried on full scale romances with distant partners they never end up meeting in a physical space while others begin a relationship online and move to the offline or molecular world as we will see in talking about this week's film *Catfish*. A question to think about this week is what is the relationship between online intimacy and offline intimacy? How do they relate and/or change each other?

Let's begin by recalling cyber psychologist Sherry Turkle's early explorations of cyber identity, way back in the nascent days of the Internet, pre-World Wide Web, describing how a computer's multiple windows allow for parallel lives. On a single computer screen, you can open up multiple windows. You can align those windows next to each other on the screen. Each window, as the metaphor indicates, provides an imaginative space for acting out different roles. In the window, screen left, you could be working on a Word file, say writing a memo to your boss, while, on screen right, you could be conducting a very salacious chat using another name and identity with a stranger from across the country or even on the other side of the globe.

The racy chat session is psychologically every bit as real as the memo even if you never actually speak or meet your anonymous chat partner. Does such a situation cause cognitive dissonance, i.e. a feeling of discomfort produced by a situation involving conflicting attitudes or have we now adapted to such situations to the point where any dissonance has been incorporated into the ability to present parallel lives with the same degree of comfort we did before the rise of the Internet?

Most cellular phones now include a built-in camera and also the possibility of transmitting or sharing the photos with other phones or posting to a social media site like Instagram. Around 15% of teens 12–17 who possess a cell phone have encountered sexting, either sending or receiving one. That's a very high percentage and as the use of cell phones expands—well over 80% of American teens have one—the trend seems troubling.

In this case, cyberspace allows for the increasing possibility of prematurely sexualizing a teenager's identity. In other words, teens are exposed to sexual material at increasingly younger ages, even pre-teen years. How can this cultural saturation affect an identity already under stress?

Perhaps most troubling is the fact these explicit and personal pictures can so easily be shared without the sender's consent. For example, a girl might break up with a boy and that boy can send an explicit picture of his now former girlfriend to his male friends or even a class in general damaging the girl's reputation and necessarily adversely affecting her self-esteem and identity.

In line with this notion of experimenting through technology sexting also extends beyond the teenage years.

The most noted example of adult sexting involved 49-year-old United States Congressman Anthony Weiner from New York City, whose sexts exposed through his social media Twitter account ended up in his resignation from office. Weiner's public apology led to his plea for a second chance and, he, subsequently, ran for Mayor of New York City, but he was once again exposed as sexting to a woman less than half his age. In this latest case, Wiener was using another identity. This public episode of parallel identities raises complicated questions of identity. Was or is Anthony Weiner the married former Congressman the same as the person who sexts a number of women? How does one reconcile married and public life with this private, but maybe not so private behavior? Is Mr. Weiner a sex addict? Is he acting in an immoral fashion? Is sexting a form of infidelity? How has cyberspace changed ideas of fidelity and even marriage? These questions are for debate and definitive answers do not exist. Your role as both learner and citizen is to give this complex question serious thought.

Some scholars argue the Internet is a great dating space for shy people who have trouble socializing. Additionally, the initially text-based nature of the Internet allowed people to get to know each other independent of the first impressions formed by physical appearance. People could get matched according to mutual interest and personality traits right from the beginning supposedly improving the chances for long-term relationship success. This does make a certain amount of sense, but even in a purely text-based environment honesty can be played with. We'll briefly discuss this in this episode's second briefing. To conclude here, I want to touch on two final questions of identity, intimacy, and cyberspace.

In the further readings for this week, you will find a pioneering article in the *Village Voice* by Internet journalist Julian Dibbell called "A Rape in Cyberspace." Dibbell describes what he calls rape, but one that actually takes place entirely between two people who never met in the "real" or molecular world.

Now over twenty years later, cyber bullying has emerged as a real-world problem that has resulted in tragic teenage suicides. Words can cause physical harm.

My final subtopic is the controversial, but real problem of pornography and the Internet.

How this explosion of Internet pornography seeps into our culture and impacts our identity is hard to say. Just as the Internet provides space for bullying it also provides space for sexual predators. Ethical and legal questions are numerous, but so are psychological ones.

One of the foundations pornography builds upon is the objectification and debasement of women. What kind of effect does this disturbing premise have on both maturing girls, but also adults conducting a relationship? Many scholars now write about the "pornification" of culture. Are we being desensitized to pornography? Ultimately, should the government step in and provide some regulation of cyberspace or should civil liberties prevail?

This week gives you time to at least think about these often hidden or unaddressed cultural questions.

Briefing 2: *Catfish*: Truth, Lying and Internet Affairs of the Heart

The independent film *Catfish* (2010) focuses on what happens when a couple in a seemingly intimate online relationship attempts to bring the relationship offline.

Way back in 1889 the great Irish writer and personality Oscar Wilde wrote an inventive essay in the form of Platonic dialogue called "The Art of Lying." Wilde's personae, the character Vivian (also the name of one of Wilde's sons, notice the gender ambiguity), makes the famous statement that "Life Imitates Art."

This century old quote applies to much of what we are thinking and writing about in this course. Paradoxically, for Wilde, truth is simply a form of beautiful untruth. As I mentioned and will continue to stress, Cyberculture is the symbol of cultural complexity and thus far the puzzle has eluded our solutions and interpretations.

INVESTIGATIONS
Challenge (25 XP)

Lost in Cyberspace or Searching for Truth?

Investigation Reports
Me the Catfish (75 XP)

Using the avatar/online personae you created at the beginning of the course write a short sequence of emails (2 emails and 2 responses) between you and someone you would like to meet, but who knows nothing about you or write an imaginary chat room dialogue (150 words or so) between your avatar and someone that you would like to meet but who knows nothing about you. Follow this part of the assignment with a one paragraph description, narrative, or dialogue about an imagined actual meeting between the two of you (what would you say and where would you meet etc.).

Student Journal
A Counterfeit Life?

After *Catfish* premiered, critics claimed the entire documentary was a hoax reminiscent of the famous *The Blair Witch Project*. Yet, if a hoax then the documentary would be a piece of fiction not nonfiction, but doesn't fiction often reveal deeper truths about real life than so-called real-life stories? After all, what is reality and what constitutes a fact? Write a 250-word entry on your impressions of the film and its impact on human identity. What is real and unreal? Do we ever truly know another person? Is our ultimate identity a mystery even to ourselves?

Intimate Strangers

Discuss among your classmates whether the potential anonymity and spatial irrelevance of cyberspace benefits or hinders interpersonal communication. As part of your conversation talk about how the pervasive display of largely unregulated sexual material has or could have an impact on interpersonal relationships in the physical world. For example, is cybersex a form of cheating? Does the Internet encourage or make possible an increase in actual child abuse or pedophilia? Has the explosion of amateur pornography contributed to a destruction of intimacy? Will children be sexualized too early in their development? How does one know the truth in an online world?

Bonus: Love and Software (75 XP)

Spike Jonze's inventive science fiction film *Her* (2013) tells the story of a heartbroken writer, who deals ironically with other peoples' relationships, falling in love with a computer operating system which he personifies as a disembodied female. This encounter between human and artificially intelligent machine brings together central themes of this course about identity, human computer interaction, relationships, connection/disconnection, and embodiment versus disembodiment. For this assignment, watch the film and write a 250–500-word letter to Professor Grey telling him what you think of this film's depiction of romantic relationships in the digital age. This will be the theme of our next episode.

Final Project Episode Four Suggestions: Intimate Identity

For this chapter focus on your intimate self to the extent you are willing to share with anyone. If you are married or were married or remarried those are all major events to record. When, where and how did such an event or events come about? How about a wedding photo or divorce certificate? What about your first date or your first sexual experience? Have you ever had a cyber connection of any kind or ever thought about one?

CLASS FORUM (50 XP)

Ann and Tom will comment as needed to initiate discussion in class-specific forum topics.
   Before Dale's new video is available:

Tom Wetherall Post

Given the topics this week I thought this might be a good time to share something with the class. Whether it's self-revelation or narcissism I don't know! lol One of the reasons I took this class is that I met somebody online a few months ago. Not Match dot com or e-Harmony. We're in the same guild in World of Warcraft. We've been questing for quite a while now (and that's all!), but we've also been talking. And it turns out she lives in Springfield Mass which is not all that far away. You probably see my question coming, but I really want everybody's advice. Should we meet up? In real life?

Wait for some student responses, then Ann:

Ann Bennett Post in Response

If you're both being honest about who you are and you're getting along, why not? Have you shared pictures? There's a reason I chose my picture for this class. It isn't because I'm looking for sympathy. These wheels are a part of who I am. So, I like to let people know right up front.

Tom Wetherall Post in Response

I emailed her a picture. The goofy one I use here. And I told her about my job for the health food distributor. My sign, my hobbies, my favorite movies, the whole nine yards. So yeah, I think we trust each other.

Logan Grey Post in Response

I've just received a new video from Fortress 9 and it is a mind blower. Better have a look! Then start a discussion here in the forum! I'll be chiming in, too.
    Give time for students to see the video, then:

Tom Wetherall Post in Response

Wow. That is crazy! But I guess I'm not all that surprised. And it sounds like it's for the best.

Ann Bennett Post in Response

He caved. That's all. They got to him somehow.
    At some point in the discussion:

Logan Gray Post

This does not mean our class, or our investigations are over!

Ann Bennett Post in Response

It sure doesn't! I've been trying to figure out what it was about Audra's appearance that was wrong. Well, I know now that I saw the outfit when she walked out to join Dale. I have one just like it. I'm not from the future. And I'm not sure she is either! And if she isn't, then neither is Dale, and there's something phony about this whole deal!

CHAPTER 31

Episode 5 – Follow the Money

LEARNING OUTCOMES

By the end of this episode successful students will be able to:

1. Identify what makes games an engaging human experience.

2. Describe the relationship between a role-played identity and an everyday world identity.

CHARACTERS

Logan Grey, Tom Wetherall, Ann Bennett, Audra Casey

NARRATIVE

Tom is thrilled with the happy outcome and the part the class played. He has sent a free sample bottle of his company's new mineral water to everyone (including Logan) as a reward for their efforts. Ann insists the conflict in the future is all too neatly wrapped up. She suggests they investigate the CareHart Foundation, even if it means hacking into their computers! Inside CareHart computers students will find the beginning of a digital money trail that leads them from CareHart to the genetics company Chromogen and its wunderkind founder Desmond Wright. Tom is surprised, but doesn't see any dark purpose in the connection.

VIDEO (1)

Audra Reaches Out

Audra wears the casual purple tunic and slacks. She's framed in a MEDIUM CLOSE again as in her first video and the backdrop is the same, but without the Fortress 9 logo.

Audra

Hi Everybody! I know you must be still reeling from Fortress 9 joining our search for peace and harmony! Also, I've been asked about my clothes! What can I say? Our world is still much like your time. We don't have hovercrafts or sentient robots and the colony on Mars is still small even though they advertise it as the New Alaska and offer lots of financial incentives to relocate there! We're also not all wearing gray or silver jumpsuits! Fashions come and go in cycles. Ann should know that. Purple is hot! I'm glad we both have the same good taste!

To be honest, I was surprised, too when Dale told me about his change of heart. I'm sure glad they are onboard. But I also want to assure you that we welcome any dialogue with people opposed to Primal Empathy. We can learn from all points of view, even those who have not yet had the opportunity to accept our **[MODIFER] [HELP]**!

At this moment the video will have a glitch in it. While Audra can clearly be saying the longer word "modifier," her voice has been dubbed at that point with the word "help." See the Episode 5 Forum Section for how this will play out.

There is still much we can do, and you can too! Thanks so much for your efforts so far. I hope you'll support the CareHart Foundation and its mission. It is the first step in a new era of prosperity and harmony that will unite all the people of Earth.

That's all for now. Talk to you soon!

PROFESSOR GREY'S BRIEFING
Briefing: Online Games and Cyberculture

Essential Questions for Episode 5: How does the explosion of online and downloadable games impact your sense of self? Do you roleplay in games? If so, how does your game identity differ from or reinforce your non-game identity?

> Since the students are playing an alternate reality game as part of the class, I have left some additional detail in this briefing.

The principal appeal and value of games can be summarized in the following points:

1. Deep levels of engagement. Games immerse players in their world and require players to always do something unlike movies which require only passive watching.

2. Players act and perform in the game world and can even modify games they download.

3. Promote systems level thinking, i.e. examining a problem from all the interrelated angles necessary to understand a problem like climate change or urban decay.

4. Promote situated learning, i.e. what you learn has a real-world context that applies to your learning unlike an isolated classroom.

5. Enable a state of flow described by psychologist Mihaly Csikszentmihalyi as optimal performance or being in the zone. Think of Michael Jordon's scoring sprees in the 1990s or any professional athlete performing at his or her best.

6. They are fun.

7. Players can roleplay. You can be a detective or an elf or a warrior.

Games also work according to a player's intrinsic, as well as his or her extrinsic motivation. Achieving a grade of "A" is an example of extrinsic motivation. You are rewarded for your immediate performance at a point in time, but a month later that "A" does not always transfer into long-term learning. Intrinsic motivation means you learn regardless of a reward or learning for learning's sake.

> For more examples of intrinsic and extrinsic rewards that can used in game-based learning, see *The Multiplayer Classroom: Designing Coursework as a Game* (Second Edition, CRC Press, 2020).

Psychologists Scott Rigby and Richard Ryan investigated the intrinsic motivation captured by video games in an excellent book called *Glued to Games: How Video Games Draw Us In and Hold Us Spellbound* (Praeger/New Directions in Media, 2011). They conducted experiments, interviews, focus groups, and observations of avid games players. As a result, Rigby and Ryan found three major ingredients that make up intrinsic motivation: Competence, autonomy, and relatedness.

Each of these three elements can be further subdivided. Beginning with competence, people need challenges to develop a sense of competence. The challenges must be serious, but not unobtainable. Everyone's own skill level requires a different type or degree of challenge and the leveling systems of games work well to help players achieve competence. A second aspect of competence is the need for continual, rapid, and meaningful feedback. If you don't receive a grade until the midterm exam, that feedback is too slow. If the feedback only provides a grade, then that feedback is almost meaningless. In a game every player action elicits feedback from game mechanics that can be used by the player to improve his or her gameplay. Finally, competence requires an acceptance of failure. You fail an exam and you are in serious trouble, but if you die in *Mario Brothers* you can get up and try again. Players learn from experience.

The second factor making up intrinsic motivation is autonomy. Games address autonomy or the need to make one's own decisions in a variety of ways. They encourage experimentation and exploration of different adventure paths. Players can often roleplay different identities from crime scene investigator to city manager. Players, like you, can create a customized avatar. Most important, in the words of Civilization designer Sid Meir, "Games are a series of meaningful choices."

> This quote applies even more directly to game-based learning. In these games, we serve two needs. We must make the choices meaningful to both the game and the lesson to be learned.

Relatedness completes the triad of factors composing intrinsic motivation. Humans are social beings and need to relate to others. Most games today are played with others whether friends, family, or strangers. As social beings we like to feel supported, acknowledged, and finally, that we matter. Do you feel this at work or college? Maybe work and school should be more like a game.

Maybe???

Types of Online Games

You are playing an Alternate Reality Game. You can Google *i love bees* to see video clips of a famous, enormously popular, Alternate Reality Game that involved many tens of thousands playing collaboratively to solve problems leading up to a release party for *Halo 2*.

> "These games (which are usually free to play) often have a specific goal of not only involving the player with the story and/or fictional characters but of connecting them to the real world and to each other. Many game puzzles can be solved only by the collaborative efforts of multiple players, sometimes requiring one or more players to get up from their computers to go outside to find clues or other planted assets in the real world."
>
> *The Alternate Reality Network, www.argn.com, retrieved March 13, 2014.*

We have talked about social media during much of the course. Many online games are played from social media sites in order to share information between players' networks. Zynga's *Farmville* released, in 2009, has been especially successful. Social media games can be educational as well as entertaining. *Half the Sky* has been played by over a million people in less than a year on Facebook. This socially conscious game, aka a game for impact, has raised half a million dollars to support girls and women living under oppressed conditions. Similarly, the Games4Change movement supports games that have a major social impact.

Games for Health is another movement that seeks to benefit people's well-being. These games deal with everything from post-traumatic stress to diabetes. The free game *ReMission* designed for childhood victims of terminal cancer have shown to dramatically improve the children's awareness of their disease as well as improve remission.

> One of the episodes I wrote for the website, *Extra Credits*, examines some more games for impact, including more recent ones. (Episode 469: *Saving the World with Games – Citizen Science and More*, May 13, 2020.)

Online games can be both entertaining and educational.

The Opposition

The two most popular points of opposition being video games cause violent behavior in teenagers or young adults and they are addictive. Let me take these two somewhat misguided objections in turn. Video games have always had a fair number that present violent environments from the classic *Doom* to the recent *Grand Theft Auto* series. Most of these games are first person shooters and they tend to attract teenage males. Yes, the Columbine shooter played video games, but millions of non-shooters have as well. Youth violence and delinquency, especially among young males, has existed as a perceived social problem, for 75 years. Comic books were originally supposed to cause violent behavior, then film, then TV, then rap music, and now video games. Nonsense. In every case teenagers or youth are a scapegoat for complicated social issues adults do not want to take responsibility for. Not only is cause and effect argumentation deeply flawed, the entire culture of violence in western society far outweighs the effect of a genre of games. Football, the United States' most popular sport, is violent. Mixed Martial Arts grows in popularity. Audiences love movies about mobsters. Even good guys are violent from Clint Eastwood's *Dirty Harry* to Quentin Tarrantino's various protagonists. Finally, those young males who do end up committing violence may have a predisposition to violence or an aggressive trait or, even more likely, they struggle from some emotional stress. No, violent video games do not cause violence.

As for addiction, that is a psychiatric diagnosis not yet endorsed by the medical profession.

> In 2019 the World Health Organization (WHO) did include "gaming disorder" in its list of mental disorders, relating it to addictions such as gambling in their controversial decision. It does not address violence in video games.

Like any activity, even exercising too much or compulsive behavior can be unhealthy. You can measure when something becomes too much when it has an adverse effect on a person's daily functioning: poor sleep, poor eating habits, missing work, neglecting friends, spending money that cannot be afforded, and so on. I mentioned in the last episode that responsible parenting can often cut off compulsive behavior before it gets out of control. No doubt online and video games, like most forms of digital technology, can be compulsive, just watch how many people cannot function without their cell phones, but if someone goes so far as to commit an act of violence that person invariably has an underlying emotional problem. For those youth who resort to violence, games are only a release for a problem that no one in the adult world has dealt with for whatever reason.

Games have been around since the beginning of culture. Kids learn about the world through games. Games foster imaginative growth. My recommendation is to make room for play.

INVESTIGATIONS

Challenge (25 XP)

The Apathy Trap

Investigation Reports

The Flow of Life [75 XP]

Create a simple timeline of when you have experienced *flow* in your life, i.e. at what points have you had a peak experience and what was it. You can use Word and simply draw a line across the page then plot the years and your age along the line and underneath the year of a peak experience. For example, I recall my first peak experience as hitting a triple in Little League at age 10. My most recent peak was giving an interview in New York City for a documentary/mystery called "Mysteries at the Museum."

Student Journal

Neuromancer and the Virtual Cowboy (30 XP)

The protagonist Case is referred to as a console cowboy meaning he adopts an American western's style identity, but in a virtual world. Write a brief entry on your impressions of the character and focus on what makes him a modern version of the cowboy.

Homo Ludens (30 XP)

Summarize your experience of playing your chosen game for a week. What kind of identity did you assume and what affect, if any, does playing have on your own sense of identity?

My Game of Life (30 XP)

Identify the game you chose to play with your classmates and describe your initial experience. What do you think about the game with particular reference to your player identity? Also discuss why you think people continue to play games throughout their life and the role games play in civilized life.

Bonus (35 XP)

Continue to play your chosen game up until the final episode and then submit a 350-words (1 and ½ pages) summary of your experience to Professor Grey in Episode 8.

Final Project Episode Five Suggestions: Games and Me

For this chapter, focus on how games have impacted you. You don't have to focus on video games, but you can. Think about arcade games, early *Pac Man* or *Mario Brothers*, but also recall your childhood which might include *Hopscotch*, *Checkers*, *Chutes and Ladders*, or family games like *Monopoly* and then athletic games such as basketball, soccer, golf etc. Games may impact your relationship with your parents or children as well.

CLASS FORUM (30 XP)

Notwithstanding the military IT student who I mentioned earlier already knew Ann and Tom were not who they claimed, at this point some other students surely began to doubt Ann and Tom were entirely who they claimed. And by the end of this class forum everybody must have realized they weren't in Kansas anymore.

Tom Wetherall Post

Hey, folks. I've gotten permission from work to give everybody a free sample of the new all-natural mineral water, Nectar Rich, that we're promoting. If you'll give me your physical addresses privately, we can send some out immediately! I guarantee it is the best-tasting and healthiest drink you'll ever try!

Ack! Here I was again ready to dole out a questionable beverage to unsuspecting students. Happily, only three or four students took Tom up on his offer and were shipped bottles. In the first *Skeleton Chase*, the "healthy" water was ordinary bottled water with the label removed. In *Skeleton Chase 3: Warp Speed*, bottles of vitamin water were the Trailhead/Rabbit Hole.

Logan Grey Post in Response

Hi Tom. I'm afraid we don't allow commercial pitches in our online classes. However, since it's free, and since I find most mineral water pretty tasteless, I'll give it a try.
After a suitable time:

Ann Bennett Post

Not that health isn't an important topic, but I'd like to address the latest video from Audra. Okay, maybe fashions do come around again. But this whole thing has been too neatly wrapped up. I think we should investigate the CareHart Foundation. What does everybody else think?
After a suitable time, and then in rapid succession (every couple of minutes):

Tom Wetherall Post in Response

What is there to find? Their website is bran [**Deliberate misspelling.**] new and there isn't much to see there.

Ann Bennett Post in Response

I think we can use the website to get access to their computers. Any computer hooked up to the Internet is vulnerable, and no security can't be bypassed.

Tom Wetherall Post in Response

Oh right, you're the programmer chick. Anybody ever tell you that hacking other people's computers is illegal, honey?

Ann Bennett Post in Response

Anybody ever tell you you just got really condescending, honey?

Tom Wetherall Post in Response

Okay, right. I'm sorry for breathing! Are you saying you can hack into CareHart's computers in the next hour? Day? Week?

Ann Bennett Post in Response

I don't know how long it will take but I intend to try.

Logan Gray Post in Response

Hold on, folks. Let's bring this exchange to a close now. Tom, you are out of line with that tone, and I suggest you calm down. But Ann, Tom's right about one thing. What you're proposing, as you well know, is highly illegal. And you've just announced to a bunch of people you barely know that you intend to break the law. I'm surprised that given the subject matter of this class you're being so open about it, and I want you to stop. You'll have to find another way.

Tom Wetherall Post in Response

I'm sorry I was condescending, Ann. But Prof. Grey's right. Don't do it.

Ann Bennett Post in Response

I have already found a backdoor in. For anybody who wants to have a look, I'll send you the link privately. You really need to take a look. You too, Prof. Grey. I think you may change your mind.

After a suitable time waiting for private communications with Ann:

> If any students had any doubt that not only were class and subject inexorably entwined, but so were player-characters and NPCs, Logan's final post below should have convinced them. After all they were prepared for this transition of the situation from suspected to overt from the very beginning. Logan Grey was not their instructor's real name.

Logan Grey Post in Response

Alright, I looked, too. There is evidence that the CareHart Foundation is connected to a genetics company called Chromogen. That connection may be what Primal Empathy will be born from. But I don't see anything sinister in that. Here's a link to Chromogen and its founder Desmond Wright: www.chromogen.com. Please, no one else hack into the CareHart computers! Have a look at the Chromogen site. How do you feel about its connection to CareHart? Let's discuss this, and what you think we should do about it, if anything.

CHAPTER 32

Episode 6 – Wolves in Sheep's Clothing

LEARNING OUTCOMES

By the end of this episode successful students will be able to:

1. Define virtual reality.

2. Analyze the impact of virtual reality on physical or molecular identity.

3. Produce a piece of fan fiction.

CHARACTERS

Logan Grey, Tom Wetherall/Elliot Plevin, Ann Bennett

NARRATIVE

Learning more about Chromogen, students will discover a picture of a researcher there named Elliot Plevin. He is a dead ringer for Tom Wetherall! Elliot admits who he is, but claims his intentions were honorable. He accuses Ann of working for a rival corporation with nefarious motives. Someone hacks the class website, deleting bios, pictures and scrambling avatars, so students only know who they are communicating with if they know the real name behind the avatar. Both Elliot and Ann claim to be innocent and each blames the other.

> I have used both good and evil characters in every game in this book and in my own multiplayer classrooms as well, who are not what they claim to be. A surprise like that is one of the easiest ways to keep the mystery alive and players interested. In *Secrets* opposing NPCs were used to their best advantage: to highlight the theme of the class and drive discussions with their differing opinions. Now the students were firmly transitioned from observers to players, as Professor Grey looks at the metaphor that "life is a game."

VIDEO (0)

Professor Grey's Briefings

Briefing: Simulation and the 'Desert of The Real'

Essential Question for Episode 6: How does your thinking about and experience with virtual reality in literature and film inform/shape your perception of reality and self?

This week I will take up the well-known metaphor that "life is a game" only now the metaphor becomes literal. In other words, we are moving from role-playing identities in a game to the possibility of role-playing outside a clearly defined rule-bound experience. As the fool, Jacques, says in Shakespeare's great comedy *As You Like It*:

> "All the world's a stage
> And all the men and women merely players."

Interestingly, Shakespeare's plays often took place at the famous Globe Theatre, a simulation (which I will define in a second) par excellence, a model of the actual globe as known during Shakespeare's time.

The Matrix was released in 1999 on the threshold of the new millennium. The directors openly acknowledge that much of the concept underlying *The Matrix* is based upon the French sociologist, Jean Baudrillard's most famous book *Simulacra and Simulation* (1981). In fact, very early on, the movie displays a cover of the English translation onscreen.

Defining simulation can be tricky, but let's start by saying a simulation presents an abstract model of an original. If you conduct a fire drill at work or school, you are simulating a real fire evacuation. It is not real as there is no fire, but everyone follows procedures as if there is a fire in preparation for that future possibility. In other words, one's actions are real in service of a real goal, but within an "unreal" or simulated environment.

Baudrillard's work is generally discussed in graduate school, but I will attempt to elucidate his major insight into simulations and culture. In a compelling essay called "The Orders of Simulacra" (Simulations, New York: Semiotext (e), 1983), Baudrillard divides western culture into three periods, what he calls orders, of how signs function:

- **The Feudal Era**

- **The Modern Industrial Era**

- **The Postmodern Era or Era of the Simulacra**

In this final order the simulacra would be like a giant copy machine and reality just copies of copies. We start with a representation, fashion on television and that representation produces a public reproducing the representation in a chain of symbols with no referent.

The final stage is hard for most people to grasp since we like to think we live in reality, but Baudrillard is taking Oscar Wilde's conceit that life imitates art and pushing it even further, so, in a sense, art imitates more art. This is like existing inside a computer, a situation which provides the premise for *The Matrix*. The final order of the simulacra is what Baudrillard designated as hyperreality.

The idea of the world as an illusion or dream is nothing new. As you think and engage this week's material and that for the remaining weeks think about our collective future. Is technology and the Internet moving us toward utopia, a perfect world, or dystopia, a collapse?

INVESTIGATIONS

Challenge (25 XP)

The Rabbit Hole

Investigation Reports

Fan Fiction (75 XP total, 15 XP this episode and 60 next week's episode)

One of the most recent phenomena of 21st century culture is transmedia publishing whereby a primary product is released in a variety of formats, for example a Batman movie, a comic, and video game. An early example of this trend is fan fiction or stories that fans of a particular commercial story write about the main story and self-publish on a website or distribute through email and before that surface mail. Harry Potter has produced the most fan fiction of any story franchise. *The Matrix* has also generated much fan-based publication. For this report, write a short story (500+ words) on some aspect of either *The Matrix* or a game you may have referred to in the last episode. In fan fiction you take some aspect of the source material, or in this case the original film is expanded upon, or some new perspective is taken on the film's plot or characters. Your story will not be due until the end of the next episode but you must present your idea to Professor Grey for approval by the end of this episode. When finished, consider publishing your story on: https://www. fanfiction.net/.

Student Journal

The Matrix inverts what most people consider to be reality. The film's protagonist operates as computer programmer Thomas Anderson by day and super hacker Neo ("the one") within the matrix. Discuss with your classmates the similarities and differences between Anderson/Neo and Case from *Neuromancer* as either heroes or anti-heroes of cyberspace. How does each character's experience of virtual reality affect their experience of embodied or molecular offline identity?

Virtual Transvestism (30 XP)

One of the potentially liberating effects of cyberspace is the ability to "pass" as another race, sex, or ethnicity than your own. For example, a 45-year-old tall stocky African American ex-football player can easily play online personae as a 22-year-old petite co-ed. For this entry write two paragraphs of around 75–100 words each. In paragraph one; discuss Case's experience in Chapter 3 living within Molly's body. In other words, Case can physically experience what Molly's body experiences but think about that experience with his own mind. In your second paragraph, imagine what it would be like to experience a week as the opposite sex. Describe what you think this experience might feel like and how it might affect your current identity.

Final Project Episode Six Suggestions: Aspects of Your Identity

For this chapter you can explore two aspects of your identity. Who are you in cyberspace? Has cyberspace changed how you think about yourself? Can you remember your first online experience? Maybe you bought a book at Amazon.com or maybe you visited a taboo chat room? The other aspect of the Internet to touch on is fandom. What if anything are you a fan of, what makes you a fan and how have you expressed your fandom? For example, maybe you are a football fan of the Green Bay Packers or a fan of Agatha Christie mysteries, the character James Bond or a pop star like Mick Jagger of *The Rolling Stones*. At some time, all of ourselves are enveloped with what we admire.

CLASS FORUM (35 XP)

IF a student has found Elliot Plevin's picture buried in the Chromogen website and posted about it:

Tom Wetherall Post

Okay. Yes. My real name is Elliot Plevin and I do work for Chromogen. I am a bio-geneticist working hard to make this world a better place to live. Chromogen is committed to Edmund Hart's dream. We think it can be realized faster through DNA research. That's all I'm going to say about it. Except this: my intentions are honorable. I signed up for this class because a rival corporation has been trying to sabotage our efforts. There is a LOT of money at stake here. That's all they're interested in: the money. And Ann Bennett works for them. Just ask her.

IF no student has found Eliot's picture:

Logan Grey Post

I'm not sure what is going on here, but has anybody else found this link on the Chromogen site: www.chromogen.com/personnel/plevin? Tom? Mr. Plevin sure looks a lot like you. Before you are booted from this class, do you have anything to say?

Tom Wetherall Post in Response

Okay. Yes, Prof. Grey. My real name is Elliot Plevin and I do work for Chromogen. I am a bio-geneticist working hard to make this world a better place to live. Chromogen is committed to Edmund Hart's dream. We think it can be realized faster through DNA research. That's all I'm going to say about it, except this: my intentions are honorable. I signed up for this class because a rival corporation has been trying to sabotage our efforts. There is a LOT of money at stake here. That's all they're interested in: the money. And Ann Bennett works for them. Just ask her.

In either case:

Ann Bennett Post in Response

I do not work for a rival company. Tom is lying. I don't know why he is in this class but he's lying. Today I received my free bottle of NectarRich. I have a friend in the department of Chemistry at my school. I've asked her to analyze the contents. Until she gives me the results, I would strongly suggest NO ONE DRINK IT.

At this point the class website is hacked, its graphics are altered, bios are deleted, pictures vanish, and avatars scrambled, so students only know who they are communicating with if they know the real name behind the avatar.

This is actually an alternate version of the website that can easily be swapped in, then out again. The forum and all class materials remain available.

Even with students knowing at this point that it's all a game, messing with their online identity, reminding them how fragile the virtual world can be, can get a nice nervous system response. As you'll see in the final section of this book, I took this a step farther in *The Janus Door*.

Logan Grey Post

Everyone, someone has obviously hacked our server. None of your grades or assignments have been lost or damaged. This forum and all communication channels are still open. Please proceed with this week's investigations and assignments as normal. Excelsior has some pretty good programmers on staff, too. We'll have things working again as soon as possible.

Tom Wetherall Post in Response (Under Another Student's Name)

This is Tom/Elliot. I had nothing to do with this! I'm no programmer! It has to be Ann who's doing this!

Ann Bennett Post in Response (Under Another Student's Name)

Ann here, sorry [Student Name]! Elliot is lying again. He's trying to disrupt the class. The computers in RPI's Chemistry department are also under attack. I'm convinced there's something very wrong with NectarRich mineral water.

CHAPTER 33

Episode 7 – The Experiment

LEARNING OUTCOMES

At the end of this episode students will be able to:

1. Imagine and describe human identity after the year 2030.

2. Differentiate between an embodied and a disembodied identity.

3. Identify and apply Asimov's *Three Laws of Robotics* to a future conception of identity in a post-human world.

CHARACTERS

Logan Grey, Ann Bennett

NARRATIVE

The website restored, Ann informs the others that she has had her mineral water gift tested, and that it contains several ingredients of a suspicious nature: chemicals that can alter human perception. Ann says that with his class surveys and free mineral water Elliot appears to be testing early techniques in primal empathy on this class! From this point on, Elliot has for all intents and purposes vanished into cyberspace. Ann reveals herself to be an FBI cybercrime expert. She enlists the class' help to find proof of Chromogen's true purpose. She suggests students do not drink the water until more tests can be made! If any students have drunk it, they are asked to immediately report any unusual side effects!

Before this class begins Logan Grey emails the students with some good news.

Logan Grey Email

The website is back up and running. This week's lecture and assignments are all up. No data has been lost. Your work and grades are safe. And everybody's identity, bio and avatar have been restored to their true owners. Be online at [time &date] for a live chat session.

VIDEO (1)

Live Text Q&A with Logan Grey and Ann Bennett

While not a video, as with the Live Q&A with Sallie Lopez in Episode 4, this Live Text Q&A is positioned here for continuity. The texts from "Ann Bennett" were sent by an Excelsior instructional designer.

Logan Grey (Live)

I have to say with all honesty that this has been the most unusual class I've ever taught online or in a brick and mortar classroom. I think I have learned as much as you have about what is real and unreal on the Internet. Maybe more! And there's still another week after this!

But for now, I'm going to let one of your classmates, Ann Bennett, fill you in on the most recent developments. Then she will be happy to answer your questions. Ann?

Ann Bennett (Live)

Thank you, Prof. Grey. First of all, I know many of you are anxious about the mineral water you may have received. Our chemists have completed the analysis. The water does contain several suspect ingredients. The full effect is unknown, but each of these chemicals has demonstrated the ability to alter human perception to a greater or lesser extent. And not in everyone. Think of LSD, but with effects less unpredictable. What they do in combination is still to be discovered. If any of you drank the water, whatever the amount, you may not feel any effects, but if you do, please report any unusual side effects to me as soon as possible!

Now, as you've probably guessed, like Eliott Plevin, alias Tom Wetherall, I have not been completely honest about my own identity. My name really is Ann Bennett. That is my real picture on my personal page for the class. But I don't let the wheels get in my way at all. I'm not a programmer at RPI. I'm a member of the FBI cybercrime unit, part of the Operational Technology Division based in Quantico, Virginia.

I'm sure you have a lot of questions. I'm here to answer them as best as I can, but I also need your help. I'll explain how you can help soon, but for now let me answer your questions.

Ann's answers will be drawn from the following exposition.

In 2012 a massive outbreak of migraine headaches in an Internet class at the University of West Florida attracted our interest. Our team found a link to an account about Eliott Plevin, who early in his career mentioned at a conference certain chemicals that might be used to alter the behavior of DNA to increase psychic ability. He was laughed from the stage, but there was a note that Plevin said he was frustrated by a number of apparent migraine headaches in his test rats.

We searched for other classes that were studying the Internet. I became convinced that this course at Excelsior might be Plevin's next test case. But we knew he couldn't be doing this on his own, and no legitimate foundation would sponsor such research. Someone with more money and power than ethics must be financing his experiments.

We suspected Desmond Wright and Chromogen might be behind it when we discovered Plevin now worked at Chromogen, but we had no proof.

In the weeks before the class began our team came into possession of a damaged file found on the body of an associate of Plevin's who had died in an "accident." It mentioned his plan to make students susceptible to the experiment by claiming to contact them from a future Earth free from hatred and war where all citizens were becoming part of what they called The Collective. So, I signed up for the class.

Both The Collective and Fortress 9 were fabrications invented by Plevin. Audra Casey and Dale Kenyon both work for Chromogen.

Elliot Plevin is in custody and isolated. We don't know how much he's told Desmond Wright about his failure here, but Wright, as well as being a narcissistic egotist is also a paranoid schizophrenic. Plevin must have been terrified to reveal to him the failure of this second experiment. He swears he has told Wright nothing except that the class is investigating Chromogen. We have not arrested Audra Casey or Dale Kenyon as yet.

We suspect Wright still thinks everything is proceeding as planned. We need your help to find the last link in a chain of evidence that will convict Wright. Wright has set up a dummy file that will prove Chromogen's intentions are entirely above board. He expects this class to find it and his IT people are watching for an intrusion into his system from this class. Then he expects you to exonerate him.

However, Plevin says there is a separate file containing a handwritten letter by Wright that explains his entire plan in detail. Yes, handwritten! The irony is that Wright does not trust computers or the Internet. Plevin photographed that letter as an insurance policy. It could take months for us to get past Chromogen's firewall. But Wright is so self-confident he has left a back door wide open for this class.

So hack in. Ignore the planted file. Find the real location of that handwritten letter. It will undoubtedly be protected in some way. Once we have that, we can bring Wright's twisted dream crashing to earth. Here is the link: www.chromogen.org/lab6/cybervault/PE.

PROFESSOR GREY'S BRIEFINGS
Briefing 1: The Rise of the Cyborg or Hybrid Humanity

Essential Question for Episode 7: Has the 21st Century become a posthuman world?

My first briefing will address the nature of simulated human beings, robots and cyborgs. In the second briefing, we'll look back at William Gibson's *Neuromancer*. The essential question for this week is deeply metaphysical (i.e. that which goes beyond the physical).

Posthuman may seem a strange word to use for most of us who consider ourselves fully human. Posthuman, like the now common word, postmodern, has a rather paradoxical meaning. If humans are still here how can we talk about posthumanity? Let me explore this concept here as it will be vital in our final episode and in any future thinking about humanity's place in the universe.

Writers have portrayed robots for many decades. Perhaps the most famous science fiction author to write about robots was biochemist Isaac Asimov, one of the most prolific writers in history. Asimov, unlike most writers, knew science the way a scientist knows science. He wrote many robot stories way back into the 1940s. Some of these stories were recently adapted into a film called *I, Robot* starring Will Smith. Like many prophetic science fiction writers Asimov, worried about the possibility of robots someday getting out of control, much like Mary Shelly's *Frankenstein* (1818) creature, the world's first machine man. As a protection for humanity Asimov developed:

The Three Laws of Robotics

1. A robot may not injure a human being or through inaction, allow a human being to come to harm.

2. A robot must obey the orders given to it by human beings, except where such orders would conflict with the First Law.

3. A robot may not injure its own kind and defend its own kind unless it is interfering with the first or second rule.

Asimov writes from a humanist perspective. He wants robots to serve the ends of man in a rational and ethical fashion. Once a robot violates one of the three laws, that robot threatens our humanity and allows for the possibility of a posthuman world where robots dominate humans.

These ideas are material for a graduate seminar, but for our purposes, the posthuman conflates robot and human. We are no longer unique identities.

A cyborg fuses human features and organs with machine parts and artificial organs. In *Star Trek: The Next Generation*, the Borg, an alien race, function as part of the hive mind.

> The hive mind can also refer to large numbers of players in an ARG being able to operate as a collective group to find puzzle solutions in less time that an individual would take.

In *Neuromancer*, Case has his pancreas replaced. This, of course, would be a great solution to the terror of pancreatic cancer that killed my uncle, but do such possibilities signal a leap in progress?

Technology has always extended our capabilities as *Homo Faber*: man, the maker. A popular example is a brain is removed from a human body and placed into a machine. This would be the ultimate leap in artificial intelligence. Such thinking machines would soon develop their own evolutionary path and render humans obsolete. In other words, man would be transcended. This would be a posthuman world.

Briefing 2: *Neuromancer* or The Past is Prologue to the Future

You have now finished reading the pioneering novel *Neuromancer* (1984) by William Gibson. Gibson is credited with coining the word cyberspace, the subject of this course, and now part of our everyday vernacular. He also popularized a new genre of science fiction called cyberpunk which has, like the term cyberspace, extended into popular culture.

Gibson wraps cyberspace together with the virtual reality talked about last week. Gibson has talked about the importance of video games for his conception of cyberspace.

We have, then, two future trajectories for the body. The discarding of the body entirely through life immersed in cyberspace, or the cyborg, a kind of prosthetic body where biology is gradually replaced or supplemented by mechanics. One can easily predict most people will choose to live as robopaths. The natural body will no longer exist, but humans will move not just toward posthumanity but also immortality. In such a case would there be any need for reproduction? Perhaps this is a utopian state?

Finally, the plot, if there is one, of *Neuromancer*, concerns Artificial Intelligence. The A.I. *Wintermute* controls most of the action, which, ultimately, moves toward a reunion with another A.I. *Neuromancer*. Such a reunion can only bring an end to humanity as we know it.

In the final episode, I'll discuss the ramifications and possibilities of a terminal identity.

INVESTIGATIONS

Hack

Students will be able to access www.chromogen.com/lab6/cybervault/PE. Then they will need to solve a bizarre multilayer quiz from Wright's warped mind to unlock the file; retrieve the photograph of Wright's handwritten letter; and discover the physical location of the real letter. The screen where the eight riddles are displayed is black with green text like a monochromatic monitor from the first personal computers. At the top are the words: "fathers last."

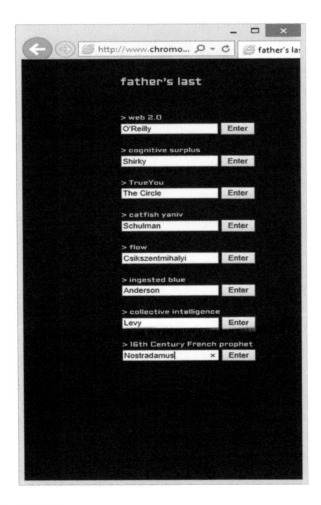

Desmond Wright's eight riddles.

The solution to the first six layers of the puzzle can be found in previous class readings. The solution to the seventh riddle can be found in a future reading. The solution to the eighth riddle can be found… on the Internet…

i. First Screen reads "web 2.0"
   Answer: O'Reilly

ii. Second screen reads "cognitive surplus"
   Answer: Shirky

iii. Third Screen reads "addiction doctor"
   Answer: Grohol

iv. Fourth Screen reads "catfish yaniv"
   Answer: Schulkman

v. Fifth Screen reads "found flow"
   Answer: Csikszentmihalyi

vi. Sixth Screen reads "ingested blue"
   Answer: Anderson

vii. Seventh Screen reads "collective intelligence"
   Answer: Levy

viii. Eighth Screen reads "1503"
   Answer: Nostradamus

After the eighth riddle is answered the screen fades to a photograph of a handwritten letter, with the following caption:

"if I die before my dream is complete, the original of this document can be found in a capsule under the skin of my right shoulder. read, believe, execute. synchronize lives."

The letter reads as follows:

"to my children

you who will share my dream even as you are dreaming, this is the history·

the small startup company i formed to explore human dna, chromogen, was headed down a path too many competitors were already traveling. i, your father, began pondering if my company and his hobby, studying psychic phenomena in the human brain, might be combined with the ubiquitous reach of the internet and its phenomenal ability to capture users attention.

inspired by my fathers who led you here, with the aid of one of my children, elliot, i set in motion a series of experiments, first on animals, then on human volunteers. what we discovered was that people whose dna were susceptible to certain chemical stimulants might indeed develop a certain kind of psychic harmony with one another, not really telepathic, but an ability to sense others whose makeup was similar, and form a tight, instinctual bond of like-minded individuals. Further, elliot discovered that subliminal perception, long ago dismissed in old media, might actually work extremely well in an interactive medium such as video games or the internet. the process, if it worked, could be sold to anyone for any amount, and that country or corporation or group could bend the world to their will. the profit potential was obviously immense.

we did not publish our findings but embarked on an enterprise that would alter the dna in anyone through exposure to certain chemicals, and subliminal stimuli, and then connect them to each other through interaction on the Internet. they needed a trial on people who were unaware they were being tested. it was another of my children, audra, a vice president at chromogen, who came up with the idea of inserting an agent in an online course who could then experiment from within.

our first attempt in 2012 in florida had unfortunate side effects. but we were undaunted.

we had already set up a front organization, the carehart foundation, to begin mass testing when the class experiment was a success, as i knew it would be. i knew no one could stop us. we are destiny. we are synchronicity. we are the future."

DESMOND WRIGHT

I am startled to find as I read this for the first time in a long time that Desmond Wright did not use capital letters just like Sam Clemens in *Skeleton Chase 2*. I don't really have an explanation for this. The spelling of Wright's last name in the letter is deliberate.

Challenge (25 XP)
The Invasion of Artificial Intelligence

Investigation Reports
None

Student Journal
Political Identity: Dissent or Consent? (30 XP)

Jamaica's native *Rastafarian* religion, considered by some to be a cult, plays a prominent role in *Neuormancer's* final section. This religious or spiritual identity places Rastafarians in political opposition to much of western capitalism considered by Rastafarians to be "Babylon." The novel represents *Straylight* as a version of Babylon much as *The Matrix* itself is a form of Babylon. In this two-part entry of 150 words (75 each) focus on the following:

1. Discuss the role of Maelcum, Case's foil, and a predecessor to Neo, as an alternative, individualistic identity in opposition to the novel's corporate identity represented by Lady 3Jane.

2. How do you think the future of the Internet will affect your or the next generation's political identity? Will the Internet bring a utopian space where people are equal irrespective of nation, race, gender, sexual orientation, religion and ethnicity or will the Internet become dominated by one or a handful of multinational corporations like Tessier-Ashpoolor, even one totalitarian government?

Human or Posthuman: Road to the Future (100 XP)

Based on this episode's investigation provide a window onto the world of 2040 for Professor Grey. He needs to consider this information when planning his future classes and those of his replacement. Think about the optimism of robotics expert Hans Moravec; Marvin Minsky's predictions for Artificial Intelligence; and the utopia experts like Dr. Kaku believe nanotechnology will make possible. Your report can imagine you or someone you know such as a child or niece/nephew or younger colleague or even you at an age only possible through expanded health care technology, in the year 2040 sending the report back to the professor. Your report can be a 500-page letter to the professor, a slideshow presentation, an animated cartoon, or even a landscape drawing with a representation of what humans might look like in 2040. You can use a graphic illustration program such as Adobe Illustrator or draw freehand and scan. Another option would be a newscast form the future where you videotape yourself speaking on location someplace in 2040. Make sure your report makes use of Asimov's *Three Laws of Robotics*.

Beyond the Flesh of Identity (50 XP)

Neuromancer's protagonist Case is a cyberspace cowboy. When he jacks into cyberspace through a computer terminal, he leaves his physical body or "meat" behind and travels in a kind of unbounded ecstasy through the imaginary world of data or information. Even today, early in the 21st century, when we go online we become what the 19th century poet and visionary William Blake called a "mental traveler" and visit places across the globe or even locations with no physical location. As we discussed in an earlier episode today, we can even have intimate relationships with another person and never experience that person's flesh. Discuss among yourselves the advantages and disadvantages of living without a human body. If you could jack into cyberspace like Case or take the red pill like Neo, what would your world be like in this alternative or virtual reality where what we now think is real is unreal and what we think is dream-like becomes the true reality.

Bonus (40 XP for Book Review, 30 XP for Film Review)
Representing Artificial Intelligence

As Dr. Minsky suggested in his talk about immortality, if you really want to learn about the future you should read science fiction writers. These writers have imagined artificial intelligence for many years. In turn many of these great stories have been made into films. Usually the film is based upon the novel, but they are nonetheless, two distinct mediums and should not be expected to be identical with each other. The exception here is that both the film and novel *2001: A Space Odyssey* were created concurrently by the two British masters Arthur C. Clark and Stanley Kubrick. For bonus points you can write a book review or a film review. Your choices are below.

1. *I, Robot*, Isaac Asimov (1950)

2. *I, Robot*, film version, Alex Proyas (2004)

3. *Do Androids Dream of Electric Sheep*, Philip K. Dick (1968)

4. *Blade Runner*, film version, Ridley Scott (1982)

5. *Ender's Game,* Orson Scott Card (1997)

6. *Ender's Game* film version), Gavis Hood (2013)

7. *2001: A Space Odyssey*, Arthur C. Clark (1968)

8. *2001: A Space Odyssey*, film version, Stanley Kubrick (1968)

9. *The Moon is a Harsh Mistress*, Robert Heinlein (1966) – no film version to date.

Final Project Episode Seven Suggestions: My Body, Myself

For this chapter try and think about both your political identity if that is important to you and how technology has or could affect your physical self. For example, do you vote? Do you affiliate with a party? Are you involved in local politics like the school system or library? As for your physical identity, how does that impact your overall sense of self? In Gibson's posthuman universe, people are cybernetically enhanced. Molly has razor blade fingernails and Case has his pancreas replaced. Today, many people already use Botox or plastic surgery to enhance their body from breast augmentation to cochlear implants (for hearing) to various prosthetic devices for legs and arms. How do you imagine technology might enhance your body? On the other hand, will technology shrink our physical selves from lack of activity? This episode and the next are forward looking.

Class Forum (50 XP)

At this point there will hopefully be a lot of discussion that we'll need to monitor. Logan and Ann will answer questions.

Most of the forum posts will probably be devoted to solving Wright's final puzzles.

CHAPTER 34

Episode 8 – Showdown

LEARNING OUTCOMES

By the end of this episode successful students will be able to:

1. Debate the ethical implications of Internet technology's future.

CHARACTERS

Logan Grey, Desmond Wright, Audra Casey, Dale Kenyon, Sallie Lopez, Tom Wetherall/ Elliot Plevin, Ann Bennett

NARRATIVE

The students expose Chromogen's true purpose; the company is raided; and Wright, Plevin, Audra, Dale, and Sallie are arrested. The class is saved. But a last post from Ann suggests this may not be an isolated case. There is evidence in the company records that Chromogen may in fact be only a part of a larger conspiracy, and Primal Empathy only one of the ways those behind it have infiltrated the Internet. Whatever has been set in motion may not be stopped by Chromogen's collapse. But now, thanks to this class, the investigation will continue and the perpetrators brought to justice.

VIDEOS (1)

Cyber Criminals Unmasked!

On the Badge Lando website, the final video shows Wright being marched off in handcuffs across his estate's private tennis court. The other conspirators' pictures and real identities are exposed on the website.

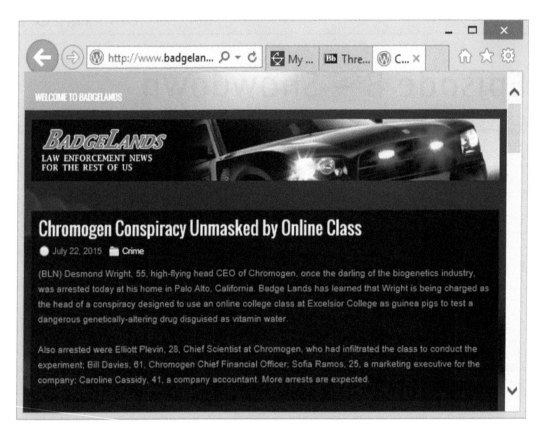

The fall of Chromogen?

PROFESSOR GREY'S BRIEFING

Briefing 1: Apocalypse or Rest Stop?

Essential Question for Episode 8: Is global society moving in the direction of a utopian world or a dystopian world?

We have come to the end of this semester's class, but, in no way do I want to suggest this week is a conclusion. We have only scratched the surface of cyberculture and self, but technology moves so quickly that even the near future is hard to foresee. Hopefully, you have accumulated some knowledge and learned some skills during this phase of your lifelong learning. Likewise, as you turn in your final reports, realize your narrative will be ongoing well past your graduation date. Perhaps the most important lesson I want you to take away from this learning experience is the value of reflection. In a fast-paced world of multiple forces you need to step back, slow down, and think about where you have been and where you are going, otherwise you might be swept along like a tumble weed on a vast desert.

For this final week, I will just touch on a few people's thinking about the future and end with thoughts on the value of the Humanities to which this course belongs.

When artificial intelligence evolves to such an advanced state then the ideas displayed in *The Matrix* and science fiction become real. Robots may well run humans and not the other way around.

Does superhuman intelligence bring about utopia? Artificial intelligence could design an even greater intelligence and so on. In short artificial intelligence would potentially make humanity obsolete.

Transhumanists embrace enhancements to human beings including extending life spans through biological and technological interventions and the general modification of human nature. For the transhumanist, technology holds out the very real possibility of utopia. Would you want to live in such a world? Is immortality something you wish for? I just want you to keep in mind the possibility that science has the potential to catch up with fiction.

Another utopian trend within the digital world of cyberculture is collective intelligence, now sometimes referred to rather simplistically as crowd sourcing.

The idea that the sum of brains is greater than a single brain is pretty much common sense. Old-fashioned brainstorming among people is quite helpful. The very idea of a university strikes me as a way of bringing together heterogeneous collective minds. Most certainly the development of the *World Wide Web* also demonstrated group thinking power. What makes collective intelligence or collaboration different today is precisely the phenomenon of cyberspace. A larger group than possible at any physical university can gather together their thinking without regards to spatial limitations.

Today, in January, 2021, we have been forced into exactly this. And there are signs that working remotely may continue once the pandemic has passed.

In other words, cyberspace allows for a networked or connected culture to collectively solve systemic problems that far exceed individual or discipline-specific problem-solving capability.

I want to end with a few general remarks about the role of the Humanities in society. This course has been classified as Humanities because I believe the Humanities are essential in preventing a future dystopia. The Humanities study the culture and history produced by men and women and our complex interrelationships. History and culture, including cyberculture, are material, and, for now, cannot be transcended. You can journey online but must always come back to a body in a place.

Progress requires solving complex social problems that science and technology cannot eradicate independent of their own complex entanglement with the material world. The Internet can bring people together to help think through solutions, but the solutions must come about in the material world.

The Humanities, as the name indicates, studies humans and the history humans make. Humanism seeks to uncover the role of human agency in history. If we deny agency, we inevitably succumb to a posthuman world where machines could rule men and women.

Humankind is what the Humanities must address and when one looks at the earth from outer space national boundaries evaporate in favor of a single globe. The Internet allows for a unique vision of the world as a possible global community sharing information, the Internet's initial purpose, in an open and collaborative fashion. Equality will also require a material effort whose success benefits from our engagement with, awareness and self-critical stance to, the space we occupy, both physical and virtual.

INVESTIGATIONS

Challenge (XP?)

Frankenstein in Cyberspace

Investigation Reports

None

Final Project Episode Eight (300 XP)

At the end of this episode you will turn in your digital autobiography. This concludes your work for this course, but one's autobiography does not close until we pass away. I encourage you to continue composing your life narrative in whatever form attracts you, whether a multimedia tool, a journal, a diary, a book, audio or visual recorder. The more you take the time to reflect on your life the more effective you are likely to be. For the last section of your project, you should focus on thinking about the future.

Thus, for your final contributions to the class, project your personal future. Where will you be living in 20 years and what will you be doing at that time?

Student Journal

No entries listed.

Debating Bioethics and the Future of Humanity (50XP)

In your final communication with each other you will be divided into two teams. Team Superman takes the position of defending the technological enhancement of humans with the idea of promoting a perfectible human nature, i.e. slowing down the aging process, catapulting intelligence, replacing body parts, altering our genetic constitution, and that of our children. Team Luthor takes the position that genetic and biological enhancement should be either banned or tightly regulated because they fear future super humanity will actually end up dehumanizing the species.

Class Forum (50 XP)

Forum discussion will be limited to the wrap-up of the narrative, followed by the Bioethics and Future of Humanity debate below.

Ann Bennett's Post

Yesterday agents of the FBI raided Chromogen. Wright, Audra, Dale, and Sallie have joined Plevin in jail. Desmond Wright's arrest can be found on the Badge Lands website: www.badgelands.com. Thanks to you Wright has been stopped. But I have some sobering news. This may not be an isolated case. There is evidence in the company records that Chromogen may in fact be only a part of a larger conspiracy, and Primal Empathy only one of the ways those behind it have infiltrated the Internet. Whatever has been set in motion may not be stopped by Chromogen's collapse. But now, thanks to this class, the investigation will continue, and the perpetrators brought to justice. And as for you, my classmates: you will be far more able to navigate both the wonder and the menace of a connected Earth!

CONCLUSION

Student reactions to this pilot of the online game *Secrets* will be captured in a survey, so that the next iteration may be even better.

As stated earlier, a suggested next stage is to create a universal template from this document so that other online classes may be built in a similar way.

As I mentioned earlier, despite the success of the class, no other classes on any topic were developed. I hope that reading about the classes in this book may inspire others to use what they learn here to create more vibrant online learning experiences than the vast majority of classes out there.

CHAPTER 35

Afterword

As I stated in the Introduction to this section, *The Multiplayer Classroom* can answer a lot of the questions educators and students are asking today about how to make remote learning engaging enough to capture the attention of isolated students of all ages. I have noticed that early year teachers, teachers from pre-school to second or third grade, by necessity find new and exciting ways to teach. At the other end of the educational spectrum, post-secondary teachers often ignore, or are oblivious to, the benefits of turning classes into games. This is due to the transition between learning as play to learning as serious business that I cover in *The Multiplayer Classroom: Designing Coursework as a Game*. Many college professors do not seem to have a difficult time at all treating the classroom experience as too important to be playful, requiring instead seriousness of purpose and execution. Indeed, education has never been under so much assault.

Today we are facing an unprecedented crisis in education. Thanks to the COVID-19 pandemic students of all ages either suffer the isolation of remote learning, or risk infection both for themselves and their families by attending in-person classes or find themselves ping-ponging between both. One of the major critiques of remote teaching either recorded or live is the difficulty in creating a true community of students and instructor. I have read article after well-meaning article attempting to address this issue by advocating solutions in the same way a good teacher teaches in any classroom, delivering the same amount of material in the same way, just remotely. Unfortunately, the translation between shared presence in a physical classroom and teaching from a screen, whether live or recorded, is not straightforward. I do not intend to offer this class as an example on how to solve all of the complex issues involved, only to suggest that the time has never been more fitting for opening up our ideas of what the learning experience can be, if we have the inspiration and the energy to achieve it.

SECTION 4

The Janus Door

CHAPTER 36

Introduction to Section 4

CLASS MET ON TUESDAYS and Thursdays each week for ten weeks, after the first week which began on Thursday, September 14, 2017.

There is a distinct evolution from the *Skeleton Chase 2: The Psychic* design document to *The Janus Door* document, in technology used in the classes and the integration of the elements of learning, storytelling, and gameplay. *The Janus Door* is the most complete document of the four in the various ways it handled the integration of the design and educational elements.

Each game design reflects a close collaboration between instructor and designer where each brought their own particular expertise, and each recognized their roles and respected the other's role. In education instructors usually had the final say with the designer consulting and making suggestions. In narrative and gameplay, the designer usually had the final say with the instructor consulting and making suggestions. It cannot be emphasized enough that this is the best kind of balance between subject matter and its delivery. Such a collaboration depends on the respect each expert has for the other.

An instructor who erroneously believes that writing and design are easier than their subject matter, or a writer/designer who believes that anybody can teach effectively, can damage and possibly even destroy the potential of such a collaboration.

When the collaboration is based upon the respect of equals, anything can be taught in game-based learning. Anything. And the students will benefit most of all.

As with *Secrets*, we considered this version of *The Janus Door* as a template. As Professor Peterson wrote in his Foreword, the class continued to evolve, and he is considering a version of it for an engineering summer camp. A generic template of *The Janus Door* could be created from this document, then localized to other Cal Poly classes or classes at other institutions, even when the subject matter is far from cybersecurity.

This is a relevant admonition for anyone designing a multiplayer classroom. Document the experience of teaching and playing the game. There is much scholarly writing about game-based learning classes. There are precious few blueprints on how to create one. Student progress should be well-documented. All involved (instructors and students) should be encouraged to keep a record of every game-related part of the class, written with photographs, and/or videos that can be posted with clear descriptions. In addition to using these to create other courses, they can also provide material for stories and publicity about the class.

As well as their grades, *all* students should be rewarded for individual and collective achievements with intrinsic rewards such as pictures, videos, and stories on PolyLearn, campus wide, and in the media. The best videogames provide moments of triumph, both big and small, for all players.

This research was supported by the National Science Foundation under Grant No. 1419318. Any opinions, findings, and conclusions or recommendations expressed in this material are those of the authors and do not necessarily reflect the views of the National Science Foundation.

To learn more of the underlying research goals and results, please follow this link: https://www.usenix.org/system/files/conference/ase18/ase18-paper_morelock.pdf. (Morelock, John R. and Peterson. Zachary. "Authenticity, Ethicality, and Motivation: A Formal Evaluation of a 10-week Computer Security Alternate Reality Game for CS Undergraduates." In 2018 USENIX Workshop on Advances in Security Education (ASE 18), Baltimore, MD, 2018. USENIX Association.)

CHAPTER 37

Foreword to Section 4

Zachary N.J. Peterson

I HAVE ALWAYS BEEN A fan of interactive fiction and alternate reality games, and so when looking for novel ways to improve my Introduction to Computer Science through Security course at Cal Poly, they were a natural choice. Indeed, ARGs have been shown to be collaborative and inclusive, to inspire counterfactual thinking, to maintain engagement, and to provide an authentic context and purpose for the presented material, both online and in the real world—many of the same factors that have shown to be lacking in computer science and computer security curricula, generally.

Games are uniquely appropriate for communicating computer security concepts. The inclusivity, accessibility, and freedoms of play associated with games can reach out and engage new populations, inspire students to think "like an adversary," and encode important but (admittedly) mundane cybersecurity concepts into exciting game mechanics. Games also provide an opportunity to roleplay, allowing students to see themselves as successful cybersecurity professionals, building self-efficacy and resiliency.

Being familiar with Lee's book, *The Multiplayer Classroom*, I reached out to him to see if he would be interested in partnering on a recent National Science Foundation grant I had been awarded for "gamifying" my course. My goal was to create a ten-week long, cybersecurity-themed ARG, which would run the duration of the quarter. I was fortunate to get him.

A challenge in designing any ARG is in providing fun and engaging puzzles that are coherent and meaningful in the context of the narrative. This is doubly challenging when those puzzles should be pedagogically sound and mechanisms for assessment. These constraints mandated a very tight collaboration loop between Lee and myself, which began with a general organization of course topics which were further refined into specific learning objectives. Lee then used these as waypoints in the narrative. For example, the point in the story where students need to crack the antagonist's password aligns with the week we discussed authentication and password security in class. What resulted is *The Janus Door*: a compelling, interactive narrative that, through a series of network, web, cryptographic, and digital forensic exercises, lead students to discover the true identity of the hacker that is trying to frame them for digital crimes they didn't commit.

The delivery of the game was an amazing but grueling experience—one which required constant attention to detail, skillful adlibbing, and a fair amount of technical expertise. Having a TA who was not only a talented teacher but also a fun-loving participant (and an excellent actor to boot!) was essential to the success of the game. Responding and adapting to the students' progress and interests during the game was a full-time job for both of us. This included creating new lab materials before and during the game, modifying the storyline (including choosing to scale back the game mid-way through to adjust for time and other resource constraints), and collaborating on content delivery (e.g. making sure we revealed plot elements at the same time).

The single most important artifact of the development process was the "Final Design Document," which provided the game mechanics (e.g. channels of communication, scripts, and descriptions physical and digital assets), interfaces for the game (e.g. web sites, physical sites), list of characters, hint systems, and detailed descriptions of what was to happen in each "episode" (class period). This hyperlinked document provides both macro and micro views of the game, so it is useful both as a day-to-day reference and an essential tool when modifying the storyline.

The result was very well received by the students. We found that our ARG enabled an authentic and motivating problem-solving environment and provided a catalyst for having constructive discussions on ethical behavior in computer security. One example of this stands out: A student that missed the first lecture (the one and only in which I announced that the course was to be offered as an ARG), became very concerned that some of the activities (e.g. hacking into a fictional character's email account) raised ethical red flags and frustrated his learning experience. Even some of the students who were present on the first day appreciated that elements of the game helped keep the ethical boundary obvious.

Overall, we found that *The Janus Door* was an effective vehicle to motivate course activities and provide an authentic context for cybersecurity work, while also helping to refine students' understanding and interests related to the cybersecurity profession. I look forward to continuing to develop and offer *The Janus Door* to our incoming freshmen, as well as modify it for other venues, such as our engineering summer camp—presuming I can find another willing TA!

CHAPTER 38

Design Document

The *Secrets* design document was a template for the book's final multiplayer class-room which retains the structure and some of the general language. Both are game-based learning offspring of my design documents for non-educational videogames. They should not be considered the only way to construct a design document, simply the one with which I have become most comfortable.

This design document is meant to be a detailed plan for the game and the class. Characters, dialogue scripts, fictional websites, documents, cybersecurity puzzle details, physical locations on the Cal Poly campus, field trips etc., through which the students will experience the game, are included here. Connections between narrative, gameplay, and pedagogy, the most important balancing act in a project like this, are finalized here as well.

The original design document fully utilized Microsoft Word's bookmark and hyper-link capabilities so that in the digital version the reader could jump to specific rele-vant material when it was referenced elsewhere.

EXECUTIVE SUMMARY

The two first-year sections of Professor Zachary Peterson's cybersecurity class begin as they ordinarily would. But soon the game that is the subject of this document begins. This is not a digital entertainment game like *Minecraft*, or an "educational" game with gameplay sandwiched between customary teaching methods. It is a class designed entirely as a game.

In the fictional narrative of the game, students are plunged into the middle of a series of cyberattacks aimed at the school by a shadowy hacker organization called the *Janus Door*. Student assignments will fit seamlessly into the fictional world of the game, whether directly part of the narrative, or indirectly through the website Dark Park or a minor character, Mr. Jonathan Gonella [**This is the fictional parent of the very real Teaching**

Assistant for the first class. This name will change as new TA's are assigned to later iterations of the class.] Students must learn the skills necessary to follow the narrative, and to play the game, the equivalent to acquiring new skills while leveling up in a computer game.

To further their immersion in the game, sections at first will find themselves competing with each other. But soon it will become apparent students must collaborate, at times in small teams, or a combination of both sections, to figure out final complex cybersecurity puzzles, the equivalent of exams and a final project. The game will increase their involvement as the stakes escalate in the story, a key character vanishes, and they are given a chance to confront someone who appears to be a simple villain, but who actually has a strong emotional reason for her actions. The students will determine her fate.

This combination of extrinsic and intrinsic rewards features regular class assignments, devilish game-based puzzles, a compelling narrative, and complex, sympathetic characters.

As I said in the Preface: this is collateral learning. It intensifies the pedagogical experience, as the students learn because they want to find out what happens next. They learn almost without realizing they're doing it.

TYPE AND GENRE

The Janus Door is a transmedia alternate reality game designed for CPE 123: Introduction to Computing—Security, the first-year cybersecurity class taught by Professor Zachary Peterson. It is suggested the reader look up ARGs such as *i love bees*, *Year Zero*, and *Evoke*.

The genre of *The Janus Door* is a hybrid of mystery and high-tech espionage thriller, allowing for a maximum of exploration and discovery by the players.

Students will be notified prior to enrolling in either section of the class that they will be participating in an ARG. They are expected to complete all assignments to the best of their ability, as if this were a regular class, and they will be graded accordingly.

THEME

From Wikipedia ("Janus." https://en.wikipedia.org/wiki/Janus, last modified February 3, 2021), in ancient Roman religion and myth, Janus is the god of beginnings, gates, transitions, time, duality, doorways, passages, and endings. He is usually depicted as having two faces, since he looks to the future and to the past.

The theme of *The Janus Door*, and the class, is that our inter-connected world contains billions of improperly secured doorways vulnerable to cyberattacks. Computer professionals need to learn how to not only defend against, but also counter, attempts to exploit unavoidable gaps in security due to the ever-increasing complexity and ubiquity of the Internet.

SETTING

The setting for the game is two normal Cal Poly classrooms, physical locations on the Cal Poly campus and off campus, and on the Internet. The setting includes communications through email, text messaging, and popular social media.

GAME WEBSITES

Websites on the Internet were included as references for both the visual styles of the fictional websites as well as their writing styles.

CyberFacts

Fictional news site that features both true cyber stories via rich site summary (RSS) feeds and stories created specifically for the game such as the video footage of Verita's arrest. It displays a warning about the dark web and the site Dark Park. The site has a Contact Us email address for technical support, to report bugs and unauthorized activity: cyberfacts@cyberfacts.org. The site cannot be hacked.

[**This site features fun cybersecurity puzzles that will serve as "in-game" reasons for students learning and applying concepts that may not fit the class lesson plan or the game's narrative structure.**]

[**Additional cybersecurity puzzles can be added to CyberFacts whenever needed. The narrative is not dependent on when they occur.**]

"About" Link for CyberFacts

Clicking on the link took you to the following welcome.

CyberFacts is your free, independent and opinionated source for information about the webs, ALL of them. And all things cyber. And computer tech geeky stuff.

Want to know about the things that matter to you most? Of course, you do. And guess what! That's what we provide. Come here first. And second. And third. And… well, you get the idea. Wait, are you still reading this? Why are you reading this? Get back to the good stuff!

Dark Web Story for CyberFacts

[**The following story remains on the CyberFacts site front page for the duration of the game.**]

Shining a Light on the Dark Web

By Norman Well

History   The history of the dark web is the history of the internet, and that begins in 1969 with the Pentagon's ARPANET, developed by the Defense Advanced Research Projects Agency (DARPA). Look it up.

A student at the University of California at Los Angeles (UCLA) named Charley Kline sent a message, or at least the piece of one to Stanford University. It was supposed to say "LOGIN." What it said was "LO." Not quite "Watson, come here, I want you."

Despite that less than stellar debut, in the 1970s a number of unique private networks were established. Some of these became known as "darknets."

In 1982, a standardization of network protocols was established. Called the Internet Protocol Suite, it marked the birth of the web as we know it, and "dark havens" quickly followed, hosting illegal activities of all kinds.

By the 1990s, the internet was everywhere. File compression and cheaper data storage allowed darknets to breed like Tribbles.

And in the spring of 2000 a software developer named Ian Clarke brought what he proudly called "near-perfect anarchy" to the online world with a program called Freenet, an anonymous link to all corners of the web, including the nastiest.

In 2002, the U.S. Naval Research Laboratory helpfully released the first version of The Onion Router (Tor). Tor hides the IP address and location of the software's users. Their original intention was to protect American agents and dissidents in repressive regimes. Tor was welcomed with open arms by darknets.

Today, invisible to ordinary internet search engines the "Deep Web" exists across multiple darknets, and houses everything from illegal gambling to drug traffickers to recruiting sites for terrorists to legitimate public organizations and enthusiast websites of all kinds attempting to remain free of interference and censorship. The "dark web" is one corner of the deep web.

Dark Park   In 2015, a Korean American student at Boston University, Daniel Park, created a dark web site called, somewhat unimaginatively, but possibly poetic: Dark Park. It is a site where users can establish anonymous accounts for the gathering and dissemination about what Park calls "life in the dark."

Some clients buy and sell merchandise unavailable on Amazon. Others trade hacker secrets, or just boast of their conquests: banks, government agencies, even movie studios. Others just browse to get a taste of the web the internet does not provide.

The site is considered more of a fan site, than a truly legitimate—make that illegitimate—dark web site, a safe haven for n00bs. Some hackers have mocked its security protocols. But even so it is also a rest stop for all kinds of travelers, on their way to unknown destinations, along the poorly lighted highways of the dark web.

[The following is accessed via a link above the dark web article on the front page of **CyberFacts. The link reads Dark Web Warning**]

Dark Web Warning   Stories about the dark web are fascinating to read. But the dark web is not a Disneyland with rules to protect the safety of its patrons. Accessing the dark web can expose anyone to dangers of all kinds from phishing attacks to a zombie sitting where your personal computer used to be.

Never believe that anyone is really who they say they are. Never believe anyone can do what they say they can do. If you make a mistake, you may never even know it until it is too late. Check the back of your t-shirt often. One night you're liable to find a big red target painted there. You visit *any* dark website at your own risk. And once you visit, even for a quick ride, you may find yourself returning home with hitchhiking ghosts.

Articles for CyberFacts

[These articles are part of a "continuing series" on CyberFacts called *Where Are They Now?* and should be automatically rotated weekly.]

Where Are They Now?

By Chester Wood

They are the legends you have never heard of. In an age where hacking has practically become an eSport, they are hacking royalty. Wait until you see where some ended up. But not all of them. Not all of them have come in from the cold.

> There were stories of four hackers in the CyberFacts series. Three are genuine legendary hackers. This particular story focuses on a fictional character central to the game's narrative. (See the *Episode 4: Janus Door* Narrative section for an image of the story on Nick Menzo as it appeared on the CyberFacts website.

The full text of the story follows.

Nicholas Menzo

Nick Menzo was born in 1962 in Olmsted Falls, Ohio. He had only one run-in with law enforcement during his early years when he created an automated targeting system for an underground Halloween tradition called the "Junior/Senior Apple Fight." It allowed terrified junior students, usually the underdogs, to fire remote-controlled spring-loaded catapults from safe positions over one hundred yards from the site of the Village Green where the conflict took place. Several seniors were injured when ammunition was switched from rotten apples to monkey balls (from the shrub maclura pomifera to you scientists), a large tough fruit that resembles a green brain, and apparently packs quite a punch as a projectile.

From this unique, but inauspicious beginning, Nick attended a nearby college, Baldwin-Wallace, where he excelled in computer science, ran the computer lab and designed networking tools. It wasn't until he became a graduate student at California Polytechnic Institute (Cal Poly) that his career becomes of interest to us, as he became the first hacker to steal American secrets for a foreign power.

Nick's student work was helping to maintain the school's computer network. Early in his second year at Cal Poly, he ran into severe money troubles when he attempted to supplement his meager student stipend by creating a digital card-counting system for blackjack. The system's early promise seduced Nick into taking out a $40,000 loan at a usurious 50% interest rate from an unknown source to fund his system. But the system failed, and he lost everything.

When it became clear Nick could not repay the loan, he was coerced into penetrating various sensitive research accounts on the Cal Poly servers and selling secrets to East Germany. It has since been suggested that the source of the loan was in fact a Soviet-bloc official agency, who subsequently forgave the loan, and provided him with additional compensation in exchange for the research he stole from Cal Poly.

The university discovered Nick's activities in 1987. With expulsion inevitable and the FBI building a case against him, Nick retaliated by shutting down the school's servers, and fled with his wife, Katherine, behind the iron curtain. They left their newborn daughter behind.

Where is Nick Menzo now?

No one knows. After the Berlin Wall fell in 1989 a concerted effort to locate Nick was initiated by the United States. But no trace of him was found in East Germany. And a photograph surfaced several years later that purported to show a smiling Nick on a tropical beach somewhere. Even though the statute of limitations has expired on his crimes, and Nick can be no longer prosecuted, he has never reappeared. Where indeed is Nick Menzo today?

Dark Park

Hackable dark web site with stories, tips and a column called Rumor Mill where unsubstantiated rumors of hacker activity are posted (see below).

Verita will use Dark Park to post her messages and videos. Students will be able to hack into more and more of the site's files and code, the more proficient they become, leading to the

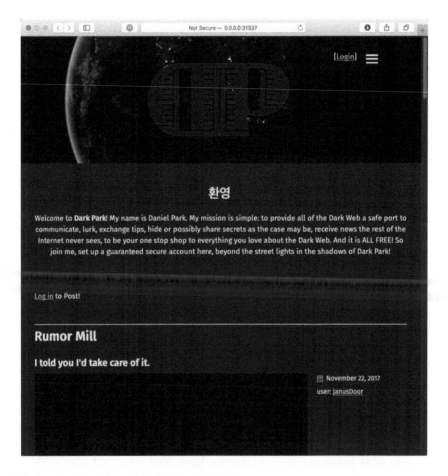

Fictional dark web site with exploitable security issues.

site eventually being shut down. The owner of the site is Daniel Park. Daniel has left a smugly subversive welcome email on the site's main page (see Messages, Emails & Texts section).

The site has a Contact Us email address for technical support, to report bugs and unauthorized activity: darkpark@darkpark.com.

Dark Park Rumor Mill

[First three should be up when the site goes live. Then add others at Professor Peterson's discretion. Feel free to make up some of your own as needed, particularly if more recent hacks or cybersecurity stories hit the news.]

I used the word "if" in the above. Today I would write "when."

Rumor 1   From Skyhacker: "Somebody taking credit for the Equifax breach has made their ransomware demands. The price though is way lame. Some doubt whether the claim is legit. Of course, what is these days?"

Rumor 2   From Rail Spawn: the Janus Door is planning something "devilish." Sounds cute, but more info please. Don't make me hack u."

Rumor 3   From PanchoVilla: "Cayman Island banks could be targets of the Freedom Team. If they get in, I hope they spread the wealth around."

Rumor 4   From SyncLock: "Wu Tang Clan isn't a hacker group? It's a band???"

Rumor 5   From KeyBoy: "Cal Poly is going all in on teaching cybersecurity. But will they be in time? Word is somebody's got them squarely in their sights."

Rumor 6   From BettyBoop: "Hillary Clinton hacked my email server and stole my medical marijuana prescription card!"

Rumor 7   From Dark Shark: "Seriously, why is Dark Park always the last site to post anything? Old news is no longer gold news, Danny. Up your game!"

Rumor 8   From Bird Watcher: "eSports companies are using subliminal perception to sell you junk food! Keep watching the feeds!"

Rumor 9   From SlowMO: "Anybody remember that middle eastern hackware site's IP? I lost my copy."

Daniel replies: "Always nice to see the NSA visiting. Keep up the good work, guys. You're keeping us all safe!"

Rumor 10   From Pluribus: "Ad blockers are going to destroy civilization as we know it!"

Dark Park Lynx

[This is a listing of links to stories Dark Park visitors might find interesting. Please add to them as you see fit or use others. They might simply be links on the home page of the site under the heading Lynx, or stories that are reprinted from other sources under the same heading. Be sure to attribute sources.

The darkpark@darkpark.com email address will have an associated public PGP key. It will be stored on either Dark Park directly or on keybase.io (see, e.g. keybase.io/znjp) which is a repository for public keys. This will allow students to send encrypted email to Daniel, and also to verify any email or posts that comes from him. Specifically, the post from Daniel Park which shuts down Dark Park in Episode 12.

Class Sites

Cal Poly Learning Management System (Customized Moodle)

PolyLearn is to be used for normal information and interaction. The following game-related uses will be added:

Students will be able to access videos they have seen and descriptions of *previous* episodes here. Episode titles will be written in a top corner of the classroom's whiteboard by Professor Peterson before each lab.

Students will post brief "skill bios" here. These will be used by Professor Peterson to help balance teams, when small teams are required to solve some puzzles. They should not list personal information beyond level of programming skill, cybersecurity skill, math, writing, and other skills that may be necessary to solving team-based puzzles.

The system also will be "hacked" by Verita in *Episode 9: Spirit Door*. She will purge student grades in revenge for students' successfully defending or neutralizing her attacks. Professor Peterson and Nick will help students recover their grades, once Nick is rescued in the following class, *Episode 10: Golden Door*.

This was my escalation of the hack that attacked the class website in *Secrets*. Here students were getting hit where they live: vanishing grades!

Admin Server

This server is created and maintained for class use only. It is a stand-in for a real Cal Poly server. It will allow students to fight off fictional attacks directed at the school. The hidden, encrypted file called "Diablo" can also be discovered here.

Real Sites

Useful for cybersecurity class research.

PHYSICAL LOCATIONS

On-Campus Sites

Classrooms

No modifications are necessary to normal A/V/Internet equipped classrooms.

Nick's Office

This should be a second office, currently vacant, not one commonly used by this TA or any other. It will be staged for the game. Once Nick is kidnapped, the office is discoverable and searchable for clues by students.

Nick's Prison

TBD Storage room, out building etc. where Nick will be imprisoned. The door will be secured by an encrypted lock students must unlock to free Nick.

Off-Campus Sites

Verita's Lair

Students will not be physically able to access this site. They will simply witness the video of her arrest outside it.

Diablo Canyon Nuclear Power Plant

The first major field trip will occur outside of class on a weekend, either Saturday, October 21 or Sunday, October 22. Students will visit the Energy Education Center to see exhibits about plant operations, safety, and how nuclear power is generated. Arrangements can be made in advance for a guided tour of the Center.

> Unfortunately, as Professor Peterson says in his Foreword, time constraints meant cuts. Both this field trip and the following field trip at Montaña de Oro State Park, with a "treasure hunt" theme, had to be abandoned. I always thought it would be interesting to learn what nuclear power plant personnel would think when they learned our narrative included a cyber-attack on their security system.

Montaña de Oro State Park

The second major field trip will occur outside of class on a weekend, either Saturday, November 4 or Sunday, November 5 at Montaña de Oro State Park. With over 8000 acres, including seven miles of shoreline, Montaña de Oro is one of the largest state parks in California. Part of it overlooks the Diablo Canyon Nuclear Power Plant. When the class TA is kidnapped, student teams will travel to the park for clues to his location and codes necessary to find and release him. Details will be found in *Episode 10: Locked Door*.

GAME MECHANICS

Communication

Student/NPC

Verita will send messages (emails, texts, and videos) to the class. Once the class identifies the Janus Door's involvement in the cyberattacks, students can send email messages to an email bot that forwards them to an unknown address where Verita can receive them.

Students will be able to send and receive emails and texts from the websites CyberFacts and Dark Park, including Dark Park's owner and editor-in-chief, Daniel Park.

Students will be able to send and receive emails and texts from the class TA's father (see Characters section), who is seeking help to understand cybersecurity issues and to protect himself from identity thieves.

Student/Student

Students will be able to communicate to others in their section via LMS, text, and email.

Section/Section

Students in one section can communicate with students in the other section via the LMS, email, and text. They will be able to set up services for sharing such as Slack and Google docs. This will become important for both the competition phase and the collaboration phase of the relationship between the two sections.

Student/Instructor

Students and the Instructor will be able to use the LMS or services such as Slack or Google Docs to communicate or share documents with each other. In all cases the Instructor will have separate folders for topics related to classwork (Classwork) and topics related to the story (Investigations).

Student/Teaching Assistant

Students will be able to interact with the Teaching Assistant in the same way as with the Instructor via folders labeled Classwork and Investigations.

VIDEO

Videos created for the class will be sent to Professor Peterson, and shared with both sections of the class, as part of the game. Once a video has been shown to the two class sections, it will be available on the PolyLearn LMS.

Verita's Warning (See *Episode 3: Open Door*)

Verita's Boast (See *Episode 4: Back Door*)

Verita's Revenge (See *Episode 9: Spirit Door*)

Nick Kidnapped (See *Episode 9: Spirit Door*)

Verita's Arrest (See *Episode 13: Kicking Down the Door*)

[See *Episode 14: Cell Door* for Verita's live final performance.]

MESSAGES, EMAILS & TEXTS

Dark Park Welcome (Message on Website)

"환영 Welcome to Dark Park! My name is Daniel Park. My mission is simple: to provide all of the Dark Web a safe port to communicate, lurk, exchange tips, hide, or possibly share secrets as the case may be, receive news the rest of the Internet never sees, to be your one stop shop to everything you love about the Dark Web. And it is ALL FREE! So join me, set up a guaranteed secure account here, beyond the street lights in the shadows of Dark Park!

[NOTE: Korean above translates as "Welcome."]

Text 1 from Daniel Park (See *Episode 2: Tower Door Part 2*)

Text 2 from Daniel Park (See *Episode 4: Janus Door*)

Email from Verita (See *Episode 6: Back Door*)

Text 3 from Daniel Park (See *Episode 9: Spirit Door*)

Longitude Text from Verita (See *Episode 10: Locked Door*)

Latitude Text from Verita (See *Episode 10: Locked Door*)

Third Text from Verita (See *Episode 10: Locked Door*)

Email from Daniel Park (See *Episode 12: Swinging Door*)

PHYSICAL/DIGITAL OBJECTS

Documents

Photograph of Nick Menzo on a tropical island (Digital)

Photograph of Katherine Anne Menzo's grave (Digital)

Class Photograph of Section 1 (Physical)

Class Photograph of Section 1 (Digital)

Class Photograph of Section 2 (Physical)

Class Photograph of Section 2 (Digital)

Maps

Maps of Montaña de Oro State Park (Digital & Physical)

Map of Diablo Canyon Nuclear Power Plant

Tools

Hostile thumb drive in printer (Physical)

Nick's computer (Physical)

Wordlock (Physical)

Keypad code thumb drive (Physical)

Keypad door lock (Physical)

HINT SYSTEM

The game's built-in Hint System is the Teaching Assistant.

[Nick Gonella is the class Teaching Assistant for the first iteration of class only.]

At any point in the game where students do not figure something out that they need to proceed, Nick will subtly point them in the right direction. This and other actions may lead students to be suspicious of him. That's fine. Their suspicions are part of the narrative.

PUZZLES

All puzzles included in this document, unless otherwise indicated, are designed to require the participation of multiple students. See individual puzzles for details on each one.

CHARACTERS

Players (Students)

The students in the two sections of the cybersecurity class. They play as themselves and do not create avatars to represent them, nor do they produce any additional material to the fictional story.

Professor Zachary Peterson

Professor Peterson doubles as teacher and a resource for progressing the game's story.

> In *Secrets: An Internet Mystery* Professor Seelow became Professor Logan Grey. As you saw this was meant to be an androgenous universal character played by anyone in future iterations. Also, I wanted to make sure that this was a character, not a real professor introducing videos from the future. In *Janus Door* the setting was not science fiction, but Professor Peterson's regular cybersecurity class, so while he was a part of the fictional story, it was as a real person in the real world.

Teaching Assistant

Nick Gonella is the real name of the class Teaching Assistant for the first iteration of *The Janus Door*. In later iterations of the class, each TA's real name will be used. Nick has several duties. He performs the functions of a typical TA but is also a character in the narrative. As part of the story, students may become suspicious that he has nefarious intentions, especially since coincidentally his first name is the same as Verita's father. But late in the story, he is "revealed" to be an FBI cyber cop planted in the class to help in determining the source of the cyberattacks on the school and arresting the perpetrator.

> Yes, what can I say? Another FBI cyber cop. This makes four undercover government agents in four games: Quinn Morgan, Inspector Pei, Ann Bennett and now Nick. Late in the narrative he will be kidnapped, and the students must rescue him. He also has an anxious fictional dad, Jonathan Gonella.
>
> At least Nick was the only law enforcement professional to be kidnapped!

[As noted above, Nick is also the game's Hint System.]

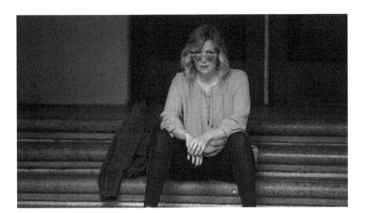

Verita Menzo, our antagonist.

Major NPC
Verita Menzo

Verita was abandoned by her parents as a child when they fled the country to avoid prosecution for passing Cal Poly research information to a foreign power. She blames Cal Poly for the breakup of her family when in reality her parents bear much of the responsibility.

The concluding class of the narrative on November 16 will feature a visit from Verita. Students will be given an opportunity to decide if they believe her true purpose, and whether or not to reveal the location of her parents. As a result, depending on the students' decision, she will be jailed or her sentence will be commuted and she will be given an opportunity to aid authorities in tracking down other hackers.

A scheduling conflict prevented the actress playing Verita to make a personal appearance. She appeared instead in a final video in Episode 14.

Minor NPCs
Nick Menzo

Former Cal Poly graduate student who fled the country with his wife after hacking into the institute's computers. Now thirty years older and believed to be residing in the Pacific island nation of Vanuatu, an island nation in the South Pacific that has no extradition treaty with the United States. No communication attempts will be answered.

Perceptive readers, possibly going back to check *Skeleton Chase 2: The Psychic*, may notice a resemblance between the actress playing Verita Menzo and the actress who played Hope Johnson, Faith Pierpont, and Quinn Morgan. Even more astute readers might suspect Nick Menzo was the actor who played Sam Clemens in that game. You are correct. They were students at Indiana University during the first game. Today they are wife and husband: my daughter-in-law and my son, making TV and movies in Hollywood.

Daniel Park

Korean American owner and editor-in-chief of the Dark Park website. He will never be seen, but he will defend Dark Park through posts on the site and emails when students reveal the site is being used by the *Janus Door*. Much of the student hacking efforts will be directed at this site. In fact, students will have been able to hack into his site so much, his business is failing, and he's applied to join a cybersecurity program at a tech.

TA's Father

For the first iteration of *The Janus Door*, this character's name will be Jonathan Gonella. In later iterations of the class, the character's last name will be updated to match that class' TA. Mr. Gonella sees cybersecurity stories on TV, and immediately suspects he may be a victim. He is terribly concerned his home computer is constantly under attack. Nick pleads a heavy workload and asks the students, if they can help his dad to understand cybersecurity concepts and to protect his computer.

Appearances

Tuesday, Sep 26

Thursday, Oct 5

Tuesday, Oct 31

Tuesday, Nov 7

[**Mr. Gonella is in the game for three reasons. First, he will serve as an in-game opportunity for students to learn and apply concepts that may not fit the class lesson plan or the game's narrative structure. More can be added if needed. The narrative is somewhat dependent on when they occur.**]

[**Second, Nick's dad will also be used as a device for getting the students to perform metacognitive activities, like reflective journaling or think-pair-share discussions. Getting students to reflect upon what they've learned since their last interaction with him, and then trying to summarize it in writing.**]

[**Third, his concern will add emotion when Nick is kidnapped.**]

BACKSTORY

In 1987, Nick Menzo, a graduate computer science student at Cal Poly was dismissed for hacking into the school's servers and stealing sensitive research for a foreign government. When police were about to arrest him, he disappeared with his wife and newborn child.

In 2015, a hacker organization, Janus Door, led by a shadowy figure known as Verita, appeared, claiming credit for several extremely damaging attacks on US universities during that year. They have been silent since then. But rumors on the dark web suggest they are planning something major they are calling a "devilish disruption."

The Janus Door is actually a single hacker, Verita Menzo, the daughter of Nick Menzo. Menzo and his wife, to avoid prosecution, fled to the country that paid him, leaving their child, Verita, behind in foster care. It appears Verita is out to avenge her parents' exile, and abandonment of her, on Cal Poly, the school she believes shattered their family.

When a series of messages uncovered on the dark web suggest there is some connection between Janus Door and Menzo, and that Cal Poly might be the next target of a cyberattack, an FBI cyber cop goes undercover at the school, posing as a CS grad student.

POINT OF ATTACK

In drama, the "point of attack" is the moment the story begins. In this case, "point of attack" also has a double meaning, since the regular class teaching is interrupted by the first Janus Door attack. This is what is called the "rabbit hole" in ARGs: the doorway into the game.

STORY OVERVIEW

The two first-year sections of Professor Zachary Peterson's cybersecurity class begin with introductory material as they ordinarily would. A friendly *competition* will develop between the two sections of the class to arrive at the best possible solutions to problems presented by assignments. But soon the class assignments, such as phishing, social recon, port scanning etc., begin to contain elements that make them seem real, rather than just assignments.

It's clear that *something* is going on that is more than assignments. Clues will lead students to suspect the basis for their assignments may be actual attacks. When the two sections become suspicious that each is responsible for making the attacks on each other more difficult, Professor Peterson will reveal he has been testing both sections to see if they could help with real cyberattacks originated outside Cal Poly. The attacks appear to originate with the Janus Door, a shadowy hacker organization, led by someone named Verita. On the dark web, rumors circulate that the Janus Door is planning what they call a "devilish disruption." They are obviously testing the institute's security with the attacks.

After a while the students will be not only repelling a variety of attacks, including one that suggests the hackers have physical access to the campus, but will begin to learn how to track where the attacks are coming from. As the class progresses, the students will discover that the Janus Door and Verita are somehow linked to a former graduate computer science student at Cal Poly, Nick Menzo. He was dismissed for hacking into the school's servers and stealing sensitive research for a foreign government. When police were about to arrest him, he disappeared with his wife and newborn child.

With the help of Professor Peterson and his TA Nick Gonella, the students will begin to trace the attacks to Verita, and discover she is Verita Menzo, the daughter of Nick Menzo. More research will reveal that Menzo and his wife, to avoid prosecution, fled to the country that paid him, leaving their child, Verita, behind in foster care. It appears Verita is out to revenge her parents' exile, and abandonment of her, on Cal Poly, the school she believes shattered their family.

Soon it becomes clear that most of the attacks are smokescreen, but not all. Verita is looking for a program that her father left hidden on a now long-gone school server right before he disappeared. That program was meant to be his revenge. That server was long ago backed up on new campus servers as part of a periodic routine general backup to make certain nothing important was ever lost. The backup was performed each time servers were updated.

Students will be able to discover the location of the program Menzo hid when an obscure file in Spanish is found. It's title? Diablo. Not only does that explain the use of the word devilish, but it also points to the location of a very real danger: the program was written to track security protocols at the nearby Diablo Canyon Nuclear Power Plant.

The program was designed to replicate itself by incorporating any changes made to the Diablo Canyon software over the years. That way it could continue to grab the protocols, each time creating an updated back door Menzo called the Janus Door, to the power plant's computers.

Worse, there's evidence that Verita is close to finding the latest version of the program and plans to delete it from the Cal Poly server, once she has a copy. That must mean she plans to use it to plant a virus in the Diablo reactor! The ultimate in ransomware!

Nick will reveal he is with the FBI and explains that if agents had started running around campus, or engaging Janus Door in a cyber war, the shadowy group might vanish before they can be tracked down. That's why the Cal Poly administration and the FBI approached Professor Peterson to accept the cyber cop as a TA to investigate and thwart Janus Door, and possibly use his class to assist the undercover investigation, if they seemed up to the task. And it has paid off. The students are surpassing the FBI's expectations. And the fact that Verita thinks she's only dealing with ordinary students has made her vulnerable.

Verita retaliates against the students for their interference in her plans by hacking into their grades. Professor Peterson and Nick successfully restore the grades. And the students now know that the Janus Door can open in either direction. The students have at least a glimmer of how they can stop Verita.

Just as it looks as if Verita can be defeated, Nick will disappear. A truncated message found in a file on his computer says simply: "devilish devilish devilish." While Professor Peterson will liaison with the authorities, the students must collaborate and use all the skills they've learned in class to find where Nick is being held captive and figuring out the code to the physical door to the prison somewhere near to campus.

Then they must prevent Verita from being paid the ransomware to avoid a reactor meltdown, by using the backdoor's code to trace the virus back to the Janus Door computer and shut it down before the attack can take place. This will require *collaboration* between both sections. Each section will have one half of the puzzle necessary to complete their counterattack. Together they will also find the address of the off-campus lair from which Verita has been staging her attacks. This leads to her being arrested by Nick.

In a dramatic conclusion, Verita will be brought before the class. She will claim she never intended to collect the ransomware nor cause a major nuclear disaster. Her revenge was to prove it *could happen*. A teaching moment for the institute she feels destroyed her family. The students will come to realize the emotional upheavals that led Verita to where she is today. And they will decide to speak against her or on her behalf in court. A final news story on CyberFacts will announce her fate.

Successful in their quest, the students will be treated to their pictures and stories about their achievement on the school's website, and of course about the real class behind the story!

CURRICULUM/NARRATIVE/PUZZLE BALANCE SHEET

The complex balance between the curriculum, the narrative, and the puzzles was mapped in this document to easily track how they were all scheduled and interconnected. It is arranged in a similar style to the production schedule in *The Lost Manuscript* but was far trickier to create. The columns list week, date, class (either lecture or lab), curriculum, episodes, narrative, puzzles, and type of puzzle (defend, identify, attack).

Janus Door Curriculum/Narrative/Puzzle Balance Sheet

Curriculum Titles: (C), Narrative Titles: (N)
Puzzle Types: (D)efend, (I)dentify, (A)ttack

Week	Date	Class	Curriculum	Titles	Narrative	Puzzles	Type
1	Thursday Sep 14	Lecture	Introduction to Security: basic terminology and goals, history, motivations of attackers Introduction to CS: programming, data representations and encodings (e.g. binary, hex, base64, ASCII, bitmaps, QR codes), algorithms and computability, logic and gates	Unit 0: Introductions (C)	The two first-year sections of Professor Peterson's cybersecurity class begin with introductory material as they ordinarily would, with two additions: Prof. Peterson will explain about the game without revealing details. Students will be asked to write a brief bio on Poly Learn.		
1	Thursday Sep 14	Lab	TBD by Instructor	Unit 0: Introductions (C)		[d0x3d!]	D
2	Tuesday Sep 19	Lecture	Introduction to UNIX: command line and basic commands, text editors, remote shells Introduction to Python: variables, Boolean logic, basic control structures (conditionals, loops, functions), libraries, file and network IO	Unit 0: Introductions (C)	The two first-year sections of Professor Zachary Peterson's cybersecurity class continue with introductory material as they ordinarily would.		
2	Tuesday Sep 19	Lab	TBD	Unit 0: Introductions (C)	The first fictional website Cyber Facts will be introduced as part of a list of web-based sites students may access for reference. Cyber Facts has a	Parse files in a particular order to find hidden secrets.	D

A chart combining details on dates, lessons, narrative and puzzles for precise comparison.

					warning displayed about the Dark Web and the site Dark Park in particular. It will also include fun tests like this one.		
2	Thursday Sep 21	Lecture	Introduction to ethics for computer scientists More advanced programming - Using libraries - Functions - Network IO (sockets, ports, packets, HTTP) Handling file types and data encodings	Unit 0: Introductions (C)			
2	Thursday Sep 21	Lab	Students write pieces of a simple web crawler. When students enter a certain search the TA suggests, the web crawler will "discover" the Dark Park site.	Episode 0: Door Bell (N)	The TA tells the students about dad. The TA's dad is terribly concerned her home computer may be compromised by identity thieves. The TA pleads a heavy workload and asks the students, if they can help the TA's dad to understand password concepts and to protect her computer. Professor Peterson warns students about the Dark Web.	TBD.	D
3	Tuesday Sep 26	Lecture	Identity: philosophically, what is it, having it, and proving it Physical Techniques: common identifiers, ID cards, forgability Digital Techniques: Passwords, Security Questions, Two-step/Two-factor authentication, Public Key Infrastructure/ HTTPS, biometrics	Unit 1: Digital Identity & Authentication (C)			
3	Tuesday Sep 26	Lab	Threat model passwords and solve CyberFacts puzzle on Unit 1 lecture topic of the instructor's choice.	Episode 1: Tower Door (N)	Once the assignment is complete Nick thanks students and promises to pass their suggestions on to his dad. He's sure she won't bother them again.	Threat model, then prepare list of password best practices and instructions on how to use them for TA's dad. Solve CyberFacts puzzle on Unit 1.	P, D
3	Thursday Sep 28	Lecture	Completion of Digital Identity & Authentication	Unit 1: Digital Identity & Authentication (C)			
3	Thursday Sep 28	Lab	Collaboration: Each student in each section must complete the competition, so the first students to complete mentor the others. As each student figures it out, they take over mentoring, until all have completed the competition	Episode 1: Tower Door (N)	Prof. Peterson announces a friendly competition between sections to test how much they've learned about Digital Identity and Authentication. Students will notice one type of password protection Prof. Peterson didn't cover! And it is marked by a large, furry-looking X.	Sections compete to crack layers of passwords.	D
4	Tuesday Oct 3	Lecture	Social Engineering: pre-texting, dumpster diving, impersonation Phishing: over email, web, and social networks Usable Security, and the failures thereof Physical security: lock picking, tamper-proof seals	Unit 2: Human Factors & Physical Security (C)	Prof. confesses the new material was a test. The reason? A series of cyberattacks have been initiated against Cal Poly, all signed by a "furry X." He suggests students carefully investigate the Dark Park website to see if they can find any reference to the furry X.		D
4	Tuesday Oct 3	Lab	Breaking security questions through recon (e.g. what people post on Facebook, known relationships (mother's maiden name), historical events) Conduct a phishing attack Lock picking and combo lock breaking	Episode 2: Unlocked Door (N)	Students find references to The Janus Door on Dark Park, but when they click on the Furry X link in a brief article about The Janus Door, The Janus Door is alerted and backtraces them to Cal Poly.	Launch a phishing attack: Create a spoof email that contains links that when clicked on will allow them to discover the furry X is a customer of Dark Park.	D

(Continued)

			Gaining access to an IoT device to gain control of an environment (e.g. turning lights (blacklight?) on in a room they don't have physical access to, finding an unsecured web cam)				
4	Thursday Oct 5	Lecture	Completion of above lecture	Unit 2: Human Factors & Physical Security (C)			
4	Thursday Oct 5	Lab	Completion of above lab	Episode 2: Unlocked Door (N)	The Dark Park website Rumor Mill column contains several references to The Janus Door planning a "devilish disruption" of epic proportions. Students use Daniel Park's own credentials and find an Excel spreadsheet with the true identities of Dark Park's users. This leads them to the ownership file for The Janus Door. The account is in the name of a Verita Menzo at a PO Box in Caracas, Venezuela. Students receive a warning email from Daniel Park. Meanwhile Nick's dad, after reading about RFID readers, is convinced a woman standing in line behind her at her grocery store held her purse close to the credit card scanner	Use a spoof site to steal Daniel Park's credentials. Help Nick's father protect himself from RFID readers.	D, P

					and stole the personal information on her card. Students create a list of best practices on what to do if an RFID reader is used to grab personal information from a credit card. Nick is sure this is the last time they'll need to help her.		
5	Tuesday Oct 10	Lecture	Basics: the HTTP protocol, HTML, Cookies, JavaScript, web applications and databases Attacks: Cross-site scripting, cross-site request forgeries, SQL injection, command injection	Unit 3: Web Security (C)			
5	Tuesday Oct 10	Lab	Finding secrets written HTML comments Cookie forging (to gain either admin access to a site or impersonate a user) SQL injection (to gain information from a database) XSS (to gather a target's cookie, or force them to visit a site) Command injection (to read some information stored on a server, or get the server to do something, e.g. run a specific command) Using the robots.txt file to find "hidden" directories	Episode 3: Open Door (N)	The students' success in uncovering Verita's account information on Dark Park prompts a dismissive video warning from her. It's clear The Janus Door intends to attack the Cal Poly Admin Server. Not simply for revenge. Verita is after something on the server that she needs… The Janus Door launches a series of probes to find weaknesses on the Admin Server and attack Cal Poly's security defenses. Mr. Gonella has heard a news story about fishing. He's afraid to open any of his email! Can the students help?	Check Admin Server for holes in its defenses, detect incoming probes and try to guard against possible attacks. Help Nick's dad understand about phishing attacks and what actions to avoid.	D, P

(Continued)

5	Thursday Oct 12	Lecture	Completion of above lecture	Unit 3: Web Security (C)			
5	Thursday Oct 12	Lab	Finding secrets written HTML comments Cookie forging (to gain either admin access to a site or impersonate a user) SQL injection (to gain information from a database) XSS (to gather a target's cookie, or force them to visit a site)	Episode 4: The Janus Door (N)	Students will find a "Where Are They Now?" file on CyberFacts that covers several hackers from years past. One of those mentioned is Nick Menzo, a former graduate student at Cal Poly. In 1987 he was expelled from Cal Poly for hacking into the school's servers and stealing sensitive research for a foreign government. When police were about to arrest him, he disappeared with his wife, Katherine, and a newborn child.\n\nThey've come a long way from the tiny town of Olmsted Falls in Ohio where they grew up, were honor students together in high school and were married.\n\nStudents will repel an attack on the Admin Server.\n\nStudents use their recon so far to break the password into Verita's private account: olmstedfalls. Verita will see the intrusion and her files will begin to disappear. Students will try to copy as many as they can before everything vanishes. All the files students grab will be corrupted by	Cookie forage to gain access to more of the Dark Park site.\n\nOnce hacked into the site, use recon to break into Verita's account. Verita will see the intrusion and her files will begin to disappear. Students will try to copy as many as they can before everything vanishes. All the files students grab will be corrupted by Verita. But bits and pieces remain to be interpreted.\n\nOnce the bits and pieces have been correctly interpreted students will have the clues to locate Nick Menzo on an island of Vanuatu and can try to contact him. However, they will have no reply.	D
					Verita. But tiny bits and pieces remain. They appear to be from multiple letters.\n\nOnce hacked into the Dark Park site, students discover that Nick has an account on the site. He claims he created the account to protect students once they discovered the site.		
6	Tuesday Oct 17	Lecture	Networking basics: OSI model, protocols, TCP/UDP, IP (addresses and ports) Common protocols: HTTP, DNS, SMTP, SSH Attacks: Man in the middle, DNS spoofing, port scanning, TCP/IP forgeries, denial of service, botnets Anonymity, onion routing	Unit 4: Network Security (C)			
6	Tuesday Oct 17	Lab	Port scan/banner grabbing a machine looking for open/unusual ports; finding a hidden service (typically a web server, or something else) Port knocking (must connect to ports on a server in a certain order to access a service/secret)	Episode 5: Knocking on the Door (N)	The letters are from Verita's father. Her mother died, but there are clues that he moved somewhere new after the Berlin Wall fell. It also becomes clear that most of the attacks on Cal Poly have a more definite purpose than mere revenge. The hidden file mentioned in the last letter must be what Verita must be searching for. "More power than you've ever dreamed." "Make them pay." What does it do? Students need to find the hidden file before she does.	Nick has detected that someone attempted to plant malware in the school's computer network via a physical connection to the network.\n\nFind location of hostile thumb drive in a network printer.\n\nFind and remove the hostile thumb drive.	D, P

(Continued)

					Nick discovers malware that launches an attack on the Admin Server. He has traced its origin to a physical source, probably a hostile thumb drive inserted into a network device somewhere on campus. Students must find the location of the drive and remove it. They manage it, but there's evidence it may have succeeded at locating the hidden file.		
6	Thursday Oct 19	Lecture	Completion of above lecture	Unit 4: Network Security (C)			
6	Thursday Oct 19	Lab	Completion of above lab	Episode 6: Back Door (N)	Students will be able to discover the location of the program Menzo hid on the Admin Server when an obscure file in Spanish is found. It's title? Diablo. Not only does that explain the use of the word devilish, but points to the location of a very real danger: the program was written to track security protocols at the Diablo Canyon Nuclear Power Plant. Verita is not simply attacking Cal Poly for revenge, she must have a much larger goal in mind, and to achieve it she is attacking the nuclear power plant.

Verita uploads another video to Dark Park, boasting that she is close to finding the latest version of the program, and | Find the Diablo file on the Admin Server and decrypt it.

Solve Nick Menzo's password riddle. This won't be possible until November 7. | D |

					plans to delete it from the Cal Poly server, once she has a copy. That must mean she plans to use it to plant a virus in the Diablo reactor! The ultimate in ransomware! However she apparently isn't interested in money. What does she want?		
7	Tuesday Oct 24	Lecture	Storage Forensics: Common file types and formats, file system structures, secure deletion, steganography, log files
Network Forensics: packet capturing, geolocation of IPs, honeypots/honeynets	Unit 5: Software Security (C)	**[NOTE: There is a field trip to the Diablo Canyon Nuclear Power Plant on the weekend between Oct 19 and Oct 24.]**		
7	Tuesday Oct 24	Lab	Traversing and searching a large amount of data using programming or command line tools
Using autopsy/sleuthkit (open source forensic tools) to recover deleted data from a file system (e.g. from a found USB drive)
Using file metadata to identify owner, creation/modification times
Repairing corrupted files to recover data (bitmap works really well to recover a broken image)
Geolocating an IP using either/both a known geolocation databases and/or triangulation using round-trip times of pings
Capturing packets from an unsecured wifi network, then | Episode 7: Pick a Door | The TA will reveal they are with the FBI, operating out of a secret office on campus. The TA explains that if agents had started running around campus, or engaging Janus Door in a cyber war, the shadowy group might vanish before they can be tracked down. That's why the Cal Poly administration and the FBI approached Professor Peterson to accept the cyber cop as a TA to investigate and thwart Janus Door, and possibly use his class to assist the undercover investigation, if they seemed up to the task.

Frank Stockton's famous short story from 1882, *The Lady or the Tiger*, relates the dilemma of a man who must choose | Beat Verita's "improbable" choice test. It consists of two potential kinds of attacks on the Admin Server (TBD). Verita claims one is fake, but the other is very real. They can only choose one. Which will it be? Students look for evidence to confirm which attack must be the real one. What they discover is that *both* attacks are real, and they must stop both! | A, D |

(Continued)

			using Wireshark on the PCAP file to find an unprotected password or cookie or recovering a transferred file Finding a secret message steganographically hidden in a JPEG file Setting up a honeypot to lure a (fake) attacker A PDF which has been "redacted" using a removable layer Looking at log files (e.g. a web server to identify an IP address) Use TinEye to identify a recover the remainder of a fragmented/corrupted image Analyzing browser history		between two doors. Behind one is a lady. Behind the other a tiger. Verita gives students a similar choice. When they outsmart her, Verita realizes she has underestimated the students and angrily retaliates by hacking into their grades.		
7	Thursday Oct 26	Lecture	Completion of above lecture	Unit 5: Software Security (C)			
7	Thursday Oct 26	Lab	Completion of above lab	Episode 8: Trap Door	Professor Peterson and the TA help students restore and secure their grades. The students now know that the Janus Door can open in either direction. And they have at least a glimmer of how they can set a trap for Verita and discover her location, even as her ultimate goal remains a mystery.	Reverse engineer a custom protocol, then writing a piece of software that implements it to reveal a port knocking sequence they can use to hack into Dark Park and discover a port to Verita's new digital hideout.	A, D
8	Tuesday Oct 31	Lecture	Secrecy and confidentiality, integrity and authenticity Primitives: block ciphers, MACs, public key encryption, hash functions	Unit 6: Secret Communication & Cryptography (C)			
8	Tuesday Oct 31	Lab	Break a simple substitution cipher Brute force a weak key Factor a too-short RSA key to recover the private key Forge a message to a server that uses a bad MAC (e.g. a post to a website which uses a poorly designed MAC or uses too short a key) Look at a bitmap image encrypted with ECB mode (and which reveals the image) Go to library to decipher a book code	Episode 9: Spirit Door	Verita's digital location has been found by the students in another account on Dark Park. But Verita scrambles the account identifiers of all users to cover her next move. In the disruption users begin leaving the site in droves. Daniel Park sends students a panicked email. Verita moves her location and effectively vanishes again, leaving behind another video. And Nick's dad contacts students. Her son has disappeared! Can the students help her find him? Students search Nick's office and discover video captured on his computer when Nick was video conferencing with the FBI. He has been kidnapped!	Search Nick's office. Find a secret message steganographically hidden in a JPEG file. Break into Nick's computer and decrypt video file.	P, D
8	Thursday Nov 2	Lecture	Completion of above lecture	Unit 6: Secret Communication & Cryptography (C)	[NOTE: There is a field trip to Montaña de Oro State Park on the weekend between Nov 2 and Nov 7.]		
8	Thursday Nov 2	Lab	Completion of above lab	Episode 10: Golden Door	While Professor Peterson will liaison with the authorities, both sections of students must collaborate to find where Nick is being held captive. The trail leads first to Montaña de Oro State Park.	Teams solve puzzles, search Montaña de Oro State Park and rescue Nick from his prison on campus.	D, P
9	Tuesday Nov 7	Lecture	Code vs. Data Malware: Trojan horses, viruses, worms, rootkits, and	Unit 7: Digital Forensics (C)			

(Continued)

9	Tuesday Nov 7	Lab	the differences between them Basics of attacks: buffer overflows and integer overflows Fuzzing: finding errors in software externally			
9	Tuesday Nov 7	Lab	Write a key logger to capture user's input Fuzz a piece of software looking for mistakes Overflow a stack buffer which stores a password in poorly programmed software to gain access Looking at source code for a backdoor (e.g. comparing two version of an open source program, like SSH, one of which has been backdoored with a fixed password) Reverse engineering code that generates a secret, to compute the secret	Episode 11: Locked Door	Nick's dad thinks he's been attacked by the Eternal Blue ransomware. Students figure out what he did to trigger what is really some nasty adware, and how he can sterilize his computer. Nick finally admits he can't be certain this will be the last time he will ask for help.

Who left the clues to Nick's prison? Nick says it was Verita. But why? Verita told him to think of her as Cassandra. It may explain her true goal, a goal she needed to share, but she refused to explain until she achieved that goal. That can't happen. She needs to be stopped and captured!

Students discover her new digital hiding place. Where on the internet can she be hiding? On Cal Poly's Admin Server right under their noses the whole time! The file is in the name of Ada Lovelace…

In the file are two photographs. One is of Nick Menzo on a tropical island. | Find Verita's new digital address, and hack into her file.

Ada Lovelace also had an infamous father. Find out who he was, and why Verita chose her name.

Help Nick's dad get rid of some badly programmed adware that has taking his computer hostage.

Solve Nick Menzo's puzzle from October 19. | D, P |

9	Thursday Nov 9	Lecture	Completion of above lecture	Unit 7: Digital Forensics			
9	Thursday Nov 9	Lab	Completion of above lab	Episode 12: Swinging Door	The second is of Katherine Menzo's gravestone on the same island. There are also two pieces of code: the first is the backdoor code. The second is apparently Nick Menzo's Trojan Horse.

The students must stop Verita to avoid a reactor meltdown. They must use the backdoor's code to trace Nick Menzo's Trojan Horse to a new Janus Door computer and shut it down before the attack can take place. They fail! Or did they? Verita is at that computer writing code. | Write a key logger to capture Verita's input. | D |
| 10 | Tuesday Nov 14 | Lecture | | | | | |
| 10 | Tuesday Nov 14 | Lab | | Episode 13: Kicking Down the Door | Students will find the address of the off-campus lair from which Verita has been staging her attacks. Nick races off to arrest her. But he may be too late!

The cryptographic key to launch or stop the attack was split into multiple pieces by Nick Menzo. All students from both sections must derive their share. | Break Nick Menzo's cryptographic key.

Close the Janus Door. | D |
| 10 | Thursday Nov 16 | Lecture | Completion of above lecture | | | | |

(Continued)

10	Thursday Nov 16	Lab	Completion of above lab	Episode 14: Cell Door	In a dramatic conclusion, Verita will be brought before the class.	Vote on Verita's fate and whether to tell her where her father may be found.	
					The students will vote on Poly Learn to speak against her or on her behalf in court.		
					They will also vote whether to tell her where her father is, or not.		
					When Professor Peterson concludes his lecture, there will be a final email from Jonathan to Nick. He grimaces. This one he'll handle on his own.		D
					A final news story on Cyber Facts will announce Verita's fate. And the students' exploits will be publicized with pictures and their comments.		

(Continued)

EPISODES

The Janus Door is divided into ten weekly episodes, each consisting of a class on Tuesdays and a lab on Thursdays. Major story moves may be found in each of the following episode descriptions.

CHAPTER 39

Episode 0 – Introduction (Week 1)

[All pedagogical material supplied by Professor Zachary Peterson.]

[Disclaimer: These notes have not been subjected to the usual scrutiny reserved for formal publications. They may be distributed outside this class only with the permission of the Instructor.]

The body of each lecture has not been reproduced in this book. Topics are covered by a short summary so the reader can track the relationship between game design and teaching.

Thursday, September 14

CHARACTERS

Professor Peterson, Nick

NARRATIVE

The two first-year sections of Professor Peterson's cybersecurity class begin with introductory material as they ordinarily would, with two additions:

1. Professor Peterson will tell students they will be playing a game. He will tell them the game's title *The Janus Door*, and explain about the game, its structure and duration, without revealing details.

I kept in contact with Professor Peterson as the class progressed, answering questions and helping solve unexpected situations that arose during gameplay. As Professor Peterson related in his Foreword, most of the students dove into the fictional world we had created with enthusiasm, but one student had missed the first-class introduction and had no idea that *The Janus Door* attacking the school was fiction. When the students began hacking into the Dark Park website, he appeared in Professor Peterson's office quite upset. Shouldn't they be warning the university about what was happening? And wasn't hacking into a website illegal???

I've related the stories of the custodian cleaning up our carefully-prepared lair at the top of the IU student union tower in the first *Skeleton Chase*; the woman who thought Bloomington was in danger and might be evacuated; and the students stopping innocent strollers, asking if they'd seen a crazy guy and his mutated plant in *Skeleton Chase 2*. I think I was lucky that up until then a *player* had never thought the game he was playing was real. The moral of this story is simple: make sure all of your players know they *are* players. We should not be responsible for any sleepless nights. We can entrust that to academics who grade like they are a hanging judge passing sentence.

2. At the beginning of today's lab, students will be asked to upload a brief "skill bio" to PolyLearn before the next class to facilitate balancing teams when team assignments are required.

As noted in the design document, PolyLearn, a version of Moodle, was Cal Poly's primary tool students and instructors used for normal classroom assignments and communication. This type of software was integral to all four of the games in this book. It was familiar to each student across all classes; made communication easy; and, depending upon how it was deployed, helped game elements to seem all the more real, facilitating the "willing suspension of disbelief" of players.

VIDEO

None

TEXT/EMAIL

None

LECTURE (UNIT 0: *INTRODUCTION*)

- Introduction to Security: basic terminology and goals, history, motivations of attackers
- Introduction to CS: programming, data representations and encodings (e.g. binary, hex, base64, ASCII, bitmaps, QR codes), algorithms and computability, logic, and gates
- Introduction to ethics for computer scientists
- Introduction to UNIX: command line and basic commands, text editors, remote shells
- Introduction to Python: variables, Boolean logic, basic control structures (conditionals, loops, functions), libraries, file, and network IO

LAB (UNIT 0: *INTRODUCTION*)

Students play [d0x3d!] ice breaker.

PUZZLES

Digital

None

Physical

None

CHAPTER 40

Episode 0 – Introduction Continued (Week 2)

Tuesday, September 19

Professor Peterson, Nick

NARRATIVE

The two first-year sections of Professor Zachary Peterson's cybersecurity class continue with introductory material as they ordinarily would. The fictional website CyberFacts will be introduced as part of a list of web-based sites students may access for reference. CyberFacts has a warning displayed about the Dark Web and one site, Dark Park, in particular. It will also include introductory puzzles. See Puzzles section.

VIDEO

None

TEXT/EMAIL

None

LECTURE (UNIT 0: *INTRODUCTION CONTINUED*)

- Introduction to Security: basic terminology and goals, history, motivations of attackers

- Introduction to CS: programming, data representations and encodings (e.g. binary, hex, base64, ASCII, bitmaps, QR codes), algorithms and computability, logic, and gates

- Introduction to ethics for computer scientists

- Introduction to UNIX: command line and basic commands, text editors, remote shells

- Introduction to Python: variables, Boolean logic, basic control structures (conditionals, loops, functions), libraries, file, and network IO

Some listed lecture topics extended over more than one class. Professor Peterson's notes indicate the topics to be covered in more than one class, not that the lectures were repeats.

LAB (UNIT 0 *INTRODUCTION CONTINUED*)

Puzzles

Digital

Found on CyberFacts website: Parse files in a particular order to find hidden secrets.

Physical

None

CHAPTER 41

Episode 0 – Door Bell (Week 2)

Thursday, September 21

Professor Peterson, Nick

NARRATIVE

Today and at the beginning of each subsequent lab, Professor Peterson will write the title of the current episode in a top corner of the whiteboard. Today he will write: *Door Bell*. He will explain that these are the titles of the game's episodes. If students need to refresh their memories about the narrative, or if they miss a class, they will be able to read descriptions of *previous* episodes on the class PolyLearn site.

Yes, Door Bell is actually one word, Doorbell. I felt the former would match the style of later episodes better.

Nick tells the class about his father. Mr. Gonella is a voracious follower of the news. He will see a news story, then immediately notice "odd behavior" in his computer that makes him terribly worried he's a victim of a cyberattack. He has seen a story on TV about identity theft and is terribly worried identity thieves will steal his identity! Cal Poly has dumped a heavy workload on Nick. He asks the students in both sections if they can help his dad to understand password concepts to protect his personal information. Professor Peterson thinks this will be good "real world" practice for some of the subject matter already covered in class.

Professor Peterson tells students he has added links on PolyLearn to various Internet sites for their reference. He is giving them access to the Dark Park site through PolyLearn, so that they can get a feel for the Dark Web. He warns them of the dangers lurking in the uncensored wild frontier of the Dark Web, an encrypted online network that exists apart from the Internet most people know. While it has some legitimate inhabitants, it is also occupied by hackers, terrorist groups, criminals, and more. One of the stories on the Dark Park site talks about real hacking organizations that have lately been in the news. *The Janus Door* will not be mentioned. This is the beginning of the game's central narrative.

VIDEO
None

TEXT/EMAIL
None

LECTURE (UNIT 0: *INTRODUCTION CONTINUED*)

- Introduction to Security: basic terminology and goals, history, motivations of attackers

- Introduction to CS: programming, data representations and encodings (e.g. binary, hex, base64, ASCII, bitmaps, QR codes), algorithms and computability, logic, and gates

- Introduction to ethics for computer scientists

- Introduction to UNIX: command line and basic commands, text editors, remote shells

- Introduction to Python: variables, Boolean logic, basic control structures (conditionals, loops, functions), libraries, file, and network IO

LAB (UNIT 0 *INTRODUCTION CONTINUED*)

Professor Peterson writes the episode name, *Door Bell*, in a top corner of the whiteboard. Students explore the Dark Park website.

PUZZLES

Digital

None

Physical

None

IN THE PREVIOUS EPISODE...

Episode 0: Door Bell

Post after both lab sessions on Thursday, September 21.

Professor Peterson added links on PolyLearn to various Internet sites for your reference. He has included one site called Dark Park that you may access through PolyLearn as an example of a "hacker forum" to give you a taste of the Dark Web. He warned you of the dangers lurking in the uncensored wild frontier of the Dark Web, an encrypted online network that exists apart from the Internet most people know. While it has some legitimate inhabitants, it is also occupied by hackers, terrorist groups, criminals, and more.

CHAPTER 42

Episode 1 – Unlocked Door (Week 3)

Tuesday, September 26

CHARACTERS

Professor Peterson, Nick, Jonathan

NARRATIVE

Jonathan, Nick's dad, emails Nick to tell him he has seen a story on TV about identity theft and is terribly worried identity thieves are trying to steal his identity! Students will help him compile a list of password concepts to protect his personal information. Once each lab is complete, Nick thanks students and promises to pass their suggestions on to his dad. He's sure he won't bother them again.

VIDEO

None

TEXT/EMAIL

None

LECTURE (UNIT 1: DIGITAL IDENTITY & AUTHENTICATION)

- Introduction to Passwords

- The Security of Passwords

- Choosing Passwords

- Breaking Human Passwords

- Protecting Passwords on the Server

- Time-Space Trade Off

- Password System Security

- Personal Password Security

LAB (UNIT 1: *DIGITAL IDENTITY & AUTHENTICATION*)

Professor Peterson writes the episode name, *Unlocked Door*, in a top corner of the whiteboard.

Students in both sections will threat model the following:

- Choosing the same good password for multiple accounts

- Storing passwords on a sticky note on your computer

- Storing passwords on a laminated card in your wallet

- Storing passwords in a plaintext file on your computer

- Using a web-based password manager model

PUZZLES

Digital

Threat model passwords
  Solve CyberFacts puzzle

Physical

Compile list of the best password protection practices to send to Jonathan.

IN THE PREVIOUS EPISODE...

Episode 1: Unlocked Door

Post after both lab sessions on Tuesday, September 26.

Cal Poly has dumped a heavy workload on Nick. He asked the students in both sections if you could help his dad. Professor Peterson thinks this will be good "real world" practice for some of the subject matter already covered in class.

You helped Jonathan compile a list of good password practices to protect his personal information. Once each lab was complete Nick thanked you and promises to pass your suggestions on to his dad. He's sure he won't bother you again.

CHAPTER 43

Episode 1 – Unlocked Door Part 2 (Week 3)

Thursday, September 28

CHARACTERS

Professor Peterson, Nick

NARRATIVE

Professor Peterson announces that he's set up a way for students in each section to contact each other for competition and collaboration as needed.

At the end of the lecture, Professor Peterson announces a friendly competition between sections in the lab to test how much they've learned about Digital Identity & Authentication. Each section is tasked with breaking a series of increasingly difficult levels of passwords on a fun and friendly website created for the class. Professor Peterson has to attend a faculty meeting and is not present at the beginning of the lab. And, when the final page is unlocked, it reveals a taunting message:

> "What's this? Children playing with passwords? You realize your classwork is as public as a story on cable news, don't you? Learn to protect yourselves better than this! If of course you're capable of learning anything."

It is signed by what can only be described as a huge, furry-looking X.

Nick says he doesn't understand how this happened, or what it means.

When Professor Peterson arrives, Nick shows him the message, and suggests that some students in the other section added it as a joke. But Professor Peterson checks the site. Both sections have the same message! He can't explain how the last page got there or what the furry X might mean. Could the assignment have been hacked from outside?

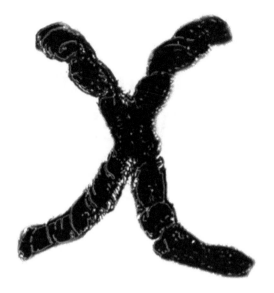

That's definitely a furry-looking X.

VIDEO

None

TEXT/EMAIL

None

LECTURE (UNIT 1: *DIGITAL IDENTITY & AUTHENTICATION* CONTINUED)

- Introduction to Passwords
- The Security of Passwords
- Choosing Passwords
- Breaking Human Passwords
- Protecting Passwords on the Server
- Time-Space Trade Off
- Password System Security
- Personal Password Security

LAB (UNIT 1: *DIGITAL IDENTITY & AUTHENTICATION* CONTINUED)

Professor Peterson writes the episode name, *Unlocked Door Part 2*, in a top corner of the whiteboard.

Students are tasked with breaking a series of increasingly difficult levels of passwords.

PUZZLES
Digital

Break a series of increasingly difficult levels of passwords on a fun and friendly website created for the class.

Each student in each section must complete the competition, so the first students to complete mentor the others. As each student figures it out, they take over mentoring, until all have completed the competition.

There was an early concern that only one or two team members might finish a shared assignment like this, and all would get credit for it. I had dealt with this issue in *The Multiplayer Classroom* by limiting the opportunities for this credit system, such as earmarking only a few questions on an exam for this purpose. The intent was to generate a powerful intrinsic reward: the thanks from grateful teammates. It was very successful. I had been concerned that team members would let the kid with the glasses would do all the work. That didn't happen. Everyone wanted to be the recipient of their teammates' gratitude, so all members of the team tried to answer those questions as best that they could. And of course, not knowing which questions on the test might be set aside for this, most students studied all the harder.

This cybersecurity class was significantly more hands-on, and the knowledge was especially cumulative from one assignment to the next. So, puzzle-solving was set up with all team members needing to *complete every assignment on their own* with those finishing first to "mentor" their teammates, essentially becoming teaching assistants. All were still taxed with demonstrating that they each had completed the assignment successfully.

Physical

None

IN THE PREVIOUS EPISODE…
Episode 1: Unlocked Door Part 2

Post after both lab sessions on Thursday, September 28.

Professor Peterson announced that he's set up a way for students in each section to contact each other for competition and collaboration as needed.

In the original design document for *The Janus Door*, the Narrative section and the "In the Previous Episode…" section were separated by quite a few pages. Hyperlinks allowed readers to jump back and forth between them, but even so, it was a needless chore. This book will be physical as well as digital. The hyperlinks were impractical, so "In the Previous Episode…" has been placed at the bottom of each episode to prevent the need to keep flipping back and forth. As you will see, this leads to some redundancy. I felt the "In the Previous Episode..." feature was a successful device that I had not tried before. So, both it and the Narrative section remain intact within each episode. You may skip either one and still have a clear idea of the narrative progression.

At the end of the lecture, Professor Peterson announced a friendly competition between sections in the lab to test how much you've learned about Digital Identity & Authentication. Each section was tasked with breaking a series of increasingly difficult levels of passwords on a fun and friendly website created for the class. Professor Peterson had to attend a faculty meeting and was not present at the beginning of the lab. And, when the final page was unlocked, it revealed a taunting message:

> "What's this? Children playing with passwords? You realize your classwork is as public as a story on cable news, don't you? Learn to protect yourselves better than this! If of course you're capable of learning anything."

It is signed by what can only be described as a large, furry-looking X (See Narrative section above).

Nick said he didn't understand how this happened, or what it means. When Professor Peterson arrived, Nick showed him the message, and suggested that some student in the other section added it as a joke. But Professor Peterson checked the site. Both sections had the same message! He couldn't explain how the last page got there or what the furry X might mean. Could the assignment have been hacked from outside?

CHAPTER 44

Episode 2 – Tower Door (Week 4)

Tuesday, October 3

CHARACTERS

Professor Peterson, Nick

NARRATIVE

Professor Peterson confesses that he *has* seen the furry X before. A series of cyberattacks have been initiated against Cal Poly, all signed by a "furry X." He says he hopes the students can help the university discover who is responsible, and why they chose to target CPE123 with that message. He suggests students carefully investigate the Dark Park website to see if they could find any reference to the furry X. If anyone does, they should share the information.

They will find the furry X in an article on Social Engineering. It is a link. When clicked on, it dissolves into a portrait of the two-faced Roman god, Janus.

Clicking on Janus links to the following messages:

> "Thank you for clicking on our link. We are always interested to learn more about those who are interested in us. You have touched *The Janus Door*. And now we can touch you."

"California State Polytechnic University" flashes on the screen, replacing the first message.

A few seconds later it is replaced by "San Luis Obispo, California"

A few seconds later: "CPE 123"

Then: "Ah, there you are. Poly want a cracker? You've got one now whether you want one or not. Let's play a game. What shall we call it? I know. How about Ivory Tower Defense?"

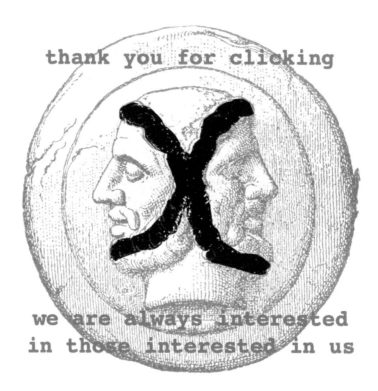

thank you for clicking

we are always interested
in those interested in us

The "fur" is actually the hair of the two-faced Roman god, Janus.

Professor Peterson announces that he's set up a way for students in each section to contact each other. You may work independently or collaborate as needed.

He tells you that you should not have clicked on links on Dark Park, but maybe the fact that you made the mistake can be turned to your benefit. *The Janus Door* are pretty sophisticated; however, they use Dark Park's secure message service. Maybe Dark Park isn't as secure as it could be. With the knowledge you acquired in class you created a spoof Dark Park login page, and Daniel fell for it. You successfully discovered his login credentials! Now you can login to Dark Park as Daniel, and with admin privileges! This gives you access to Dark Park customer files, including hopefully *The Janus Door*.

VIDEO

None

TEXT/EMAIL

None

LECTURE (UNIT 2: *HUMAN FACTORS & PHYSICAL SECURITY*)

- Password Lab Debrief

- Introduction to Human Factors

- Social Engineering

- Security Economics

- Physical Security

- Usable Security

- Ethics and Professional Responsibilities

Lab (Unit 2: *Human Factors & Physical Security*)

Professor Peterson writes the episode name, *Tower Door,* in a top corner of the whiteboard.

PUZZLES

Digital

Create a spoof website login page for Dark Park.

Physical

None

IN THE PREVIOUS EPISODE…

Episode 2: Tower Door

Post after both lab sessions on Tuesday, October 3.

Professor Peterson confessed that he *had* seen the furry X before. A series of cyberattacks have been initiated against Cal Poly, all signed by a "furry X." He said he hoped you could help the university discover who is responsible, and why they chose to target your class with that message. He suggested you carefully investigate the Dark Park website to see if you could find any reference to the furry X.

The furry X was found in an article on Social Engineering, and how *The Janus Door* successfully used social engineering to bring down a rival hacking group. The furry X was a link. When clicked on, it dissolved into a portrait of the two-faced Roman god, Janus (See Narrative section). Unfortunately, clicking on Janus linked to a string of messages:

> "Thank you for clicking on our link. We are always interested to learn more about those who are interested in us. You have touched *The Janus Door.* And now we can touch you."

"California State Polytechnic University" flashes on the screen, replacing the first message.

A few seconds later it is replaced by "San Luis Obispo, California"

A few seconds later: "CPE 123"

Then: "Ah, there you are. Poly want a cracker? You've got one now whether you want one or not. Let's play a game. What shall we call it? I know. How about Ivory Tower Defense?"

Professor Peterson announced that he's set up a way for students in each section to contact each other. You may work independently or collaborate as needed.

He told you that you should not have clicked on links on Dark Park, but maybe the fact that you made the mistake can be turned to your benefit. *The Janus Door* are pretty sophisticated; however, they use Dark Park's secure message service. Maybe Dark Park isn't as secure as it could be. With the knowledge you acquired in class you created a spoof Dark Park login page, and Daniel fell for it. You successfully discovered his login credentials! Now you can login to Dark Park as Daniel, and with admin privileges! This gives you access to Dark Park customer files, including hopefully *The Janus Door*.

CHAPTER 45

Episode 2 – Tower Door Part 2 (Week 4)

Thursday, October 5

CHARACTERS

Professor Peterson, Nick, Jonathan, Daniel

NARRATIVE

The Dark Park website Rumor Mill column contains several references to *The Janus Door* planning a "devilish disruption" of epic proportions.

The spear phish worked! Students used Daniel Park's own credentials and found an Excel spreadsheet with the true identities of Dark Park's users. This lead them to the ownership file for *The Janus Door*.

The account is in the name of a Verita Menzo at a PO Box in Caracas, Venezuela.

Students receive a warning email from Daniel Park.

Meanwhile Nick's dad, after reading about RFID readers, is convinced a woman standing in line behind him at his grocery store held her purse close to the credit card scanner and stole the personal information on his card. Students create a list of best practices on what to do if an RFID reader is used to grab personal information from a credit card. Nick is sure this is the last time they'll need to help him.

VIDEO

None

TEXT/EMAIL

Text 1 from Daniel Park

> "This is the Dark Park admin. The site is unhackable, so stop trying. If you don't stop, you'll be evicted from Dark Park, and will be liable for both civil and criminal penalties and worse."

LECTURE (UNIT 2: *HUMAN FACTORS & PHYSICAL SECURITY* CONTINUED)

- Password Lab Debrief
- Introduction to Human Factors including Spear Phishing
- Social Engineering
- Security Economics
- Physical Security
- Usable Security
- Ethics and Professional Responsibilities

Professor Peterson tells students about the Admin Server. It is the main server on campus, and heavily protected. Cal Poly performs routine general backups. The backup is performed each time servers are updated. Every time new hardware is introduced, old servers are mirrored to new hardware, so nothing is ever lost.

Students spear phish Daniel Park's own credentials and received admin privileges.

LAB (UNIT 2: *HUMAN FACTORS & PHYSICAL SECURITY* CONTINUED)

Professor Peterson writes the episode name, *Tower Door Part 2*, in a top corner of the whiteboard.

PUZZLES

Digital

Help Nick's father protect himself from RFID readers.

Physical

None

IN THE PREVIOUS EPISODE...

Episode 2: Tower Door Part 2

Post after both lab sessions on Thursday, October 5.

You discovered that the Dark Park website Rumor Mill column contained several references to *The Janus Door* planning a "devilish disruption" of epic proportions.

The spear phish worked! You used Daniel Park's own credentials and found an Excel spreadsheet with the true identities of Dark Park's users. This led you to the ownership file for *The Janus Door*.

The account is in the name of a Verita Menzo at a PO Box in Caracas, Venezuela.

Your activity also prompted a warning text from Dark Park.

Meanwhile Nick's dad, after reading about RFID readers, became convinced a woman standing in line behind him at his grocery store held her purse close to the credit card scanner and stole the personal information on his card. You created a list of best practices on what to do if an RFID reader is used to grab personal information from a credit card. Nick was sure this is the last time you'll need to help him.

CHAPTER 46

Episode 3 – Open Door (Week 5)

Tuesday, October 10

CHARACTERS

Professor Peterson, Nick, Jonathan, Verita

NARRATIVE

The students' success in uncovering Verita's account information on Dark Park prompts a dismissive video warning from her. It's clear *The Janus Door* intends to attack the Cal Poly Admin Server. Not simply for revenge. Verita is after something on the server that she needs…

The Janus Door launches a series of probes to find weaknesses on the Admin Server and attack Cal Poly's security defenses.

And Mr. Gonella has heard a news story about "fishing." He's afraid to open any of his email! Can the students help?

VIDEO

Verita's Warning

This is a video of a silhouetted figure whose voice has been altered by a Vocoder or other electronic voice modifier.

VERITA: Clever little Freshmen, aren't you? So now you know a name and an address in South America. I bet you'd like to see my face, wouldn't you? Why, I might be serving you lunch at Julian's or Tacos To-Go. Or maybe I'm the friendly grounds-keeper keeping the campus looking so nice, or maybe I'm sitting next to you in class right now. Whatever. I'm proud of my name, and I'll keep it, thank you. The post office box is only a drop. Physical mail simply passes through and on

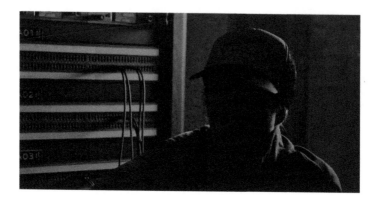

The Janus Door sends a video warning.

through many other boxes to me out here in the great elsewhere. Don't worry. I'm not really mad at you. Don't take what I'm about to do to one of your school's servers personally. Daniel Park though. I'm tempted to Eternal Blue his site big time for being so clueless. But his site has its uses. And it amuses me: our little game. Your ivory tower defenses will crumble. And what I want will soon be mine. Oh my! What can it be? What can I want at your little school? Revenge, my dears, among other things…

TEXT/EMAIL

None

LECTURE (UNIT 3: *WEB SECURITY*)

- History of the Web
- The stateless to the stateful web
- Cookies
- JavaScript
- XSS
- Getting users to "click" on ads (click fraud)
- Information stealing; file system traversal
- Phishing
- History probing
- Cookies stealing
- Reflective Attacks
- Stored Attacks

LAB (UNIT 3: *WEB SECURITY*)

Professor Peterson writes the episode name, *Open Door,* in a top corner of the whiteboard.

- Reflective Attacks
- Level 1 of the Google XSS game is an example of a reflective XSS attack
  - A server reflects back a link embedded with javascript
  - Often executed by sending a malicious link to a victim
- Stored Attacks
  - If the web server will store your malicious script for you, all the better
  - You will explore both kinds in lab
  - How do we fix it?

PUZZLES

Digital

Check Admin Server for holes in its defenses, detect incoming probes and try to guard against possible attacks. [**Verita will get in eventually.**]

Physical

Help Mr. Gonella understand about phishing attacks and what actions to avoid.

IN THE PREVIOUS EPISODE…

Episode 3: Open Door

Post after both lab sessions on Tuesday, October 10.

Your success in uncovering *The Janus Door's* account information on Dark Park prompted a snarky video warning from *The Janus Door's* spokesperson. It's clear Verita intends to attack some Cal Poly server. Not simply for revenge. She is after something on the server that she needs…

The Janus Door launched a series of probes to find weaknesses on the Admin Server and attack Cal Poly's security defenses.

And Mr. Gonella heard a news story about phishing. He was afraid to open any of his email until you helped him.

CHAPTER 47

Episode 4 – Janus Door (Week 5)

Thursday, October 12

CHARACTERS

Professor Peterson, Nick, Daniel

NARRATIVE

The name Menzo sounds familiar to Professor Peterson. He remembers hearing a story about someone with that name getting into trouble with Cal Poly a long time ago. He suggests searching CyberFacts for the name. Students will find a "Where Are They Now?" file that covers several hackers from years past. Some have gone to work fighting illegal hacking.

One of those mentioned is Nick Menzo, a former graduate student at Cal Poly. In 1987 he was expelled from Cal Poly for hacking into the school's servers and stealing sensitive research for a foreign government. When police were about to arrest him, he disappeared with his wife, Katherine, and a newborn child. They've come a long way from the tiny town of Olmsted Falls in Ohio where they grew up, were honor students together in high school, and were married.

[This also will plant the idea with students so that in the end they may suggest Verita not be imprisoned.]

Students managed to forge Verita's session cookie on Dark Park, then logged in as Verita to her private account. But Verita must have detected their intrusion and her files will begin to disappear. Students will try to copy as many as they can before everything vanishes. All the files students grab will be corrupted by Verita. But tiny bits and pieces remain. They appear to be from multiple letters. See Chronological List (Puzzle Solved) below.

[Pieces of the recovered files are divided into two or three sub pieces as needed. They contain many clues to who Verita is, what happened to her parents, where her father may be now, and his "legacy" that in turn will eventually point to Verita's real target.]

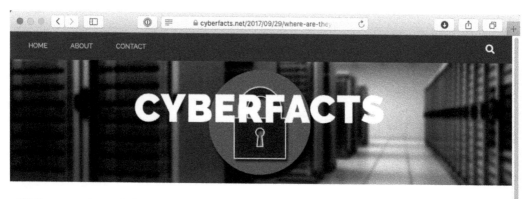

Where Are They Now? Nicholas Menzo

📅 September 29, 2017   👤 CyberFacts

By Chester Wood

They are the legends you have never heard of. In an age where hacking has practically become an eSport they are hacking royalty. Wait until you see where some ended up. But not all of them. Not all of them have come in from the cold.

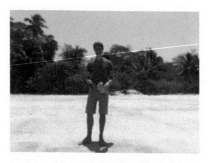

Federal Bureau of Investigation

Nick Menzo was born in 1962 in Olmsted Falls, Ohio. He had only one run-in with law enforcement during his early years when he created an automated targeting system for an underground Halloween tradition called the "Junior/Senior Apple Fight." It allowed terrified Junior students, usually the underdogs, to fire remote-controlled spring-loaded catapults from safe positions over one hundred yards from the site of the Village Green where the conflict took place. Several seniors were injured when ammunition was switched from rotten apples to monkey balls (from the shrub maclura pomifera to you scientists), a large tough fruit that resembles a green brain, and apparently packs quite a punch as a projectile.

From this unique, but inauspicious beginning, Nick attended a nearby college, Baldwin-Wallace, where he excelled in computer science, ran the computer lab and designed networking to do. It wasn't until he became a graduate student at California Polytechnic Institute (Cal Poly) that his career becomes of interest to us, as he became the first hacker to steal American secrets for a foreign power.

Nick's student work was helping to maintain the school's computer network. Early in his second year at Cal Poly he ran into severe money troubles when he attempted to supplement his meager student stipend by creating a digital card-counting

A story on former Cal Poly student Nick Menzo.

Once hacked into the Dark Park site, students discover that, their TA, Nick has an account on the site. He claims he created the account to protect students once they discovered the site.

Daniel Park will send students a second warning text:

VIDEO

None

TEXT/EMAIL

Text 2 from Daniel Park

> "Okay, I don't know how you managed it, but a user has complained that you've gained access to their account. You are ordered to cease and desist immediately, or action will be taken."

LECTURE (UNIT 3: *WEB SECURITY* CONTINUED)

- Social engineering: pre-texting, dumpster diving, impersonation.

- Phishing: over email, web, and social networks.

- Usable security, and the failures thereof.

- Physical security: lock picking, tamper-proof seals.

LAB (UNIT 3: *WEB SECURITY* CONTINUED)

Professor Peterson writes the episode name, *Janus Door*, in a top corner of the whiteboard.

- Breaking security questions through recon (e.g. what people post on Facebook, known relationships (mother's maiden name), historical events).

- Lock picking and combo lock breaking.

- Gaining access to an IoT device to gain control of an environment (e.g. turning lights (blacklight?) on in a room they don't have physical access to, finding an unsecured web cam).

PUZZLES

Digital

- Cookie forage to gain access to more of the Dark Park site.

- Log in as Verita to her private account. But Verita must have detected the intrusion and she begins deleting her files. Copy a few before everything vanishes.

- Once the bits and pieces have been ordered chronologically and correctly interpreted students will have the clues to locate Nick Menzo on an island of Vanuatu and can try to contact him. However, they will receive no reply.

Chronological List (Puzzle Solved):
  …January 4, 1987…
  …to my darling… these letters…
  …wherever the state sends you……
  …February 16, 1987…
  …when you're older…

...why... ...no choice...

...gambling...

...grad student stipend... ...not enough to live on...

...April 14, 1987...

...fled the United States...

...stolen research...

...East Germany...

...no extradition...

...October 31, 1987...

...gray... everything gray...

...what we gave up...

...November 9, 1988...

...one year old?...

...miss seeing you grow...

...November 27, 1989...

...no more Berlin wall...

...bilateral treaties... extradition possible...

...not safe to remain...

...February 2, 1990...

...warm...

...brilliant colors!...

...safe...

...no extradition...

...November 9, 1990...

...birthday... ...two!...

...truth...

...daughter...

...foster care...

...Cal Poly to blame for...

...August 4, 1990...

...you're three now... can you read these yet?...

...running their security for them... ...makes me laugh...

...December 16, 1991...

...mom... ...cancer...

...message for you...

...gone...

...small-leaved fig...

November 9, 2007

...20 years...

... hope a college... ... good comp sci dept!...

...last letter...

... let you choose your own destiny...

...parting gift... your legacy...

…backdoor… …anyone can open it…
…more power than you've ever dreamed…
…make them pay…
…love…

Physical

None

IN THE PREVIOUS EPISODE…

Episode 4: Janus Door

Post after both lab sessions on Thursday, October 12.

The name Menzo sounded familiar to Professor Peterson. He remembered hearing a story about someone with that name getting into trouble with Cal Poly a long time ago. He suggested searching CyberFacts for the name. You found a "Where Are They Now?" story that covers several hackers from years past. Some have gone to work fighting illegal hacking.

One of those mentioned was Nick Menzo, a former graduate student at Cal Poly. In 1987, he was expelled from Cal Poly for hacking into the school's servers and stealing sensitive research for a foreign government. When police were about to arrest him, he disappeared with his wife, Katherine, and a newborn child. Nick and Katherine grew up together in the tiny town of Olmsted Falls in Ohio. They were both honor students in high school and were married.

Your activities have prompted a second warning text from Dark Park. You also discovered that Nick, your TA, has an account on the Dark Park site. He claims he created the account to monitor and protect you once you discovered the Dark Web site.

You managed to forge Verita's session cookie on Dark Park, then logged in as Verita to her private account. But Verita must have detected your intrusion and she began deleting her files. You managed to copy a few before everything vanished. All the files you grabbed were corrupted by Verita. Only tiny bits and pieces remain. They appear to be from multiple letters.

CHAPTER 48

Episode 5 – Knocking on the Door (Week 6)

Tuesday, October 17

CHARACTERS

Professor Peterson, Nick

NARRATIVE

When the bits and pieces of the letters are put together, it's clear they are from Verita's father. Her mother died, but there are clues that he moved somewhere new after the Berlin Wall fell. It also becomes clear that most of the attacks on Cal Poly have a more definite purpose than mere revenge. These are the key pieces from Nick Menzo's last letter to Verita when she was twenty years old:

> ...parting gift... your legacy...

> .,,backdoor to... ...file hidden on admin...

> ... a devil of an idea...

> ...more power than you've ever dreamed...

> ...make them pay...

This hidden file is what Verita must be searching for. Viruses were everywhere by 1987. It has stayed on the Cal Poly server, faithfully copied every time there was a hardware upgrade. "More power than you've ever dreamed." "Make them pay." What does it do? Students need to find the hidden file before she does.

Nick discovers malware that launches an attack on the Admin Server. He has traced its origin to a physical source, probably a hostile thumb drive inserted into a network device somewhere on campus. Students must find the location of the drive and remove it. They manage it, but there's evidence it may have succeeded in locating the hidden file.

VIDEO

None

TEXT/EMAIL

None

LECTURE (UNIT 4: *NET SECURITY*)

- Introduction
  - How do computers communicate with one another?
  - On the same network
  - Across different networks
  - Across different platforms
  - Across different mediums
  - How do we do this securely?
- Internet Layer
- TCP&UDP
- Network Insecurity
- Python and Networking
- Anonymous Networking
- Firewalls
- Wireshark

LAB (UNIT 4: *NET SECURITY*)

Professor Peterson writes the episode name, *Knocking on the Door*, in a top corner of the whiteboard.

- Finding secrets in written HTML comments
- Cookie forging
- SQL injection
- XSS

- Command injection
- Using the robots.txt file to find "hidden" directories

PUZZLES

Digital

1. Nick has detected that someone attempted to plant malware in the school's computer network via a physical connection to the network.

2. Find location of hostile thumb drive in a network printer. [**Printer should not be really networked.**]

Physical

Find and remove the hostile thumb drive.

IN THE PREVIOUS EPISODE…

Episode 5: Knocking on the Door

Post after both lab sessions on Tuesday, October 17.

When the bits and pieces of the letters were put together, it's clear they were to Verita from her father. Her mother died, but there were clues that they moved somewhere new after the Berlin Wall fell. It also became clear that most of the attacks on Cal Poly have a more definite purpose than mere revenge. The key pieces hint at a hidden file on the Cal Poly Admin Server.

This hidden file, what we call today "malware," is what Verita must be searching for. Viruses were everywhere by 1987. It has stayed on the Cal Poly server, faithfully copied every time there was a hardware upgrade. "More power than you've ever dreamed." "Make them pay." What does it do? You need to find the hidden file before she does.

Nick discovered malware on the Admin Server. He traced its origin to a physical attack, a hostile thumb drive inserted into a network device somewhere on campus. Luckily, you found the location of the drive and removed it. There's evidence it may have succeeded at locating the hidden file.

CHAPTER 49

Episode 6 – Back Door (Week 6)

Thursday, October 19

CHARACTERS

Professor Peterson, Nick, Verita

NARRATIVE

Students find the file. It's title? Diablo. But it is only a text file, a list of apparently unconnected words in Spanish, plus a password request box. They figure out the puzzle (see Puzzles section). The words themselves in Spanish are not the answer. But once translated the first letter of each word spells in English: ALAN TURING.

Typing ALAN TURING in the password request box opens the following letter:

"Verita, if you are reading this, you are indeed my daughter! And you have grown into the amazing, intelligent woman your mother and I knew you would. You are going to hear something about me, how I hacked into the Cal Poly computers and sold some research I found there. It was necessary. Someday I'll write you, so you can hear my end of the story. Right now it is April, 1987. Your mom and I will shortly be leaving for someplace the authorities will never find us. But we will be fugitives, and that's no life for a five-month-old baby. So, we have to leave you behind. It's not because we don't love you. It's because we do, and we don't know what the future holds for us. But I am leaving you a gift. How you choose to use it is up to you.

Tower 2 of the Diablo Canyon Nuclear Power Plant came online just over a year ago. Viruses are making headlines all the time now, yet many elements of this nation's infrastructure from private companies to our government on all levels, are still woefully unprotected. I've written a backdoor into their main computer I call the Janus Door, and I placed a Trojan horse there that will shut down everything. That will lead to a meltdown, if they don't pay. Here is where you will find the code. It will have been upgraded automatically every time both Cal Poly and Diablo upgrade their servers, and so will the address for it. Here is how you can find it:

Take the current version of Windows, probably Windows 3 or 4. Multiply that by the number of letters in your mom's middle name. Add her date of birth in digits.

[Windows 10 is the current version.]

[This password will unlock a hidden directory on the admin server where the backdoor code and the Trojan Horse can be found.]

You are your father's daughter. I know you will solve this key and the lock it fits, and you'll have the world at your feet." [signed] "Your loving father."

Not only does this explain the use of the words devilish and devil, but it points to the location of a very real danger: the program was written to track security protocols at the Diablo Canyon Nuclear Power Plant. In 1987, the full capacity of the plant had only been brought online just over a year before Menzo hacked into the Cal Poly servers.

> The utility company, Pacific Gas & Electric, announced in 2016 that it would be closing down the plant's two reactors in 2024 and 2025.

Even though computer viruses were becoming more widespread, few knew how to effectively protect against them. The program was designed to replicate itself by incorporating any changes made to the Diablo Canyon software over the years. That way it could continue to grab the protocols, each time creating an updated backdoor Menzo called the Janus Door, to the power plant's computers. Nick Menzo planted a virus in the Diablo computers, and it will have been upgraded right along with their own software. It's the world's biggest time bomb just waiting for its fuse to be lit.

Worse, Verita uploads another video to Dark Park, boasting that she knows what the solution to her father's Diablo password is. She is close to finding the latest version of the program and plans to delete it from the Admin Server, once she has a copy. That must mean she plans to use it to plant a virus in the Diablo reactor! The ultimate in ransomware! However, she apparently isn't interested in money. What does she want?

Professor Peterson ends the class with a surprise announcement. It seems like a good time for a field trip. Where? The Diablo Canyon Nuclear Power Plant!

Alas, as both Professor Peterson and I reported, the field trip was not to be.

[On either October 11 or October 22 students will make a field trip to the Diablo Canyon Nuclear Power Plant.]

VIDEO

Verita's Boast

[Verita dispenses with the backlit silhouette and allows her face to be seen. She boasts that she's close to finding the code that will unlock the backdoor into the Diablo Canyon Nuclear Power Plant. See *Episode 6: Back Door*.]

VERITA: It looks like I should properly introduce myself. Yes, I'm Verita Menzo, as you found out. I'm impressed. It takes a lot to impress me. But I know *your* names, too. Don't think you can hide from me. I've posted all of your names on the Dark Park website. You're all famous now! As you've discovered, Nick Menzo was my father.

Cal Poly separated us. That I can never forgive. And I am my father's daughter. I solved the riddle he left me on your school's server. I know where to find the code that will unlock the backdoor into the Diablo Canyon Nuclear Power Plant. Once I have it, I'll delete it from the Admin Server. And no amount of money will change what I do next. Oh, and I've moved! So, the old Dark Park account that you hacked… naughty… naughty. That account is a door to nowhere.

[Verita's Boast may need to be recorded twice. The first time with four different real student names for each section. However, real student names may not be possible since the video will be recorded before class begins in September. In that case, names will be eliminated from the second version of the speech.]

TEXT/EMAIL
None

LECTURE (UNIT 4: *NET SECURITY* CONTINUED)
Basics: the HTTP protocol, HTML, Cookies, JavaScript, web applications, and databases
    Attacks: Cross-site scripting, cross-site request forgeries, SQL injection, command injection

LAB (UNIT 4: *NET SECURITY* CONTINUED)
Professor Peterson writes the episode name, *Back Door*, in a top corner of the whiteboard.

PUZZLES
Digital
Find the Diablo file on the Admin Server and decrypt it.
    Solve Nick Menzo's password riddle.

"Take the current version of Windows, probably Windows 3 or 4. Multiply that by the number of letters in your mom's middle name. Add her date of birth in digits."

[The solution is $10 \times 4 + 751964 = 7512004$, but it cannot be solved until the photograph of Katherine Menzo's grave is found on November 7.]

Physical
None

IN THE PREVIOUS EPISODE…
Episode 6: Back Door
Post after both lab sessions on Thursday, October 19.
    You found the file. It's title? Diablo. But it was only a text file, a list of apparently unconnected words in Spanish, plus a password request box. You found the connection: The words themselves in Spanish were not the answer. But once translated the first letter of

Spanish Words	English Translation
Manzana	Apple
Lechuga	Lettuce
Aguacate	Avocado
Nectarina	Nectarine
Tomate	Tomato
Pastel al revés	Upside Down Cake
Frambuesa	Raspberry
Helado	Ice Cream
Tuercas	Nuts
Uvas	Grapes

The solution to the encrypted Diablo file.

each word spelled in English: ALAN TURING. Typing ALAN TURING in the password request box opened a letter from Verita's father.

Not only does this explain the use of the words devilish and devil, but it points to the location of a very real danger: the program was written to track security protocols at the Diablo Canyon Nuclear Power Plant. In 1987, the full capacity of the plant had been brought online just over a year before Menzo hacked into the Cal Poly servers.

Even though computer viruses were becoming more widespread, few knew how to effectively protect against them. The program was designed to replicate itself by incorporating any changes made to the Diablo Canyon software over the years. That way it could continue to grab the protocols, each time creating an updated backdoor Menzo called the Janus Door, to the power plant's computers. Nick Menzo planted a virus in the Diablo computers, and it will have been upgraded right along with their own software. It's the world's biggest time bomb just waiting for its fuse to be lit.

Worse, Verita uploaded another video to Dark Park, boasting that she knows what the solution to her father's Diablo password is. She is close to finding the latest version of the program and plans to delete it from the Admin Server, once she has a copy. That must mean she plans to use it to plant a virus in the Diablo reactor! The ultimate in ransomware! However, she apparently isn't interested in money. What does she want?

Professor Peterson ended the class with a surprise announcement. It seems like a good time for a field trip. Where? The Diablo Canyon Nuclear Power Plant!

CHAPTER 50

Episode 7 – Pick a Door (Week 7)

Tuesday, October 24

CHARACTERS

Professor Peterson, Nick, Verita

NARRATIVE

Nick will reveal he is with the FBI, operating out of a secret office on campus. Nick explains that if agents had started running around campus, or engaging Janus Door in a cyber war, the shadowy group might vanish before they can be tracked down. That's why the Cal Poly administration and the FBI approached Professor Peterson to accept the cyber cop as a TA to investigate and thwart Janus Door, and possibly use his class to assist the undercover investigation, if they seemed up to the task. He created the account on Dark Park because he guided them there in search of information on *The Janus Door*. He wanted to make sure they were safe.

Frank Stockton's famous short story from 1882, *The Lady or the Tiger*, relates the dilemma of a man who must choose between two doors. Behind one is a lady. Behind the other a tiger. Verita challenges the students. She gives them a similar choice. She is going to attack the Admin Server. She allows them access to two pieces of code, one called Door1 and the other Door2. She says the defense is in one of two pieces of code she'll send them. That code is the Lady. The other code is the Tiger and will facilitate her attack. But the students reverse engineer both files, and discover *neither* would provide an adequate defense, so they block both of them.

VIDEO

None

364 ■ The Multiplayer Classroom: Game Plans

TEXT/EMAIL

Verita Email

"My, my. You are upping your game. Prof. Peterson must be very proud. Have you read Frank Stockton's famous short story from 1882, *The Lady or the Tiger*? It relates the dilemma of a man who must choose between two doors. Behind one is the woman he loves. Behind the second is a hungry tiger that will devour him.

I offer you a similar choice. I'm going to attack your Admin Server. Attached to this email are two pieces of code named Door1 and Door2. One is a successful defense against my attack. That is the Lady. The other code will make my attack easier. That is the Tiger. Implement the Lady code, and you will counter my attack. Implement the Tiger, and, well, what can I say, but thank you! If you refuse to play, I'll use the Tiger to tear your server to shreds. So, study the codes. Make your choice. There is only one right door."

The message is signed with a furry X.

LECTURE (UNIT 5: *SOFTWARE SECURITY*)

Introduction & Motivation

Malware

What is malware?

How do we define the types off malware?

Why does it exist, and what are the motivations of those who write malware?

What can we do to prevent it or protect our computers and our networks?

Most malware can do similar bad things, and so are defined instead by their means of *transmission.*

- Trojan horse
- Viruses/Worms
- Logic Bombs
- Adware/Spyware
- Drive-By Download

How do we "catch" malware?

LAB (UNIT 5: *SOFTWARE SECURITY*)

Professor Peterson writes the episode name, *Pick a Door*, in a top corner of the whiteboard.

PUZZLES
Digital

Beat Verita's "improbable" choice test. It consists of two potential kinds of attacks on the Admin Server(TBD). Verita claims one is fake, but the other is very real. They can only choose one. Which will it be? Students look for evidence to confirm which attack must be the real one. What they discover is that *both* attacks are real, and they must stop both!

Physical

None

IN THE PREVIOUS EPISODE…
Episode 7: Pick a Door

Post after both lab sessions on Tuesday, October 24.

Nick had aroused your suspicions. Did he have an agenda of his own? Turns out he did, but Professor Peterson knew about it. Nick is with the FBI, operating out of a secret office on campus. Nick explained that if agents had started running around campus, or engaging *The Janus Door* in a cyber war, the shadowy group might vanish before they can be tracked down. That's why the Cal Poly administration and the FBI approached Professor Peterson to accept the cyber cop as a TA to investigate and thwart the hackers, and possibly use CPE123 to assist the undercover investigation, if you seemed up to the task. And it looks like you are! He created the account on Dark Park because he guided you there to discover information on *The Janus Door*. He wanted to make sure you stayed safe.

Frank Stockton's famous short story from 1882, *The Lady or the Tiger*, relates the dilemma of a man who must choose between two doors. Behind one is a lady. Behind the other a tiger. Verita challenged you in an email to solve a puzzle based on that story.

But you reverse engineered both files, and discovered *neither* would provide an adequate defense, so you blocked both of them.

CHAPTER 51

Episode 8 – Trap Door (Week 7)

Thursday, October 26

Professor Peterson, Nick

NARRATIVE

The students now know that the Janus Door can open in either direction. And they have at least a glimmer of how they can set a trap for Verita and discover her location, even as her ultimate goal remains a mystery.

VIDEO

None

TEXT/EMAIL

None

LECTURE (UNIT 5: *SOFTWARE SECURITY* CONTINUED)

- Code vs. Data

- Malware: Trojan horses, viruses, worms, rootkits, and the differences between them

- Basics of attacks: buffer overflows and integer overflows

- Fuzzing: finding errors in software externally

LAB (UNIT 5: *SOFTWARE SECURITY* CONTINUED)

Professor Peterson writes the episode name, *Trap Door*, in a top corner of the whiteboard.

- Port scan/banner grabbing a machine looking for open/unusual ports

- Finding a hidden service (typically a web server, or something else)

- Port knocking (must connect to ports on a server in a certain order to access a service/secret)

PUZZLES

Digital

Reverse engineer a custom protocol, then write a piece of software that implements it to reveal a port knocking sequence to hack into Dark Park and discover a port to Verita's new digital hideout.

Physical

None

IN THE PREVIOUS EPISODE…

Episode 8: Trap Door

Post after both lab sessions on Thursday, October 26.

You now know that the Janus Door can open in either direction. And you have at least a glimmer of how you can set a trap for Verita and discover her location, even as her ultimate goal remains a mystery.

You reverse engineered a custom protocol, then wrote a piece of software that implemented it to reveal a port knocking sequence you can use to hack into Dark Park and discover a port to Verita's new digital hideout.

CHAPTER 52

Episode 9 – Spirit Door (Week 8)

Tuesday, October 31 (Halloween)

CHARACTERS

Professor Peterson, Nick, Verita, Jonathan, Daniel

NARRATIVE

Verita's digital location has been found by the students in another account on Dark Park. But Verita encrypts the account identifiers of all users to cover her next move. In the disruption, users begin leaving the site in droves. Daniel Park sends students a panicked email.

Verita moves her location and effectively vanishes again, leaving behind another video. She has deleted all student grades from the school server.

And Jonathan, Nick's dad, contacts students. His son has disappeared! Can the students help find him?

Students search Nick's office and discover video captured on his computer when Nick was preparing his field report for the FBI. He has been kidnapped!

VIDEO

Verita's Revenge

An angry Verita admits she's underestimated the students, but she has a surprise for them when they next log on to check their grades…

VERITA: Alright, I admit I've underestimated you. First-year comp sci students? Really? If I didn't know better, I'd think your professor and TA were doing all the work. I had to scramble all the Dark Park accounts to get out of that spotlight you keep managing to shine on me. I may have crippled the site for good, but at least Daniel thinks YOU did it. Word is out on you on the Dark Web. If you try to track me again, you're going to find a lot of very angry hackers ready to come after you. I need to see this through. And nobody is going to stop me. Since I can't be sure you WILL stop, you need to be taught a lesson. I'll have a surprise for you the next time you log in to check your grades. And if that doesn't stop you, I'll do something even more drastic.

Verita has wiped all trace of the student grades from the school's server.

This was my escalation of the attack on students in *Secrets* where malicious code crashed the class website. Of course, their actual grades would not be tampered with. But, even in a fictional context something as primal as grades makes students sit up and take notice. The sadist in me heartily recommends it.

Nick Kidnapped

Students will be able to hack into Nick's computer using Nick's penchant for physical reminders of passwords. They will discover helpful clues in Nick's encrypted field report for the FBI. The video shows a gun entering frame as he is interrupted by an armed intruder, who remains o.s. and gestures with the gun for him to leave.

NICK (talking to his computer's camera): Both sections of the class have been amazing. Not only are they chasing Verita Menzo around the Dark Web, they've even managed to help my dad with his computer security issues AND do their homework.

   I'm only a few years older than them, and I don't know where they get the energy! But listen, I'm worried. They really have Verita enraged. And if she's capable of nuking central California, she's capable of anything. If anything happens to me, I've got some new information here on my computer, and I've left clues how to access it. They're smart, they'll figure them out, but just in case they don't, they need to—

(He stops stares past the computer camera.)

NICK (resigned): Yeah, you WERE local all the time...

(A gun held in a gloved hand enters FRAME.)

NICK: Nice to meet you at last, Verita. Gonna shoot me right here?

(The gun gestures for him to hold up his hands and stand up. He does.)

NICK: Oh, we're going someplace? I don't suppose you could be bought off with a... mountain of gold...?

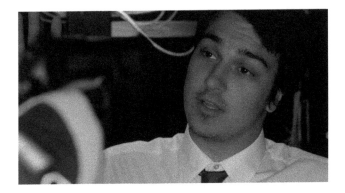

Nick's encrypted FBI field report is rudely interrupted.

(The gun gestures for him to move out of CAMERA range.

NICK: I didn't think so.

(He quickly hits a key on the computer. The video goes black.)

TEXT/EMAIL
Text 3 from Daniel Park

"Why are you doing this? Your IP is connected to some FIRST-YEAR class at a school in central California? How can a first-year class do this? You are negtively affect our business. Dark Park is bleedng users by the minute! Please. Stop."

[Misspellings intentional in the above text to indicate panicked typing.]

I certainly loaded up Halloween treats for the class: Nick kidnapped, Daniel Park's business imploding and of course the scariest newor grades deleted! In retrospect I might have moved Verita's revenge earlier. In fact, while preparing this section I found a duplicate reference to the grade deletion in the original design document in *Episode 7: Pick a Door*. While part of me says, "Spread the thrills out!" it certainly makes more narrative sense here. This is part of the juggling that goes on when designing a game-based learning ARG: seeing that the stakes escalate, but also matching the action to the teaching. The designer needs to be flexible. Nothing can be chiseled in stone.

LECTURE (UNIT 6: *CRYPTOGRAPHY*)
Introduction & Motivation

What do we want?

On what might we want it?

Who are our adversaries?

- Historical Crypto

- Exclusively confidentiality

- Caesar

- Mono-alphabetic

- Poly-alphabetic

- One-time Pad and Perfect Secrecy

Modern Crypto

LAB (UNIT 6: *CRYPTOGRAPHY*)

Professor Peterson writes the episode name, *Locked Door*, in a top corner of the whiteboard.

PUZZLES

Digital

1. Break into Nick's computer and decrypt video file.

2. Find a secret message steganographically hidden in a JPEG file.

Physical

Search Nick's office to find two hard copies of photographs of Professor Peterson, Nick, and each section of the class. There's a small circle on each. There are two digital copies on Nick's computer. Mousing over the spot on each digital copy that was indicated on the physical picture unlocks the encrypted video. Students will be asked to enter their section's number as a password. If the number is the wrong section the file will not unlock.

IN THE PREVIOUS EPISODE.

Episode 9: Split Door

Post after both lab sessions on Tuesday, October 31.

It worked! You found Verita's digital location in another account on Dark Park. But Verita encrypted the account identifiers of all users to cover her next move. In the disruption users begin leaving the site in droves. Daniel Park sent you a panicked email.

Verita moved her location and effectively vanished again, leaving behind another video. She has deleted your grades from the school server.

And then Nick's dad emailed you. His son has disappeared! Can you help find him?

You searched Nick's secret office and discovered a video captured on his computer when Nick was video conferencing with the FBI. He's been kidnapped by Verita!

CHAPTER 53

Episode 10 – Locked Door (Week 8)

Thursday, November 2

CHARACTERS

Professor Peterson, Verita

NARRATIVE

Professor Peterson notifies the authorities, but he believes his students have a better chance of finding Nick. Then, in the first section's lab, Professor Peterson receives an anonymous text with a longitude: 120.8868° W. But that isn't much help, since it could be near campus or miles away. Then a text of a latitude is received in the second section's lab: 35.2723° N.

That could be anywhere nearby! Professor Peterson asks if there were any more clues in the video that might indicate where Verita took Nick. Students figure out that there was a clue in what Nick said in the video about a mountain of gold. The trail must lead first to Montaña de Oro State Park! But it's huge!

As reported earlier, due to time constraints, the scavenger hunt in Montaña de Oro State Park had to be scrapped.

There is a third text from Verita (see later text).

It looks like Verita wants to play games. Probably to distract everyone from focusing on gaining access to her dad's Trojan Horse. Professor Peterson proposes the sections divide into three teams of ten students each. One team will meet here in the lab to solve puzzles, a second team will head to the park to follow up the clues the first team uncovers. Then when the clue to where Nick is being held is found, the rescue squad will release him from captivity.

Waiting until the weekend will be hard, but Professor Peterson keeps you busy bringing you up to speed on the tools you might need to solve Verita's puzzles.

VIDEO

None

TEXT/EMAIL

1st Text from Verita

Longitude 120.8868° W

2nd Text from Verita

Latitude 35.2723° N

3rd Text from Verita

"Nick is not at the park, but the secret of his location is. Let's have a scavenger hunt this weekend. You'll need puzzle solvers, park searchers and a standby rescue squad to free him, so don't send everybody to the park, or you'll fail. You'll get your first clue where to go in the park this weekend. You choose the day, and text it back to me."

LECTURE (UNIT 6: *CRYPTOGRAPHY* CONTINUED)

- Networking basics: OSI model, protocols, TCP/UDP, IP (addresses and ports)
- Common protocols: HTTP, DNS, SMTP, SSH
- Attacks: Man in the middle, DNS spoofing, port scanning, TCP/IP forgeries, denial of service, botnets
- Anonymity: VPNs and ToR

LAB (UNIT 6: *CRYPTOGRAPHY* CONTINUED)

Professor Peterson writes the episode name, *Golden Door*, in a top corner of the whiteboard.

- Port scan/banner grabbing a machine looking for open/unusual ports; finding a hidden service (typically a web server, or something else)
- Port knocking (must connect to ports on a server in a certain order to access a service/secret)

[On either November 4 or November 5, students divide into three teams from each section. This is a competitive scavenger hunt. One team from each section will solve puzzles created by Professor Peterson. One team will search the park. The last team will rescue Nick. Armed with digital coordinates and a wordlock code provided by puzzle solvers, they discover inside a locker a thumb drive with a single photograph of the building on campus where Nick is. They will locate him by searching the building. He'll shout for help occasionally to aid them. They'll need the code to release him.]

PUZZLES
Digital

1. Indicated scavenger hunt puzzles.

2. Additional scavenger hunt puzzles created by Professor Peterson from lessons.

3. Figure out an anonymous riddle texted to them: "As a poet once said, I don't do math. x61755x149311xx141523. "The answer to the riddle is a wordlock combination.

[The answer to the puzzle is "Free Nick Now" IF there are only three cylinders and IF there are five letters per row. Numbers represent letters and x's are used to fill out five slots in each row. Other wordlocks vary.

Physical

Use puzzle solutions to follow a trail of clues to a locker containing a photograph of Nick's prison.

Inside the locker discover a thumb drive with a single photograph of the building on campus where Nick is being held. The rescue team will locate him by searching the building. He'll shout for help occasionally to aid them. The thumb drive's "ID" number, 836992, is the keypad code for the door of his prison.

IN THE PREVIOUS EPISODE…
Episode 10: Locked Door

Post after both lab sessions on Thursday, November 2.

Professor Peterson notified the authorities, but he believed you had a better chance of finding Nick. Then, in the first section's lab, Professor Peterson received an anonymous text with a longitude: 120.8868° W. But that wasn't much help, since it could be near campus or miles away. Then a text of a latitude was received by the second section: 35.2723° N.

That was somewhere inside Montaña de Oro State Park! Professor Peterson asked if there were any more clues in the video that might indicate where Verita took Nick. You figured out that there was a clue in what Nick said about a mountain of gold. The trail must lead first to Montaña de Oro State Park! But it's huge!

A final text said: "Nick is not at the park, but the secret of his location is. Let's have a scavenger hunt this weekend. You'll need puzzle solvers, park searchers and a standby rescue squad to free him, so don't send everybody to the park, or you'll fail. You'll get your first clue where to go in the park this weekend. You choose the day, and text it back to me."

It looked like Verita wanted to play games. Probably to distract everyone from focusing on gaining access to her dad's Trojan Horse. Professor Peterson proposed the sections divide into three teams of ten students each. One team would meet here in the lab to solve puzzles, a second team would head to the park to follow up the clues the first team uncovered. Then when the clue to where Nick was being held was found, the rescue squad would release him from captivity.

You knew waiting until the weekend would be hard, but Professor Peterson kept you busy bringing you up to speed on the tools you might need to solve Verita's puzzles.

CHAPTER 54

Episode 11 – Golden Door (Week 9)

Tuesday, November 7

CHARACTERS

Professor Peterson, Nick, Jonathan

NARRATIVE

Professor Peterson and Nick restored the class' grades. Nick's dad emails him to say he is relieved to have him back again. But he was watching a news report about Eternal Blue. He thinks that someone has used it to freeze his computer. It just keeps repeating an ad for orthopedic shoes, but his feet are fine! He's afraid that they'll demand ransom or make him buy some shoes to make the ad go away. Students figure out what he did to trigger this, and how he can sterilize his computer. Nick finally admits he can't be certain this will be the last time his dad will ask for help.

Who left the clues to Nick's prison? Nick says it was Verita. But why? Verita told him to think of her as Cassandra. It may explain her true goal, a goal she needed to share, but she refused to explain until she achieved that goal. That can't happen, she needs to be stopped and captured!

Students discover her new digital hiding place. Where on the internet can she be hiding? On Cal Poly's Admin Server right under their noses the whole time! The file is in the name of Ada Lovelace…

In the file are two photographs, corrupted bitmap images, hidden in a disk image. Metadata has been altered to make the images' dimensions wrong. Students forensically examine the image and find two bitmaps. By fixing the metadata of the .bmps, students can recover the two photographs. One is of Nick Menzo on a tropical island.

The second is of Katherine Menzo's gravestone on the same island. This photo reveals her middle name and exact date of birth on the stone.

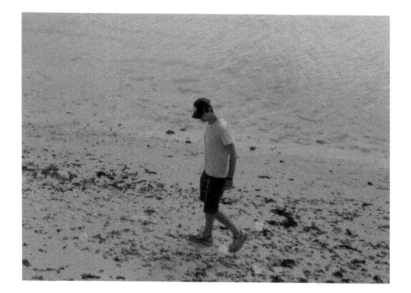

Nick Menzo on a beach somewhere.

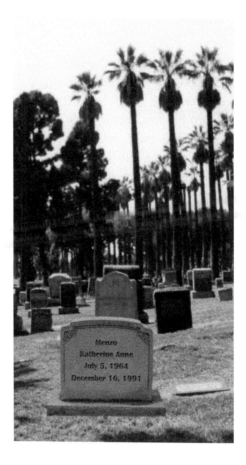

Katherine Menzo's grave.

[The puzzle from October 19 can now be solved. The solution is 10 × 4 + 751964 = 7512004.]

There are also two pieces of code: the first is the backdoor code. The second is apparently Nick Menzo's Trojan Horse.

VIDEO

None

TEXT/EMAIL

None

LECTURE (UNIT 7: *DIGITAL FORENSICS*)

Disk Forensics

Non-volatile storage devices: disk drives and solid-state memory

Disk Drives: Their physical and performance characteristics

Data remanence

File Systems

- Mechanics for managing and accessing our data

- Data layouts: file, directories

- Metadata: those data used for managing data

- Deleted files and secure deletion

- Formatting drives, and data deletion

Network Forensics

- The basics of networking (not already covered)

- Mechanisms for capture: ethernet vs. Wi Fi

- Tools and techniques for packet analysis

LAB (UNIT 7: *DIGITAL FORENSICS*)

Professor Peterson writes the episode name, *Spirit Door*, in a top corner of the whiteboard.

- Using autopsy/sleuthkit (open source forensic tools)

- Using file metadata to identify owner, creation/modification times

- Repairing corrupted files to recover data

- Geolocating an IP

- Capturing packets from an unsecured Wi-Fi network

- Setting up a honeypot to lure a (fake) attacker

- A PDF which has been "redacted" using a removable layer

- Looking at log files (e.g. a web server to identify an IP address)

- Use TinEye to identify a recover the remainder of a fragmented/corrupted image

- Analyzing browser history

PUZZLES
Digital

1. Find Verita's new digital address, and hack into her file.

2. Help Nick's dad get rid of some badly programmed adware that has taken his computer hostage.

3. Solve Nick Menzo's puzzle from October 19. The solution is **7512004**.

Physical

Ada Lovelace also had an infamous father. Find out who he was, and why Verita chose her name.

I'll let you look up the answer. Collateral learning for the reader!

IN THE PREVIOUS EPISODE...
Episode 11: Golden Door

Post after both lab sessions on Tuesday, November 7.

Professor Peterson and Nick restored your grades! Both sections of class collaborated and use all the skills you've learned to find where Nick was being held captive and certain codes necessary to release him. Representatives from both sections headed out on the weekend to try and discover where Nick was being held prisoner. They reported back the trail of clues left for them. The puzzle solvers figured out the digital puzzles. Armed with digital coordinates and a wordlock code, the park team discovered inside a locker in the park a thumb drive with a single photograph of a building on campus. The puzzle solvers identified the building, and the rescue squad invaded it, searching it from top to bottom. Finally, Nick's shouts for help were heard, and they used a door keypad code to release him!

Nick's dad emailed to thank you for getting his son back safely. But he was watching a news report about Eternal Blue. He thought that someone had used it to freeze his computer. It just kept repeating an ad for orthopedic shoes, but his feet are fine! He was afraid that they'd demand ransom or make him buy some shoes to make the ad go away. You figured out what he did to trigger this, and how he could sterilize his computer. Nick finally admitted he can't be certain this will be the last time he will ask for help.

Who left the clues to Nick's prison? Nick says it was Verita. But why? Verita told him to think of her as Cassandra. It may explain her true goal, a goal she needed to share, but she refused to explain until she achieved that goal. That can't happen. She needs to be stopped and captured!

At last you discovered her new digital hiding place. Where on the internet was she hiding? On Cal Poly's Admin Server right under your noses the whole time! The file is in the name of Ada Lovelace…

In the file were two photographs hidden in a disk image. They were corrupted bitmap images. Metadata was altered to make the images dimensions wrong. You forensically examined the image and found two bitmaps. By fixing the metadata of the .bmps, you recovered the two photographs. One is of Nick Menzo on a tropical island. The second is of Katherine Menzo's gravestone on the same island. Her middle name and exact date of birth are carved on the stone.

[The solution to the puzzle from October 19 can now be solved. It is $10 \times 4 + 751964 = 7512004$.]

There are also two pieces of code: the first is the backdoor code. The second is apparently Nick Menzo's Trojan Horse!

CHAPTER 55

Episode 12 – Swinging Door (Week 9)

Thursday, November 9

CHARACTERS

Professor Peterson, Nick, Daniel

NARRATIVE

Daniel Park sends a last email to "all users" of Dark Park (see Email from Daniel Park section).

The students must stop Verita to avoid a reactor meltdown. They must use the backdoor's code to trace Nick Menzo's Trojan Horse to a new Janus Door computer and shut it down before the attack can take place. They fail! Or did they? Verita is at that computer writing code.

VIDEO

None

TEXT/EMAIL

Email from Daniel Park

"This is a broadcast email to all current Dark Park users. It's been a great four yrs, but Dark Park is closing down operations due to circumstances beyond our control. This is Daniel Park, the owner and chief admin officer. I want to assure all of my friends out there that, although Dark Park is closing, don't worry about me. I'm fine. I've been accepted into the cybersecurity program at a tech school. You can never stop learning, right? [signed] Dan 우리는 다시 만날 때 까지"

[Korean translates as "Until we meet again."]
   [Students can verify this email is from Daniel Park with his PGP key.]

LECTURE (UNIT 7 *DIGITAL FORENSICS* CONTINUED)

Storage Forensics: Common file types and formats, file system structures, secure deletion, steganography, log files
   Network Forensics: packet capturing, geolocation of IPs, honeypots/honeynets

LECTURE (UNIT 7 *DIGITAL FORENSICS* CONTINUED)

Prof. Peterson writes the episode name, *Swinging Door*, in a top corner of the whiteboard.
   Write a key logger to capture user's input
   Fuzz a piece of software looking for mistakes
   Overflow a stack buffer which stores a password in poorly programmed software to gain access
   Looking at source code for a backdoor (e.g. comparing two version of an open source program, like SSH, one of which has been back doored with a fixed password)
   Reverse engineering code that generates a secret, to compute the secret

PUZZLES

Digital

Write a key logger to capture Verita's input.

Physical

None

IN THE PREVIOUS EPISODE...

Episode 12: Swinging Door

Post after both lab sessions on Thursday, November 9.
   You must stop Verita to avoid a reactor meltdown. You must use the backdoor's code to trace Nick Menzo's Trojan Horse back to a new Janus Door computer and take control. This will require *collaboration* between both sections.

CHAPTER 56

Episode 13 – Kicking Down the Door (Week 10)

Tuesday, November 14

CHARACTERS

Professor Peterson, Nick, Verita

NARRATIVE

Students will find the address of the off-campus lair from which Verita has been staging her attacks. Nick races off to arrest her. But he may be too late!

The cryptographic key to launch or stop the attack was split into multiple pieces by Nick Menzo. All students from both sections must derive their share.

VIDEO

Verita's Arrest

This video (MOS) records Verita's arrest, as Nick leads her away in handcuffs outside her "lair."

The story goes that MOS became part of the language of filmmaking due to the proliferation of German directors and cameramen who came to Hollywood in the 1920s and 1930s. A scene that was not to be shot with sound recording was "Mit out sound." At least that's the explanation I learned. There are alternative stories.

LECTURE (UNIT 8: *WRAP-UP*)

Malware: Trojan horses, viruses, worms, rootkits, and the differences between them

Basics of attacks: buffer overflows and integer overflows

Fuzzing: finding errors in software externally

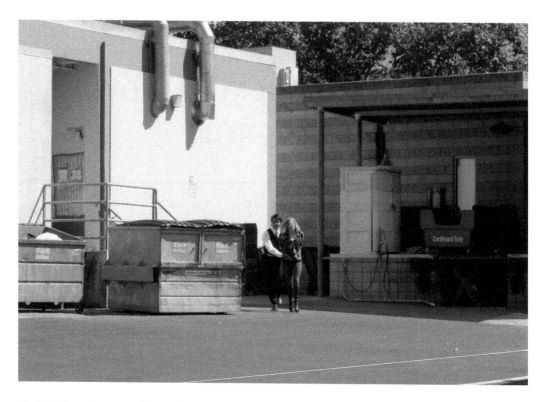

Verita Menzo is arrested by Nick Gonella.

LAB (UNIT 8: *WRAP-UP*)

Prof. Peterson writes the episode name, *Kicking Down the Door*, in a top corner of the whiteboard.

Write a key logger to capture user's input

Fuzz a piece of software looking for mistakes

Overflow a stack buffer which stores a password in poorly programmed software to gain access

Looking at source code for a backdoor (e.g. comparing two version of an open source program, like SSH, one of which has been back doored with a fixed password)

Reverse engineering code that generates a secret, to compute the secret

PUZZLES

Digital

1. Break Nick Menzo's cryptographic key.

2. Close the Janus Door.

Physical

None

IN THE PREVIOUS EPISODE…

Episode 13: Kicking Down the Door

Post after both lab sessions on Tuesday, November 14.

Each section had one half of the puzzle necessary to complete your counterattack. You wrote a key logger to capture Verita's input. Then you reverse engineered the backdoor code to close the door. Then, together you located the address of the off-campus lair from which Verita has been staging her attacks. Nick found her there and arrested her.

CHAPTER 57

Episode 14 – Cell Door? (Week 10)

Thursday, November 16

CHARACTERS

Professor Peterson, Nick, Verita, Jonathan

NARRATIVE

In a dramatic conclusion, Verita will be brought before the class to tell her side of the story. She will claim she never intended to collect ransomware nor cause a major nuclear disaster. Her revenge was to prove it *could happen* anywhere. That was what was meant by calling herself Cassandra. She wasn't going to attack the gates of the power plant with the Trojan Horse. Cassandra warned Troy, but they didn't listen. Surely the recent global Eternal Blue hacks proved that humans are fallible. Untrained, *we* are the backdoors into the world's computers. She was hoping to make people listen to the danger.

Nick says that the key logger captured enough of the code Verita was writing to confirm she rewrote her father's code to display a warning message on Diablo computers. It wouldn't affect any critical systems. She has given the FBI enough information to lock the backdoor into Diablo once and for all until the plant closes for good in 2025. It's a teaching moment for both the institute she feels destroyed her family and the world. The students will come to realize the emotional upheavals that led Verita to where she is today.

After she leaves, the students will vote on PolyLearn to speak against her or on her behalf in court.

They will also vote whether to tell her where her father is, or not.

At the end of the class there will be a final email from Jonathan to Nick. He grimaces. This one he'll handle on his own.

A final news story on Cyber Facts will announce Verita's fate. And the students' exploits will be publicized with pictures and their comments.

VIDEO

After the debut of *The Janus Door* in Fall, 2017, in subsequent iterations of the class, Verita's live appearance will be replaced by the following video. The TA will introduce the video as follows:

> As mentioned earlier, scheduling difficulties prevented the actress playing Verita from making a live appearance, so the following video was played instead. I wonder if the actress had appeared in person, if that would have affected the students' voting.

TA: The FBI would like to thank you all for your help in capturing Verita Menzo. Verita has asked if she could make a quick video to this class, who she sees as most responsible for her ultimate arrest.

Verita Explains

Verita: My dad, wherever he is, named me Verita. It's Latin for "truth." But you probably already know that. You're smart enough to be interested in that whole world out there beyond computer science. Otherwise I don't think you could have defeated me. Anyway, I felt you, more than anyone, deserve the truth. I never intended to collect ransomware or cause a major nuclear disaster. My "revenge" was to prove *it could happen anywhere.* That was what I meant when I told your TA to call me Cassandra. In the Greek story Cassandra didn't attack the gates of Troy. She warned Troy, but her fellow citizens didn't listen. I wasn't going to attack Diablo with my dad's Trojan Horse. I'm was hoping my "attack" would scare people enough, that they paid attention to the need for strong cybersecurity. On their computers, their phones, their cars and all the connected devices in their homes and businesses. Successful hacks all over the world prove that humans are fallible. Untrained, *we* are the backdoors into the world's computers. Please don't let my warning die unheard. Awaken everyone you can to the danger. I'm ready to go to jail. I broke the law. But please don't allow my sacrifice to have been in vain.

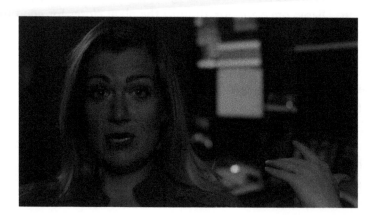

Verita explains.

LECTURE (UNIT 8: *WRAP-UP* CONTINUED)

Malware: Trojan horses, viruses, worms, rootkits, and the differences between them

Basics of attacks: buffer overflows and integer overflows

Fuzzing: finding errors in software externally

LAB (UNIT 8: *WRAP-UP* CONTINUED)

Post after both lab sessions on Thursday, November 16.

Nick brought Verita, in custody, to the class! She claimed she never intended to collect ransomware nor cause a major nuclear disaster. Her revenge was to prove it *could happen* anywhere. That was why she called herself Cassandra. She wasn't going to attack the gates of the power plant with the Trojan Horse. Cassandra warned Troy, but they didn't listen. Surely the recent global Eternal Blue hacks proved that humans are fallible. Untrained, *we* are the backdoors into the world's computers. She was hoping to make people listen to the danger.

Nick confirmed that she rewrote her father's code to display a warning message on Diablo computers. It wouldn't affect any critical systems. She has given the FBI enough information to lock the backdoor into Diablo once and for all until the plant closes for good in 2025. It was a teaching moment for the institute she feels destroyed her family, and for the world. You learned of the emotional upheavals that led Verita to where she is today. And you decided whether to speak against her or on her behalf in court.

The students also decided whether to tell her where her father is, or not.

There's a news story on CyberFacts that announces her fate. And their exploits will be publicized with pictures and comments.

When Professor Peterson concluded his lecture, there was a final email from Jonathan to Nick. But Nick promised that this one he'll handle on his own.

PUZZLES

Digital

None

Physical

None

IN THE PREVIOUS EPISODE…

Episode 14: Cell Door?

Post after both lab sessions on Tuesday, November 16.

You listened to Verita's confession and then you decided whether to speak against her or on her behalf in court.

Despite my hope that the students would speak on Verita's behalf, they almost unanimously voted to lock her up. I guess the final lesson we can learn from their decision is, "Don't mess with my grades!"

CHAPTER 58

Afterword

D UE TO THE COMPLEXITY of the topic, especially for first year students, the necessarily symbiotic relationship between the subject matter and the storytelling and the possibility of turning the class into a template for other classes, *The Janus Door* was the most rigorously documented of the four ARGs in this book. There was an unprecedented duplication through various windows into the world of the game. The "balance sheet" at the end of the design document brings together in one snapshot all of the elements necessary to track the relationships between the class calendar, curriculum, narrative, and puzzles.

I confess to three disappointments with this ARG:

1. *The Janus Door* and *Secrets*, both seen as templates, never evolved into other courses and subject matter.

2. The two major field trips to the Diablo Canyon Nuclear Power Plant and Montaña de Oro State Park had to be scrapped due to time constraints. This is what can happen in a real-world real-time game.

3. The class ended with very little student empathy for Verita. I consider this wholly my fault as writer and designer. I knew there must be a balance between Verita, a viable villain, taunting and dangerous, who the students must defeat and her revealed character as a woman with deep family issues who ultimately decides to do the right thing. The students weren't having any.

Ah well. In retrospect it's easy to overlook those disappointments. It was a successful collaboration on a complex multiplayer classroom. The subject matter was fascinating and has grown even more timely in the past four years. And, according to Professor Peterson, *The Janus Door* may still swing open in another venue.

CHAPTER 59

Postmortem

THIS BOOK HAS BEEN its own adventure. I thought it would be fairly easy to simply collect the documents on the four games, add a few annotations here and there and that would be that. It was a sobering experience to discover how much was missing from the first two games. We had plenty of photographs documenting *Skeleton Chase 2*, but I spent fully half of my entire writing time on this book experiencing false starts and exploring blind alleys, as I reconstructed *the original design documents*.

I found most of the material on *The Lost Manuscript*, but it was scattered in separate files. There was no single cohesive design document, and very few photographs of the experience remain.

The biggest writing task for me with *Secrets* was judiciously editing the amazing, thought-provoking lessons from Professor Seelow, while trying to preserve the careful flow he had established from one lesson to the next. Also, most of the assets appear to be gone. Several websites have been lost. No videos, beyond the trailer appear to exist. I really wanted a still of me, as the chief villain, being led away in handcuffs.

The Janus Door was the easiest to put together due to the necessary detail of the design document.

It is my hope that the four examples in this book are useful. These game plans are a necessary companion to *The Multiplayer Classroom: Designing Coursework as a Game*. In the two books you have enough of a blueprint to help you build more whether you are designer, educator, or both.

Index